Proceedings of the North American Symposium

on Bovine Respiratory Disease

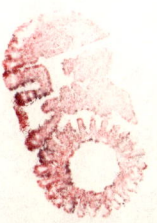

Published for the
Texas Agricultural Experiment Station,
the College of Veterinary Medicine, Texas A&M University,
and the Regional Research Technical Committee,
NC 107 Bovine Respiratory Diseases

Sponsors of the
North American Symposium
on Bovine Respiratory Disease

BOVINE RESPIRATORY DISEASE

A Symposium

Editor
Raymond W. Loan
Associate Dean
College of Veterinary Medicine
Texas A&M University
College Station, Texas
USA

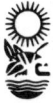

TEXAS A&M UNIVERSITY PRESS

College Station

Library of Congress Cataloging in Publication Data

North American Symposium on Bovine Respiratory Disease
(1983): Amarillo, Tex.)
Proceedings of the North American Symposium on Bovine
Respiratory Disease.

Includes bibliographical references.
1. Cattle—Diseases—Congresses. 2. Respiratory organs—
Diseases—Congresses. 3. Communicable diseases in ani-
mals—Congresses. 4. Cattle—Diseases—Prevention—Con-
gresses. 5. Respiratory organs—Diseases—Prevention—Con-
gresses. 6. Communicable diseases in animals—Prevention—
Congresses. I. Loan, Raymond W. (Raymond Wallace), 1931–
. II. Title. III. Title: Bovine Respiratory Disease. [DNLM:
1. Cattle diseases—Congresses. 2. Respiratory tract diseases—
Veterinary—Congresses. SF 967.R4 N867p 1983]
SF967.R47N67   1983   636.2′08962   83-40491
ISBN 0-89096-187-5

Manufactured in the United States of America
FIRST EDITION

Contents

Preface

It has been over fifteen years since the last symposium on bovine respiratory disease in 1967. For all our efforts during the intervening time, bovine respiratory disease still costs the cattle industry between 250 and 750 million dollars annually. From the outset in the planning of this North American Symposium on Bovine Respiratory Disease, it was the clear intent that the Symposium should represent the highest level of science and technology as it applies now and in the future to the bovine respiratory disease problem. The underlying idea of the Symposium was to set the stage for the next decade of research.

Topics for the Symposium were selected, not on the basis of their important past contributions to our understanding of the disease, but with an eye to the potential of the subject matter in future bovine respiratory disease research. In keeping with this, invited speakers were asked to assume a high level of technical knowledge concerning the disease on the part of the participants and to emphasize the newer "cutting edge" knowledge and technology.

The Symposium came about through the efforts of three organizations: The Texas Agricultural Experiment Station;

the College of Veterinary Medicine, Texas A&M University; and the Regional Research Technical Committee, NC-107, Bovine Respiratory Disease. The Academy of Veterinary Consultants supported the Symposium through adoption of this Symposium as a part of their official program for the year. In addition, Philips Roxane, Inc., Eli Lilly Laboratories, the UpJohn Company, Fort Dodge Laboratories, Norden Laboratories, Beecham Laboratories and CEVA Laboratories contributed financial support for the poster sessions and the publishing of the Proceedings of the Symposium.

The Symposium was introduced with a session on management and economics in the bovine respiratory disease complex. This was followed by presentations and discussions of immune and resistance factors, pathogenesis and cause and prevention. Finally, the Symposium was concluded with a presentation on projections into the future by Dr. Robert F. Kahrs. The Organizing Committee felt that it was especially important that participants gain an appreciation of management and economic factors which impact on the industry and the disease. The economic structure of the beef cattle industry greatly influences methods which can be used for the control of bovine respiratory disease. Certainly the stocker/feeder calf marketing system in North

America influences this.   Preconditioning programs, vaccination programs and special marketing programs effective in some areas of the country may not be effective in other areas of the country.   In some areas the delivery of herd health-management procedures to cow-calf operations on small remote farms with a minimum of livestock handling equipment presents formidable problems.

The Organizing Committee set out to achieve a suitable blend of management and economic factors with the highest level of research technology applicable to the bovine respiratory disease complex.   It is the hope of the Committee that the scientist will find this record of the Symposium useful in research into methods for better control of the disease and that the feedlot disease consultant will find it useful in feedlot practice.

Organizing Committee

Raymond W. Loan, D.V.M., Ph.D.; Chairman
College of Veterinary Medicine
Texas A&M University
College Station, Texas 77843

Ernst L. Biberstein, D.V.M., Ph.D.
Department of Veterinary Microbiology and Immunology
School of Veterinary Medicine
University of California/Davis
Davis, California 95616

Joseph M. Cummins, Jr., D.V.M., Ph.D.
Texas A&M Research and Extension Center
6500 Amarillo Boulevard West
Amarillo, Texas 79106

Merwin L. Frey, D.V.M., Ph.D.
Department of Veterinary Science
University of Nebraska
Lincoln, Nebraska 68583

Robert W. Fulton, D.V.M., Ph.D.
Department of Parasitology, Microbiology and Public Health
College of Veterinary Medicine
Oklahoma State University
Stillwater, Oklahoma 74078

David E. Reed, Ph.D.
Veterinary Medical Research Institute
Iowa State University
Ames, Iowa 50011

Ronald F. Slocombe, B.S.V.S., Ph.D.
Department of Pathology
Veterinary Clinical Center
Michigan State University
East Lansing, Michigan 48824

Paul C. Smith, D.V.M., Ph.D.
Department of Microbiology
College of Veterinary Medicine
Auburn University
Auburn, Alabama 36849

G. B. Thompson, Ph.D.
Texas A&M Research and Extension Center
6500 Amarillo Boulevard West
Amarillo, Texas 79106

Acknowledgments

The following companies contributed financial support for the Poster Sessions and publication of the Symposium Proceedings:

Philips-Roxane, Inc.
2621 North Belt Highway
St. Joseph, Missouri 64502

Lilly Research Laboratories
Greenfield Laboratories
P.O. Box 708
Greenfield, Indiana 46140

The UpJohn Company
Agricultural Division
Kalamazoo, Michigan 49001

Fort Dodge Laboratories
Research and Development
Fort Dodge, Iowa 50501

Norden Laboratories, Inc.
601 West Cornhusker Highway
Lincoln, Nebraska 68521

Beecham Laboratories
501 Fifth Street
Bristol, Tennessee 37620

CEVA Laboratories, Inc.
10551 Barkley, Suite 500
Overland Park, Kansas 66212

The Organizing Committee expresses appreciation to Ms. Carolyn K. Wallace for assistance in editing manuscripts, for developing the layout and for typing the final text, to Dr. Donald H. Lewis for assistance in implementing computer text processing, and to the staff of the Biomedical Learning Resources Center of Texas A&M University for technical assistance.

Appreciation is also extended to session chairmen, speakers and participants who together made this Symposium a success.

Participants

Lorne A. Babiuk, Ph.D.
Professor, Department of Veterinary Microbiology
Western College of Veterinary Medicine
University of Saskatchewan
Saskatoon, Saskatchewan, Canada S7N 0W0

James L. Bittle, D.V.M.
Department of Molecular Biology
Scripps Clinic and Research Foundation
10666 North Torrey Pines Road
La Jolla, California 92037

Neville P. Clarke, D.V.M., Ph.D.
Director, Texas Agricultural Experiment Station
Texas A&M University System
College Station, Texas 77843

N. Andy Cole, Ph.D.
USDA Conservation and Production Research Laboratory
P.O. Drawer 10
Bushland, Texas 79102

Glynn H. Frank, D.V.M., Ph.D.
National Animal Disease Center
P.O. Box 70
Ames, Iowa 50010

Robert W. Fulton, D.V.M., Ph.D.
Professor,   Department   of   Veterinary   Parasitology,
Microbiology and Public Health
College of Veterinary Medicine
Oklahoma State University
Stillwater, Oklahoma 74048

Dallas P. Horton, Jr., D.V.M., M.S.
Owner, Horton Feedlot and Research Center
5100 East County Road 70
Wellington, Colorado 80549

George J. Jakab, Ph.D.
Associate Professor, Environmental Health Sciences
School of Hygiene and Public Health
Johns Hopkins University
Baltimore, Maryland 21205

Robert F. Kahrs, D.V.M., Ph.D.
Dean, College of Veterinary Medicine
University of Missouri
Columbia, Missouri 65211

Raymond W. Loan, D.V.M., Ph.D.
Associate Dean, College of Veterinary Medicine
Texas A&M University
College Station, Texas 77843

C. W. McMillan
Assistant Secretary for Marketing and Inspection Services
U.S. Department of Agriculture
Washington, D.C. 20250

John L. Merrill
Chairman, Research Committee
National Cattlemen's Association
Route 1, Box 54
Crowley, Texas 76036

Delbert G. Miles, D.V.M., M.S.
Veterinarian, Miller Feed Lots, Inc.
P.O. Box 937
LaSalle, Colorado 80645

Donald O. Morgan, D.V.M., Ph.D.
USDA, Agricultural Research Service
Plum Island Animal Disease Center
P.O. Box 848
Greenport, New York 11944

Michael B. A. Oldstone, M.D.
Department of Immunopathology
Scripps Clinic and Research Foundation
10666 Torrey Pines Road
La Jolla, California 92037

David E. Reed, Ph.D.
Professor, Veterinary Medical Research Institute
Iowa State University
Ames, Iowa 50011

Harland W. Renshaw, D.V.M., Ph.D.
Associate Professor, Department of Veterinary Microbiology
and Parasitology
College of Veterinary Medicine
Texas A&M University
College Station, Texas 77843

N. Edward Robinson, M.R.C.V.S., B.S.V.S., Ph.D.
Professor, Department of Physiology
College of Veterinary Medicine
Michigan State University
East Lansing, Michigan 48824

Bruce D. Rosenquist, D.V.M., Ph.D.
Professor, Department of Veterinary Microbiology
College of Veterinary Medicine
University of Missouri
Columbia, Missouri 65211

James A. Roth, D.V.M., Ph.D.
Associate Professor, Department of Veterinary Microbiology
and Preventive Medicine
College of Veterinary Medicine
Iowa State University
Ames, Iowa 50011

Paul C. Smith, D.V.M., Ph.D.
Professor and Chairman, Department of Microbiology
Auburn University
Auburn, Alabama 36849

R. G. Thomson, D.V.M., Ph.D.
Professor, Department of Veterinary Pathology
Western College of Veterinary Medicine
University of Saskatchewan
Saskatoon, Saskatchewan, Canada S7N 0W0

Edward Uvacek, Jr., Ph.D.
Extension Economist, Livestock Marketing and Professor,
Agricultural Economics
Texas A&M University
College Station, Texas 77843

Bruce N. Wilkie, D.V.M., Ph.D.
Professor, Department of Veterinary Microbiology and
Immunology
Ontario Veterinary College
University of Guelph
Guelph, Ontario, Canada N1G 2W1

Don E. Williams, D.V.M., M.S.
General Manager, Hitch Feedlot
P.O. Box 1442
Guymon, Oklahoma 73942

Lemuel J. Wilson
President, Lemmy Wilson Livestock, Inc.
P.O. Box 627
Newport, Tennessee 37821

Proceedings of the North American Symposium

on Bovine Respiratory Disease

Management, Marketing and Medicine

Dallas Horton, M.S., D.V.M.

Horton Feedlot & Research Center
5100 East County Road 70
Wellington, Colorado 80549

Many scientists feel that the old axiom of stress plus virus plus *Pasteurella* is still the etiology of shipping fever. I would like to propose to you today that the real etiology of shipping fever is the antiquated method we use to market calves. It has been estimated the average number of middlemen between the rancher and the consumer is about fifteen. Many calves, from the day they are removed from the dam (weaned) until they reach the feedlot, travel 800 to 1,000 miles and have seen more auction markets, truck rides and new country than the rancher who raised them. Then we ask ourselves after they have been through a journey such as this, why do they have respiratory disease and a 10 percent to 15 percent death loss? The question should be: why is the other 85 percent still alive?

I predict this marketing approach will change on the larger ranches in the Western states in the next ten years. Retained ownership by the rancher will occur mainly because of marketing and financial reasons and side benefits will be control of respiratory diseases through vaccination before weaning, holding the calves on the ranch until the stress of weaning is over, the use of good nutrition programs the first and second weeks post-weaning, and genetic selection. Research by the author has shown, with improved genetics which increases weaning weights, a 1 percent reduction in the incidence of disease occurs with every fifteen-pounds increase in weaning weight. Also our research has shown that for each one-day delay in vaccination, you can expect a 1 percent increase in the incidence of respiratory disease. A rancher with retained ownership can obviously markedly influence the genetics of his herd and, along with his veterinarian, can also influence the time and selection of vaccination.

As mentioned earlier, the real economic benefit to the rancher will be in the marketing arena. Retaining ownership will allow him to market his cattle in the late Spring and early Summer at fifteen to sixteen months of age to 1,100 to 1,150 pounds finished weight rather than in the Fall as 450- to 500-pound calves. A seasonal review of marketing shows that over the last twenty years, 85 percent of the time the market is higher in the Spring than in the Fall. The reason for this is 85 percent of all ranchers sell their calves in the Fall, thus repeatedly depressing the price with volume. Conversely, the seasonal high is usually late Spring and early Summer. Therefore, retained ownership will allow the rancher the opportunity to sell at a higher market versus a lower one.

The genetic improvement of a rancher's herd, resulting in improved weaning weights with current marketing methods, has resulted in a discount rather than a premium. On the average, 500-pound calves have brought five cents to ten cents per pound less than 400-pound calves because they were heavier.

Our research has shown the genetically superior heavier calf will have a better average daily gain and feed conversion, less death loss, and a superior carcass; therefore, showing the heavier calf is worth more, not less. Obviously, if we are going to improve the performance of feedlot cattle with genetics, we must have a marketing system that provides the rancher a premium for making them better rather than discounting these superior calves.

So far this paper has addressed calves raised on large Western ranches. Obviously, a large percentage of the feeder cattle in this country are raised in the Southeast on small farms with only ten to fifteen head raised on each farm. Control of disease through retained ownership for these cattle is not a reality.   Therefore, vaccines primarily for *Pasteurella* are going to have to be developed and administered as soon as is feasible, along with backgrounding and improved nutrition programs, in the Southeast before the long haul west. Also, medicated water and feed or the injection of long-acting medication while cattle are healthy, rather than waiting until the herd is ill, will markedly aid in respiratory disease control.

In summary, control of respiratory disease of calves raised on small farms in the Southeast will be through discovery of new and improved products in the field of immunology, backgrounding immediately after weaning, and the earlier use of medicinal agents via injection, feed or water.   Control of respiratory disease on large western ranches will come primarily from changes in marketing, namely retained ownership.

The Economics of the Cattle Industry

Edward Uvacek, Jr., B.S., M.S., Ph.D.

Agricultural Extension Service, Texas A&M University
College Station, Texas 77843

The livestock and meat industry is dynamic and constantly changing. The driving forces of change have been the consumer who desires a different, better quality or less expensive product; the scientist who discovers a new technique of production, processing and marketing; and the businessman who turns changes in consumer tastes, preferences or technological innovations into a profit. Some might add to this list a myriad of government policies that prevent packers from getting involved in meat retailing, import regulations or changes in nutrition education policies. The effects of such changes are seldom isolated at only one level of the market system. Changes at each level, in fact, have a tendency to create a chain reaction effect that causes ripples--or more frequently waves--throughout the entire system.

In a market-oriented economy, consumers are the driving force. When consumers change their meat-buying or preparation habits, the effect is felt throughout the whole livestock and meat industry. Consumer changes may be recorded in population, income levels or tastes and preferences. They also react directly to changes in price--both the absolute price and the price relative of beef to other meats and foods.

Through the 1950's, probably the most important change was in the number of consumers, reflecting America's continuous population growth. In the 1960's, the dominant force of change shifted from population growth to income levels and geographic shifts in the population. Higher incomes meant increased ability to buy meat as people consumed more meat per capita, ate more meat away from home and ate higher priced cuts of meat. Movements of the U.S. population to the West Coast early in the decade increased the demand for more fed beef and stimulated the location of the large cattle-feeding business in the Southwest. Toward the end of the 1960's and in the first part of the 1970's, the feeding industry of the Southern Great Plains matured to satisfy the growing consumer demand for fed cattle. During the late 1970's and early 1980's, consumer demand for convenience foods and a growing but variable price disparity between beef, poultry and other meat items appeared to take over as the driving force of consumer change.

The supermarket, combining the concepts of self-service and large-scale centralized buying of meat, brought with it a new era of meat marketing. Each consumer was offered a cafeteria of individually packaged meat cuts in a self-service supermarket meat case. Supermarket meat purchasing agents desired consistent quality and uniform size of cuts. To satisfy these requirements, all meat was purchased to certain specifications. While the small butcher shop bought five or ten carcasses per week, the retail chain store bought two or three thousand carcasses each week. Thus, the need for rigid specification buying was obvious and it soon became an accepted method of communicating the supermarket's perception of consumer meat demands to packers.

Meat packers, a functional level located between the producer and retailer market segments, responded to this new array of market forces from producers and retailers. In general, most packers located their plants where the livestock was produced and where other resources such as water, sewage and labor were abundant and cost-competitive. Packer changes came in response to the demands of the retail food supermarkets and the away-from-home eating market. As supermarkets and fast-food outlets developed their own brands and became more important market forces, the packer brands found the competitive battle much more intense.

Scale economies also played an important role. In the early to mid-20th century, industry trends were characterized by a relatively small number of very large multi-species packing plants located at or near the large central livestock markets of the Midwest. Since then, these large plants have been superseded by a trend toward decentralization and specialization. Initially, specialization resulted in a separation of the slaughtering and processing functions of the packer. Subsequently, packing plants became even more specialized to the degree of slaughtering only a single species of livestock or even a single livestock type (fed steers or cows) within a species.

Along with increased specialization within the packing industry, there was a substantial shift in the geographic location of the slaughter of the different species. While Chicago, St. Paul and Kansas City were once the major slaughtering centers for the industry, these markets have now given way to new plants located in other production areas such as the Southern Plains.

A major consequence of this relocation of the industry and the move toward increased specialization, was the decreasing importance of the old-line packers such as Armour, Swift, Cudahy and Wilson. This demise was accompanied by a rise of some new industry giants like Iowa Beef Processors, MBPXL, Monfort of Colorado and American Beef.

Since World War I, declines have occurred in the U.S. farm population. The number of livestock producers disappearing has been even more pronounced. Along with this adjustment in numbers, have come locational shifts and a dramatic increase in the scale of operations--particularly in the livestock feeding function. Cattle feeding became largely a separate enterprise from cattle raising. The rise of the cattle feedlot was accompanied by a geographic shift in the location of cattle feeding from the farmer-feeder of the Midwest, to the commercial feedlot in the Plains states.

The emergence of the custom feedlot of the Southern Plains resulted from a combination of forces including climatic advantages, tax shelters, a source of low-cost feedgrains, biomedical advances allowing confinement feeding and massive economies of scale. The large capital requirements associated with feedlot operation then resulted in a need to separate cattle ownership from the feeding function. This unique financial structure also provided ranchers and farmers with the alternative of integrating vertically into the feeding function.

Producer adjustments were far from independent of those that occurred at other levels of the market system.   The cattle industry began tailoring its production and feeding to the demands of consumers and retailers for the degree of leanness and uniformity desired.   Such changes obviously had implications for producers of breeding stock throughout the United States and, for that matter, the world.

Technological innovations have occurred continuously throughout the livestock industry from breeding through food preparation.   These changes have made the industry highly dynamic.   The past has been shaped by such new innovations as cross breeding, artificial insemination, refrigeration, the refrigerated rail car, mechanical deboning, the home freezer, cryovac packaging, the 18-wheeler, antibiotics, assembly-line processing and, the most recent, boxed beef. The bulk of these technologies were adopted quite slowly, however, and the industry structure evolved through several decades.   While historically the acceptance of new technology has been slow, it is anticipated that the adoption of new ideas will rapidly accelerate in the future.

FED CATTLE MARKETINGS, 1982

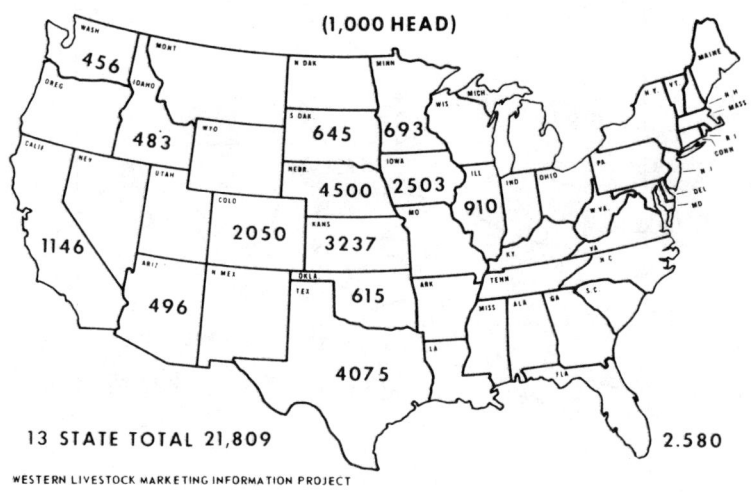

(1,000 HEAD)

13 STATE TOTAL 21,809   2.580

WESTERN LIVESTOCK MARKETING INFORMATION PROJECT

COW NUMBERS JANUARY 1, 1954 TO 1983

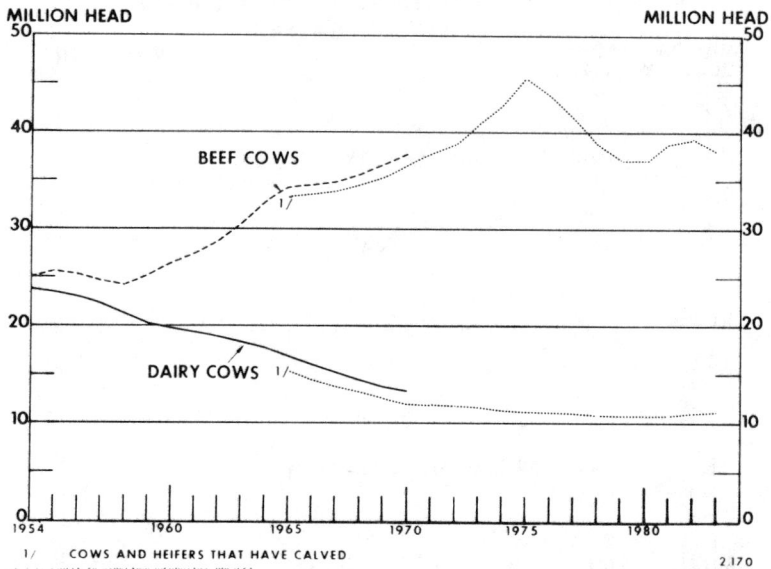

1/   COWS AND HEIFERS THAT HAVE CALVED

2.170

CATTLE ON FARMS BY CYCLES

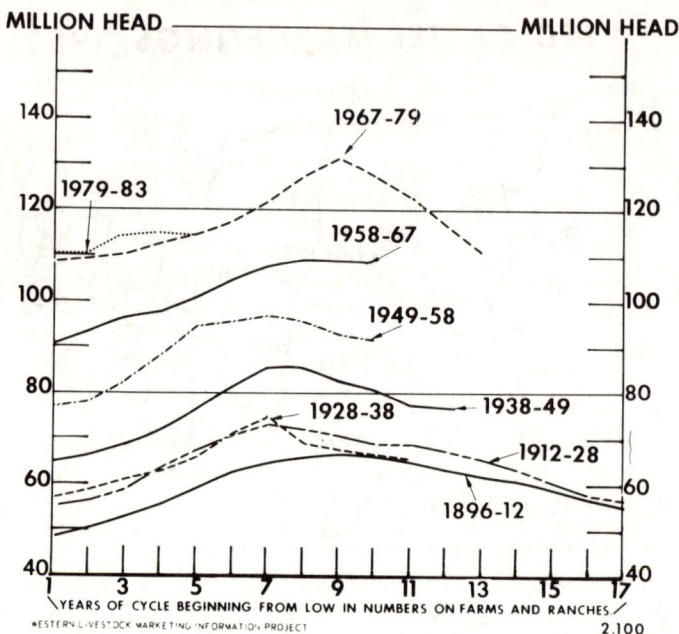

WESTERN LIVESTOCK MARKETING INFORMATION PROJECT

2.100

FED CATTLE MARKETINGS BY SIZE OF FEEDLOT
13 STATES 1964-1982

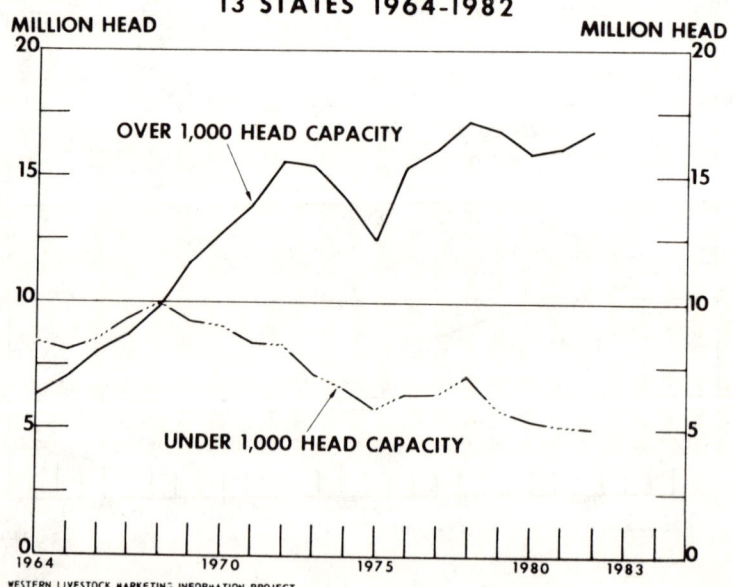

WESTERN LIVESTOCK MARKETING INFORMATION PROJECT

2.592

BEEF COWS THAT HAVE CALVED
JANUARY 1, 1983
(1,000 HEAD)

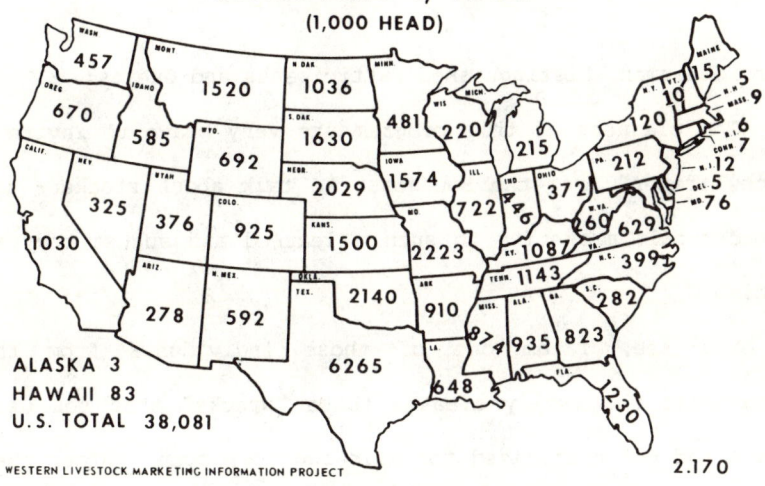

ALASKA 3
HAWAII 83
U.S. TOTAL 38,081

WESTERN LIVESTOCK MARKETING INFORMATION PROJECT

2.170

FED CATTLE MARKETINGS (13 STATES), 1960 - 1982

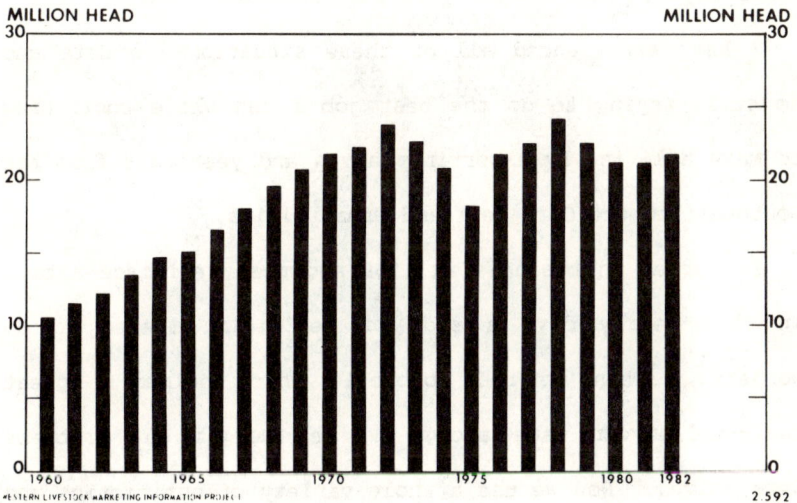

WESTERN LIVESTOCK MARKETING INFORMATION PROJECT

2.592

Stocker-, Feeder-Calf Marketing

Lemuel J. Wilson

President, Lemmy Wilson Livestock, Inc.
P.O. Box 627
Newport, Tennessee 37821

Mr. Chairman, Distinguished Participants and Guests:

The planners of this program are very brave to invite a "cow trader" from the Southeast to talk about stocker- and feeder-calf marketing to such a learned and august body as this.

You see, I am one of those individuals from the Southeast who really creates those "wrecks" that you deal with and get criticized for allowing to happen. After they get through with you people, then the blame comes to the order-buyer.

I have experienced all of these situations to date and am still trying to do the best job I can while continuing to make a living by exporting calves and yearlings from the Southeast to the Corn Belt and Great Plains.

I started in business in 1959 and must reminisce a bit. In those early days a shot of penicillin seemed to do wonders. Then we had combiotic which helped a great deal--terramycin came along and we thought our problems were solved. Now we use a whole variety of antibiotics and still have the same problems.   Sometimes it seems more severe now than in earlier years.

I became very enthusiastic about preconditioning in the Southeast and built a very expensive facility to prove it. That has been a SAD STORY.

I just knew that I could really solve these respiratory problems before we stressed the cattle by transporting them long distances. However, they can get just as sick at my place as they do in Texas, New Mexico or Kansas.   As a matter of fact, I have more trouble than the good caretakers do out here.

Now, I know many of you are saying the thing to do is build immunity in the calves before they leave the farm, and I agree that would be good.   But I am kind of reminded of a "high powered" vet who came to my preconditioning facility to solve my health problems.   He said it was very simple, just do like the broiler people: put 1,200 calves in at one time, precondition them, move them all out, start again.   Now, obviously he has never tried to get an order every six-eight weeks for 1,200 head of Southeast calves and get them all bought in 24 hours and have all of them in condition to ship at the same time.

As you well know, we are basically dealing with cow herds of around 25 head and the degree of management is not very good. These producers use their cow-calf operation like a savings account. When they need money they sell a calf or two or three. There is virtually nothing to be done for that animal until I get my hands on him in my facility--about 12-24 hours after he leaves the farm gate.

Now, this is where I really want to put it to you! Our research efforts need to be directed toward building some effective, fast *immunity* at this point in the marketing process. Now, I realize this is very easy to say and at present impossible to accomplish. But there is enough brain power at this meeting to get started toward such a breakthrough in bovine respiratory diseases--*FAST EFFECTIVE IMMUNITY*--I want to drive it home.

As far as treating sick calves, we really do a lot of guessing and shotgunning these days. Why can't we have a timely technique that would tell us what antibiotic would be most effective in each case? There must be a way to develop such a procedure.

Genetic engineering is a popular subject these days and I would like to add my two cents. From my standpoint, I would like to see some work done toward selecting for the calves that don't get sick. I don't care how efficient the animal is, if he dies or becomes a chronic, it is all in vain. I have never experienced a load of calves where they *all* got sick. Now, 90 percent might, but not all. Why not? What is different about the ones that never get sick?

Well, as you expected I don't have any answers, just a lot of questions. But I truly would like to stimulate your thinking toward *Fast, Effective Immunity,* and *Easy, Reliable Sensitivity* for the best antibiotics, and genetic knowledge related to our *respiratory problems.*

Feeder-calf marketing in the Southeast hasn't really changed much in the 24 years I have been in business. We are developing some good marketing techniques for the farmers that have as much as one load that we can trade as a marketable unit. I have been selling yearlings and calves this way for years and our volume increased 322 percent this year over last year. But this will always be a small part of the total volume marketed in the Southeast because of the herd size.

I sincerely want to express my thanks to you for this opportunity to get acquainted with many of you during this meeting. I have the greatest respect for a symposium of this kind because we desperately need the answers to bovine respiratory disease—a condition that will not be cured without your continuing efforts and dedicated service.

Thank you very much.

A Critical Evaluation of Preconditioning

N. Andy Cole, Ph.D.

Conservation and Production Research Laboratory
Agricultural Research Service, U.S. Department of Agriculture
P.O. Box 10
Bushland, Texas 79012

Summary

Preconditioning has been highly publicized for many years as a program to reduce the incidence of bovine respiratory disease. Much of this publicity, however, has been based on uncontrolled surveys and testimonials. The purpose of this manuscript is to review the available controlled data on preconditioning of feeder calves. A review of the controlled data indicates that preconditioning will do the following:

1. have no effect on farm weight gains compared to calves left with their dams,

2. will not affect market-transit shrink,

3. will not affect feedlot performance if calves are fed longer than 100 days,

4. will reduce feedlot morbidity about six percentage units, and

5. will reduce feedlot mortality about 0.7 percentage

units but will tend to increase mortality at the farm.

Although theoretically sound, the practice of preconditioning will not, in general, reduce sickness sufficiently to repay the cost of the program. Future reseach should concentrate on methods to revise the preconditioning concept so that it will be more economically feasible to the cattle industry.

Introduction

Preconditioning of feeder calves to reduce feedlot morbidity has been highly publicized for many years. In brief, preconditioning can be described as a comprehensive management system designed to immunize calves against some major pathogens involved in the bovine respiratory disease complex and to reduce the stressors encountered by feeder calves at marketing. As defined by the American Academy of Bovine Practitioners (1), preconditioning consists of the following elements, all done at the farm-of-origin and certified by a veterinarian:

1. calves weaned at least three weeks before sale,

2. calves trained to eat from a feed bunk and to drink from a trough,

3. calves treated for parasites,

4. calves vaccinated for blackleg, malignant edema,

parainfluenza-3 virus (PI-3), infectious bovine rhinotracheitis virus (IBR), *Pasteurella,* and sometimes bovine viral diarrhea virus (BVD) and *Haemophilus somnus,*

5. calves castrated and dehorned, and

6. calves identified with an ear tag.

Terms such as backgrounding and preweaning are sometimes confused with preconditioning. Backgrounding, while similar to preconditioning, is generally accomplished by obtaining calves from several sources rather than from a single cow-calf operation. Before shipment to the feedlot, backgrounded calves are normally fed a growing ration or grazed on pasture for 30 to 90 days at a location close to the source of the cattle. Preweaning consists of weaning and feeding calves as in preconditioning but vaccinations and treatments for parasitism are not done.

Information from uncontrolled surveys and testimonials has suggested that preconditioning of feeder calves will do the following:

1. increase on-farm weight gain,

2. reduce market-transit shrink,

3. improve feedlot performance,

4. reduce feedlot morbidity and mortality, and

5. increase profits for producer and feeder.

The purpose of this manuscript is to summarize the controlled research data in which preconditioned calves are compared to an equal group of non-preconditioned calves. Included in this review are several studies in which calves were preweaned only.   The use of these studies will be discussed later in the manuscript. Due to the known effects of farm-of-origin on calf health and performance (2, Table 1), experiments in which controls and preconditioned calves originated from different farms were omitted from this review.

Table 1. Influence of farm-of-origin on calf weight gains and feedlot morbidity[a]

Farm	Weight gain at farm, kg		Feedlot morbidity, %	
	Control	Preweaned	Control	Preweaned
A	9	8	62	38
B	40	25	25	0
C	9	13	83	86
D	14	17	17	43
E	26	31	25	44
13 farm mean	15	20	53	51

[a] J. B. McLaren et al., unpublished data.

Observations

On-Farm Weight Gains and Marketing Transport Weight Losses

The effects of preweaning and feeding on calf weight gains at the farm-of-origin are presented in Table 2 (3-11).

Table 2. Influence of preweaning or preconditioning on weight gains at the farm-of-origin

Reference	Days	Weight gain, kg Control	Weight gain, kg Treated	DMI[a] kg/hd
Meyer et al., 1971[b*]	45	36	39	–
Meyer et al., 1971[c*]	45	18	10	–
McArthur et al., 1973[d]	30	10	11	–
Wieringa et al., 1974[b*]	20	13	10	114
Pate and Crockett, 1978[b*]	28	10	10	116
Cole et al., 1979[b]	30	15	20	136
Cole et al., 1982[b]	30	29	34	118
Cole et al., unpublished[b]	30	27	21	–
Strohbehn et al., 1981[b*]	84	71	71	–
Hutcheson et al., unpublished[b*]	30	14	17	137
Trial average (10)[e]		24.3	24.3	–
Preconditioned(6)[*]		27.0	26.2	–
Preweaned (4)		20.2	21.5	–
DMI only (5)		16.2	18.2	124

[a] Total dry matter intake of preweaned calves.

[b] Greater than 50% concentrate, fed ad libitum.

[c] Greater than 50% concentrate, limit fed.

[d] Primarily pasture.

[e] Value in parentheses is number of trials included in the means.

[*] Totally preconditioned. References without asterisk are preweaned only.

Preweaned calves gained on the average about the same weight as calves left with their dams with a range of five kilograms more to eight kilograms less than unweaned control calves. Studies at Oklahoma (12) and Florida (13) indicate that calves require about twelve days to regain their initial weight after weaning. Thus, during a 28-day preconditioning period, only the last sixteen days will actually produce an increase in calf weight. Preweaned calves required about 8.3 kilograms of feed dry matter for each kilogram of weight gained at the farm-of-origin (Table 3) (5-8,11).

Table 3. Feed/gain of preweaned calves at farm-of-origin

	Total		Extra[a]	
Reference	Gain, kg	Feed/Gain	Gain, kg	Feed/Gain
Wieringa et al., 1974[*]	10	11.4	−3	—
Pate and Crockett, 1978 [*]	10	11.6	0	—
Cole et al., 1979	20	6.8	5	27.2
Cole et al., 1982	34	3.5	5	23.6
Hutcheson et al., unpublished[*]	17	8.0	3	45.7
Five trial average	18.2	8.26	2.4	51.7

[a] Increase in gain over calves left with their dams.

[*] Totally preconditioned. References without asterisks are preweaned only.

However, if the weight gains are compared to unweaned calves left with their dams, preweaned calves required about 52 kilograms of feed dry matter for each kilogram increase in weight gain over unweaned calves.

It has been observed that on some farms preweaned calves will significantly outgain control calves left with their dams, while just the opposite is true on other farms (Table 1) (2). These farm differences could be due to differences in grass conditions and cow milk production. One may assume that when grass is in short supply or of poor quality and cows are milking poorly, preweaned calves could outperform calves left with their dams. However, when plenty of high-quality grass is available and cows are milking well, preweaned calves would probably perform more poorly than calves left with their dams.

The effects of preweaning and feeding on market-transit weight losses are presented in Table 4 (6-11,14,15). When unweaned control calves and preweaned calves were subjected to the same marketing channels, weight losses were similar. Trials at this station (7,8,11) indicate that preweaned calves will consume more feed at the order-buyer facility than freshly weaned calves and thus lose less weight during marketing (auction and order-buyer). During transit, however, preweaned calves lose more weight probably due to

their greater gut-fill. The difference in composition of
weight loss (i.e., gut-fill or tissue-shrink) during
marketing and transit has not been compared in control and
preweaned calves.

Table 4. Effects of preweaning or preconditioning on market-transit
         weight losses

| Reference | Hrs in transit | Weight loss | | | |
| | | Control | | Treated | |
		kg	%	kg	%
Knight et al., 1972[*]	3[a]	—	5.7	—	4.4
Wieringa et al., 1976[*]	128[b]	24	11.4	24	11.4
Pate and Crockett, 1978[*]	30	21	10.0	28	12.4
Pate and Crockett, 1978[*]	3	6	2.7	12	5.4
Cole et al., 1979	26	23	10.8	25	11.4
Cole et al., 1982	26	29	13.0	27	12.5
Cole et al., unpublished	26	32	14.3	29	13.7
Strohbehn et al., 1981[*]	3[a]	7	2.9	8	3.3
Hutcheson et al., unpublished[*]	28	—	6.7	—	6.2
7 or 9 Trial average		20	8.6	22	9.0

[a] Estimated from length of haul.

[b] Calves were fed and watered 3 times while in transit.

[*] Totally preconditioned. References without asterisks are preweaned only.

Feedlot Performance and Health

During the first 30 to 45 days in the feedlot, preweaned calves generally consume more feed and gain more weight than control calves (Table 5) (3,5,7-9,11,14,16,17). By 100 days in the feedlot, however, control and preweaned calves have similar daily gains (Table 6) (3-9,11,14,16,17). Preweaned calves had a significant (P<0.05) advantage in feedlot daily weight gain (advantage, 0.06 kilogram) in only one of eleven trials reviewed (17), and that trial was only 90 days long. Only seven trials were available to study the effects of preweaning or preconditioning on feedlot feed conversion (kilograms feed dry matter consumed/kilograms weight gained) (Table 6) (3-9,11,14,16,17).

Table 5. Performance of preweaned or preconditioned calves during the first
30 to 45 days in the feedlot

Reference	Daily gain, kg		Dry matter intake, kg	
	Control	Treated	Control	Treated
Meyer et al., 1971[*]	1.07	1.31	—	—
Knight et al., 1972[*]	0.89	0.95	—	—
Woods et al., 1973[b*]	0.50	0.84	—	—
Wieringa et al., 1974[*]	0.98	0.95	—	—
Cole et al., 1979	1.04	1.14	5.5	6.0
Cole et al., 1982	1.12	0.95	7.0	7.6
Cole et al., unpublished	1.08	1.31	6.7	8.0
Strohbehn, 1981[*]	0.67	0.92	8.3	8.1
Hutcheson et al., unpublished[*]	1.16	1.31	6.6	7.0
Trial average	0.94	1.08	6.8	7.3

[*] Totally preconditioned. References without asterisks are preweaned only.

Table 6. Influence of preweaning or preconditioning on feedlot performance

Reference	Days fed	Daily gain, kg		F/G[a]	
		C[b]	T[b]	C[b]	T[b]
Meyer et al., 1971[*]	252	.97	.97	7.85	8.00
Knight et al., 1972[*]	204	1.15	1.15	—	—
Woods et al., 1973[b*]	130	.50	.54	—	—
McArthur, 1973	210	1.09	1.12	—	—
Wieringa et al., 1974[*]	30	.98	.95	—	—
Pate and Crockett, 1978[*]	200	.92	.97	8.31	8.34
Cole et al., 1979	211	1.15	1.10	5.89	6.40
Cole et al., 1982	186	.98	.97	8.10	8.50
Cole et al., unpublished	184	1.10	1.10	6.90	7.50
Strohbehn, 1981[*]	90	.94	1.00	8.94	8.68
Hutcheson et al., unpublished[*]	56	1.13	1.22	6.80	6.50
7–11 Trial average		.99	1.01	7.54	7.70
Less than 100 days		.89	1.00	7.87	7.59
More than 100 days		.98	.99	7.41	7.75
Preconditioned[*]		.94	.97	7.98	7.88
Preweaned		1.08	1.07	6.96	7.47

[a] Kg of feed dry matter per kg weight gain.

[b] C = control, T = preweaned or preconditioned.

[*] Totally preconditioned. References without asterisks are preweaned only.

In five of seven trials, preweaned calves had poorer feed conversions than control calves. In the two trials in which preweaned calves had an advantage in feed conversion (11,17), the feeding period was less than 100 days. Studies of calf growth and body composition (18) suggest that preweaned calves tend to have poorer feed conversions than control calves due to a greater rate of fat deposition during the last few weeks at the farm and the first few weeks at the feedlot. Billingsley et al. (19) demonstrated that feedlot gains were inversely proportional to weight gains during the last 30 days at the farm-of-origin. Pate and Crockett (20) reported that preconditioned calves had a greater fat thickness (8 millimeters versus 10 millimeters) and kidney fat (3.5 percent versus 3.7 percent) than control calves after 200 days in the feedlot.

In the seven trials reviewed, preconditioning reduced feedlot morbidity about six percentage units or about 23 percent compared to controls (Table 7) (6-9,11,14-17,21). Preweaning alone produced a reduction in morbidity similar to total preconditioning--17 percent versus 23 percent, respectively. Preconditioned calves had a higher morbidity rate than control calves in only one of ten trials (14). In that trial, the preconditioned calves were vaccinated at weaning.

Table 7. Influence of preweaning or preconditioning on feedlot
          morbidity

Reference	Control	Treated
Knight et al., 1972[a][*]	16.4	20.2
Knight et al., 1972[b][*]	16.4	9.6
Woods et al., 1973[a][*]	23.8	21.5
Woods et al., 1973[b][*]	73.0	63.0
Wieringa et al., 1976[*]	12.0	4.0
Pate and Crockett, 1978[*]	23.0	7.0
Cole et al., 1979	53.3	51.1
Cole et al., 1982	53.7	51.6
Cole et al., unpublished	51.1	28.9
Hutcheson et al., unpublished[*]	20.9	17.2
Strohbehn, 1981[*]	NR[c]	NR
10 Trial average	34.4	27.4 (−20%)
Preconditioned (7)[*]	26.5	20.4 (−23%)
Preweaned (3)	52.7	43.9 (−17%)

[a] Vaccinated at weaning.

[b] Vaccinated 30 days before weaning.

[c] Not reported, but no difference between controls and preconditioned
calves (Strohbehn, personal communication).

[*] Totally preconditioned. References without asterisk are preweaned
only.

Preconditioning reduced feedlot mortality about 0.7 percentage units in the trials reviewed. Preweaning alone reduced feedlot mortality about 0.37 percentage units. Two trials have reported on-farm death losses of 1.0 percent to 1.9 percent in preconditioned calves due to bloat, acidosis and surgical infections. Although few trials report the effects of preconditioning or preweaning on morbidity and mortality at the farm-of-origin, it is apparent from several trials (3,6,17) that when calves are preconditioned, the cow-calf producer will have more health problems, especially if he is unfamiliar with feeding calves.

Economics

A list of reasonable costs to precondition a calf is presented in Table 9 (3). Of the total cost of $38.76, about 50 percent is feed and about 20 percent is labor. These cost figures assume the producer has facilities to work cattle, to feed calves separated from the cows and to store and handle feed.

When the cow-calf producer chooses to precondition calves, he must decide if he will wean them at the usual time and then feed them for 28 days or if he will wean them 28 days earlier than normal and sell them at the usual time. If he weans the calves early, he cannot expect to sell heavier calves since they will gain about the same amount of weight as calves left on the cow. If he holds them an extra 28 days, he can expect to sell about an 18-kilograms heavier calf (Table 2, 28- and 30-day data only) (3-11). If the producer weans his calves early, he will require a bonus price of about $21.00/100 kilograms ($9.69/cwt) to break even (Table 10). If he holds his calves an extra 28 days, he will need a bonus price of about $5.50/100 kilograms ($2.51/cwt) to break even.

Using the data from Tables 6 (3-9,11,14,16,17), 7 (6-9,11,14-17,21) and 8 (6-9,11,14-17,21), the economics of using preconditioned calves in the feedlot (Table 11) or in a stocker program (Table 12) were calculated assuming the feeder or stocker paid the break-even bonus required by the cow-calf producer. In the feedlot (Table 11), preconditioning would reduce feed and medicine costs minimally, but the higher purchase price along with the additional interest cost would result in a net loss to the feeder approximately equal to the bonus he paid for the calves. In a 120-day stocker program (Table 12), preconditioned calves may be heavier than non-preconditioned calves after 120 days but their higher purchase price would result in a higher break-even cost for the stocker.

Table 8. Influence of preweaning or preconditioning on calf mortality

| Reference | Control | Preweaned or Preconditioned | | |
		Farm	Feedlot	Total
Knight et al., 1972[a][*]	2.5	—	0.0	0.0
Knight et al., 1972[b][*]	2.5	—	1.9	1.9
Woods et al., 1973[a][*]	1.4	—	0.8	0.8
Woods et al., 1973[b][*]	0.0	—	1.3	1.3
Wieringa et al., 1976[*]	0.0	—	0.0	0.0
Pate and Crockett, 1978[*]	2.5	1.0[c]	0.0	1.0
Cole et al., 1979	3.3	0.0	2.2	2.2
Cole et al., 1982	1.1	0.0	1.1	1.1
Cole et al., unpublished	0.0	0.0	0.0	0.0
Strohbehn, 1981[*]	NR[d]	1.9[c]	NR[d]	NR
Hutcheson et al., unpublished[*]	1.2	0.0	1.2	1.2
Trial average	1.45	(0.26)	0.85	0.95
Preconditioned	1.44	(0.36)	0.74	0.88
Preweaned	1.47	0.0	1.10	1.10

[a] Vaccinated 30 days before weaning.

[b] Vaccinated at weaning.

[c] Deaths due to bloat, acidosis, or surgical infection.

[d] Not reported, but no difference between controls and preconditioned calves (Strohbehn, personal communication).

[*] Totally preconditioned. References without asterisks are preweaned only.

Table 9. Estimated cost to precondition a calf for 30 days
excluding facility costs

Item	Amt/Head	$/Unit	$/Head
Feed	127 kg	0.165 ($150/ton)	20.96
Vaccines	—	—	3.00
Wormer	1 dose	1.20	1.20
Grubacide	1 dose	0.50	0.50
Labor	2 hr[a]	4.00	8.00
Veterinarian	.05 hr[a]	50.00	2.50
Antibiotic	10%	10.00/head	1.00
Death loss	0.4%	70.00/cwt	1.12
Interest	15%	—	.48
			38.76

[a] Meyer et al., 1971.

Table 10. Economics of preconditioning calves: cow-calf producer

Item	Unit price, $	Value or cost, $	
		Early weaned	Normally weaned
Calf, 182 kg	1.54	280.28	280.28
Preconditioning	—	38.76	38.76
Total cost, $	—	319.04	319.04
Sold: 182 kg calf	1.54	280.28	—
Sold: 200 kg calf[a]	1.54	—	308.00
Difference[b], $	—	38.76	11.04
Bonus $/kg[b]	—	0.213	0.055
($/cwt)[b]	—	(9.69)	(2.51)

[a] Gain of 18 kg over 28 days (Table 2).

[b] Bonus required for cow-calf producer to break even financially.

Table 11. Economics to the feeder of feeding preconditioned calves
to 500 kg[a][b]

Item	Normal 182 kg	Preconditioned 182 kg	Preconditioned 200 kg
Calf cost	280.28	280.28	308.00
Bonus paid	0.00	38.76	11.04
Subtotal, $	280.28	319.04	319.04
Feed cost	418.71	413.46	390.06
Medicine	3.98	3.06	3.06
Death loss	4.06	2.73	2.73
Interest	63.65	68.56	67.04
Subtotal, $	490.40	487.81	462.89
Total cost, $	770.68	806.85	781.93
Increase over controls, $	—	36.17	11.25

[a] Cost figure: calf — $1.54/kg ($70/cwt); feed — $0.165/kg ($150/ton); medicine — $15/head treated; interest — 15% on 100% of cattle and 50% of feed.

[b] Control calves: daily gain = 0.94 kg; F/G = 7.98; morbidity = 26.5%; mortality = 1.44%. Preconditioned calves: daily gain = 0.97 kg; F/G = 7.88; morbidity = 20.4%; mortality = 0.74%.

Table 12. Economics of using preconditioned calves in a 120-day stocker program

Item	Normal 182 kg	Preconditioned 182 kg	Preconditioned 200 kg
Calf cost	280.28	280.28	308.00
Bonus	0.00	38.76	11.04
Subtotal, $	280.28	319.04	319.04
Pasture	40.00	40.00	40.00
Medicine	3.98	3.06	3.06
Death loss	4.06	2.73	2.73
Interest	15.02	16.93	16.93
Supplement	12.00	12.00	12.00
Subtotal, $	75.06	74.72	74.72
Total cost, $	355.34	393.76	393.76
Final wt, kg[a] (lb)	295 (649)	302 (664)	320 (704)
Break-even price: $/kg[b]	1.20	1.30	1.23
($/cwt)	(54.75)	(59.27)	(55.93)
Increase over controls: (S/cwt)		4.52	1.18
Total, $		30.01	8.31

[a] Daily gains of .94 and 1.0 kg for normal and preconditioned calves, respectively.

[b] Price required by stocker to break even.

Conclusions

Throughout this review it was sometimes necessary to use data from calves that were preweaned only and not totally preconditioned. The author has attempted to separate data from preconditioned and preweaned calves whenever possible. The deficiency of data on preconditioned calves in some areas, however, has necessitated the combining of this data. A comparison of preweaning alone and preconditioning is presented in Table 13. There is little difference in farm gain, shrink, feedlot gain, morbidity and mortality when preweaning and preconditioning are compared. The efficacy of vaccination for the prevention of bovine respiratory disease has recently been reviewed and questioned (22). The similarity between results of preweaning and preconditioning in this review would tend to substantiate the conclusions of Martin (22). In addition, several studies (6,10) have used a factorial arrangement of treatments to compare various aspects of preconditioning (preweaning, vaccination, et cetera) and, in general, the trials have shown little or no difference in vaccinated and non-vaccinated calves.

Table 13. Comparison of preweaning only (PW) vs. a total preconditioning (PC) program

Item	Comparison to controls		Difference
	PW	PC	
Farm gain, kg	+1.0	−1.0	−2.0
Shrink, %	−.2	+.6	−.8
Feedlot ADG, kg	−.01	+.03	+.04
Feed/gain[a]	+.51[a]	−.10[a]	+.61[a]
% BRD	−8.8	−6.1	−2.7
% Death, FL	−.37	−.70	+.33
% Death, total	−.37	−.56	+.19

[a] Shortage of data and differences in length of trials make this comparison questionable.

Table 14. A comparison of survey data vs. controlled data regarding preconditioning

Item	Survey	Controlled
Farm gains	+10–30 kg	N.E.[a]
Shrink	−5%	N.E.
Feedlot gains	+???	N.E.
Feedlot F/G	−???	N.E.
Morbidity	−20–30%	−6%
Mortality, FL	−0–1.7%	−0.7%
Mortality, total	−	−0.6%
Bonus price	$3–7/cwt.	Uniform groups

[a] N.E. = no effect.

The results of controlled experiments and surveys on preconditioning are very contradictory (Table 14). Although surveys often report improved feedlot performance in preconditioned calves, these reports are often speculative since there is no true control group with which to compare. Both controlled studies and surveys report that preconditioned calves will gain ten to thirty kilograms during the last 28 days at the farm-of-origin. Many surveys, however, fail to consider that unweaned calves left with their dams will gain a similar amount of weight. Most surveys compare preconditioned calves that did not pass through an order-buyer facility to groups of calves that passed through an order-buyer facility (i.e., normal calves). This may account for the differences in shrink, morbidity, and mortality noted between surveys and controlled studies. Most surveys report that preconditioned calves will sell for $6.60 to $15.40/100 kilograms ($3.00 to $7.00/cwt) more than non-preconditioned calves. Studies in Tennessee indicate that calf prices can be increased $4.40 to $11.00/100 kilograms ($2.00 to $5.00 cwt) simply by sorting them into uniform groups (2). Although several surveys suggest that preconditioning can be profitable to the producer and feeder, these surveys often do not take into account all the costs involved. Although surveys and testimonials can be good sources of preliminary information that may lead to controlled experiments, it is apparent that their results can sometimes be misleading. After twenty years of publicity and debate, the concept of preconditioning should be evaluated on the basis of controlled experimentation rather than on testimonials. The concept of preconditioning is theoretically sound; however, it is apparent from the controlled data available that modification and improvement of the preconditioning program is needed before it is ready to be used by the majority of the U.S. beef cattle industry.

References

1.   Anon:Report of the panel for the symposium on immunity to the bovine respiratory disease complex. J Am Vet Med Assoc 152:713-719, 1968.

2.   McLaren JB, Billingsley RD, Orr CL, Damron WS, McCurley JR, Moody EL:Unpublished data, Dept of Anim Sci, Univ of Tenn, Knoxville.

3.   Meyer KB, Beeson WM, Armstrong TH:Observations on the preconditioning of feeder cattle.   Indiana Cattle Feeders Day, Purdue Univ, pp. 5-8, March 1971.

4.   McArthur JAB:Early weaning of beef calves.   Oregon State Univ, 15th Ann Beef Cattle Day Rept No. 384, pp. 35-38, 1973.

5. Wieringa FL, Curtis RA, Radostits OM:The effect of preconditioning on weight gain and shrinkage in beef calves. Can Vet J 15:309-311, 1974.

6. Pate FM, Crockett JR:Value of preconditioning beef calves. Univ of Florida Agric Exp Stn Bulletin No. 799, 1978.

7. Cole NA, Irwin MR, McLaren JB:Influence of pretransit feeding regimen and post-transit B-vitamin supplementation on stressed feeder steers. J Anim Sci 49:310-317, 1979.

8. Cole NA, McLaren JB, Hutcheson DP:Influence of preweaning and B-vitamin supplementation of the feedlot receiving diet on calves subjected to marketing and transit stress. J Anim Sci 54:911-917, 1982.

9. Cole NA, Hutcheson DP, McLaren JB:Unpublished data. USDA-ARS, Bushland, Tx; Texas A&M Univ Agric Res, Amarillo, Tx; and Univ of Tenn, Knoxville, respectively.

10. Strohbehn DR, Willham RL, Rouse G:Effect of calf management on growth rate of crossbred calves up to sale time as feeder calves. Iowa State Univ Coop Ext Serv, Ames, Iowa, A.S. Leaflet R329, 1981.

11. Hutcheson DP, Cummins JM, Cole NA, Ross JE, Thorm J:Unpublished data. Texas A&M Univ Agric Res, Amarillo, Tx; USDA-ARS, Bushland, Tx; and Univ of Missouri, Columbia, respectively.

12.   Pope LS:Cow herd management and preconditioning. Preconditioning seminar, Univ of Wyoming, Laramie, pp. 13-14, June 1968.

13.   Pate FM, Crockett JR:Effect of limited creep feeding beef calves on postweaning performance.   Univ of Florida, IFAS AREC, Belle Glade Res Rep EV-1973-3, 1973.

14.   Knight AP, Pierson RE, Hoerlein AB, Collier JH, Horton DP, Pru JB:Effect of vaccination time on morbidity, mortality, and weight gains of feeder calves. J Am Vet Med Assoc 161:45, 1972.

15.   Wieringa FL, Curtis RA, Willoughby RA:The influence of preconditioning on plasma corticosteroid levels, rectal temperatures and the incidence of shipping fever in beef cattle.   Can Vet J 17:280-286, 1976.

16.   Woods GT, Pickard JR, Cowsert C:A three-year field study of preconditioning native Illinois beef calves sold through a cooperative association - 1969 to 1971. Can J Comp Med 37:224-227, 1973b.

17.   Strohbehn DR:Effect of management on growth and efficiency of crossbred calves as feeder calves after sale time.   Iowa State Univ Coop Ext Serv, Ames, Iowa, A.S. Leaflet R330, 1981.

18.   Byers FM:Effects of limestone, monensin, and feeding level on corn silage net energy value and

composition of growth in cattle.   J Anim Sci 50:1127-1135, 1980.

19.   Billingsley RD, McLaren JB, Moody EL, Damron WS, Orr CL, Cole NA:Market-transit shrink and post-transit performance of steers of different feeder grades. Tenn Farm and Home Sci 119:9, 1981.

20.   Pate FM, Crockett JR:Feeding calves at weaning. Florida Beef Cattle Short Course, Univ of Florida, May 1974.

21.   Woods GT, Mansfield ME, Webb RJ:A three-year comparison of acute respiratory disease, shrink, and weight gain in preconditioned and non-preconditioned Illinois beef calves sold at the same auction and mixed in a feedlot. Can J Comp Med 37:249-255, 1973a.

22.   Martin SW:Vaccination: is it effective in preventing respiratory disease or influencing weight gains in feedlot calves? Can Vet J 24:10-19, 1983.

Feedlot Health Management

Delbert G. Miles, M.S., D.V.M.

Miller Feed Lots, Inc.
P.O. Box 937
LaSalle, Colorado 80645

Summary

Calves are received and processed within 24 hours after arrival. The calves are closely observed for general appearance and feed consumption. If too many animals are "pulled" due to sickness or if feed consumption drops to an unacceptable level, the entire pen is taken back to the processing area for mass medication. The cattle are given one of the following:

1. LA® 200,

2. benzathine-penicillin G procaine,

3. infectious bovine rhinotracheitis (IBR) vaccine intramuscularly with one of the above antibiotics, or

4. Levasole® injectable with one of the above antibiotics.

This procedure reduces sick "pulls" and increases consumption within 24-72 hours. The use of IBR along with a long-acting antibiotic seems to be the most beneficial.

Introduction

Several thousand head of calves are received into Miller Feed Lots, Inc. each Fall. The origin of these calves varies from unweaned sale-barn calves to preconditioned ranch calves. The problem with bovine respiratory disease (BRD) varies as much as the origin of the cattle. Economics of the operation do not allow high-quality scientific studies, therefore conclusions are drawn from observations, not statistically significant studies.

Procedure

Newly-arrived cattle are processed within 24 hours. Processing includes:

1. parainfluenza$_3$ (PI-3), infectious bovine rhinotracheitis (IBR), bovine virus diarrhea (BVD), *Leptospira pomona* vaccine,

2. *Clostridium chauvoei, Cl. septicum, Cl. sordellii, Cl. novyi* Type B and Type D toxoid,

3. Levasole® (levamisole phosphate) injectable solution 13.65 percent,

4. Ralgro® implants,

5. GX-118® (prolate) dip, and

6. ear tag with lot number and lettering to identify source of cattle.

Long-stem hay is placed in the bunk on arrival. Purina Receiving Chow is fed twice daily after processing until calves are consuming 3 percent of their body weight. If additional feed is required, the cattle are offered ration A which contains corn silage and/or ground hay, dry rolled corn, dry or liquid protein supplement, Rumensin® and Tylan® .

The calves are checked twice a day by cowboys on horses for the first 30 days after arrival. Sick cattle are placed in satellite hospitals and hauled to the main hospital in trailers at Lot Number 1. At Lot Number 2, the calves are driven to the main hospital. The cattle are individually identified in the hospital by ear tags. A treatment card is filled out and includes information concerning disease condition, temperature and drugs administered. Antibiotics used in order of preference are: oxytetracycline, erthromycin, sulfadimethoxine, penicillin and tylosin. Tripelennamine hydrochloride injection (Re-Covr®) is also administered the first two-three days. If the temperature or general appearance indicates a poor response, the antibiotic is changed.

The general appearance of the pen, daily sick "pulls" and feed consumption is closely monitored. If one or more of these criteria become unacceptable, the entire pen is returned to the processing area and medicated. One of the following mass medications is administered:

1. LA® 200,

2. benzathine penicillin G procaine in aqueous suspension,

3. intramuscular IBR and one of the above antibiotics, or

4. Levasole® injectable and one of the above antibiotics.

The regimen selected depends on recorded temperatures and responses to various antibiotics in the hospital. High temperatures normally dictate intramuscular IBR and an antibiotic. Temperatures of 103-105° F along with poor general appearance and/or poor feed consumption dictates Levasole® injectable and an antibiotic.

Observations

The observations and responses of six pens of cattle received during the Fall of 1982 are summarized in Graphs I-VI. Lot Number 293 (Graph I) contained 224 steers weighing 581 pounds. Twenty milliliters of LA® 200 was given on day 12 because the feed consumption dropped from 19 pounds dry matter/head to 9 pounds and morbidity was high. Feed consumption declined to 5 pounds on day 13, but started increasing on day 14 with a peak of 18 pounds/head on day 17. Sick "pulls" continued high through day 16. Intramuscular IBR administered at the time of LA® 200 administration may have slowed the sick "pulls" sooner.

Graph II summarizes the responses of Lot Number 294. The lot contained 196 steers with a pay weight of 531 pounds. On day 13, 20 milliliters of LA® 200 was administered due to to high morbidity and a decline in feed consumption from 19 pounds dry matter/head to 5 pounds. Dry-matter feed consumption increased to 18 pounds by day 17 and sick "pulls" declined dramatically.

Lot Number 303 (Graph III) contained 99 heifers weighing 447 pounds off the truck. Dry-matter feed consumption was erratic after arrival and dropped to 10 pounds dry matter/head on day 21. Twelve milliliters Levasole® injectable and 13 milliliters benzathine penicillin G procaine in aqueous suspension were administered on day 21. Feed consumption improved on day 22 but declined on day 27. The spike in dry matter feed consumption on day 19 is probably due to the bunk checkers not allowing for the large number of "pulls" on day 18.

Lot Number 311 (Graph IV) consisting of 98 steers weighing 522 pounds off the truck had a peak dry-matter feed consumption of 22 pounds but this dropped to 12 pounds on days 11 and 13. Levasole® injectable (13 milliliters) and 12 milliliters benzathine penicillin G procaine in aqueous suspension were administered on day 13. The general appearance improved and feed consumption increased to 18 pounds dry matter on day 17. Morbidity was not a problem in this lot.

Graph V summarizes Lot Number 315 consisting of 175 steers with a pay weight of 541 pounds. The general appearance and a dry matter feed consumption drop of 4 pounds/head day dictated mass medication. Ten milliliters of benzathine penicillin G procaine in aqueous suspension and 6 milliliters of Levasole® injectable were administered on day 18. The 50 percent dose of Levasole® injectable did not seem to give as dramatic a response as the full dose had been giving, but feed consumption did improve to previous levels after five days.

Graph VI summarizes Lot Number 909 consisting of 212 steers with a pay weight of 562 pounds. This pen was put together over a two-week period with the last steers being added on day 15. Sick "pulls" were high from day 15 to day 26. Intramuscular IBR and 14 milliliters of benzathine penicillin G procaine in aqueous suspension were administered on day 26. Morbidity declined dramatically and dry matter feed consumption increased.

Death losses for the six lots are also shown in Graphs I-VI.

Conclusions

1. The perceived results may be figments of our imaginations.

2. The movement and disruption of the cattle may contribute to, or be responsible for, the changes seen.

3. If bovine respiratory disease is a factor as evidenced by high temperatures, coughing, depression and labored breathing, infectious bovine rhinotracheitis (IBR) vaccine seems to greatly enhance chances for a positive response.

4. Long-acting antibiotics are beneficial but need to be supplemented with IBR or Levasole® injectable.

5. If depressed feed consumption is the primary

problem, a full dose of Levasole® injectable and a long-acting antibiotic seem to be very beneficial.

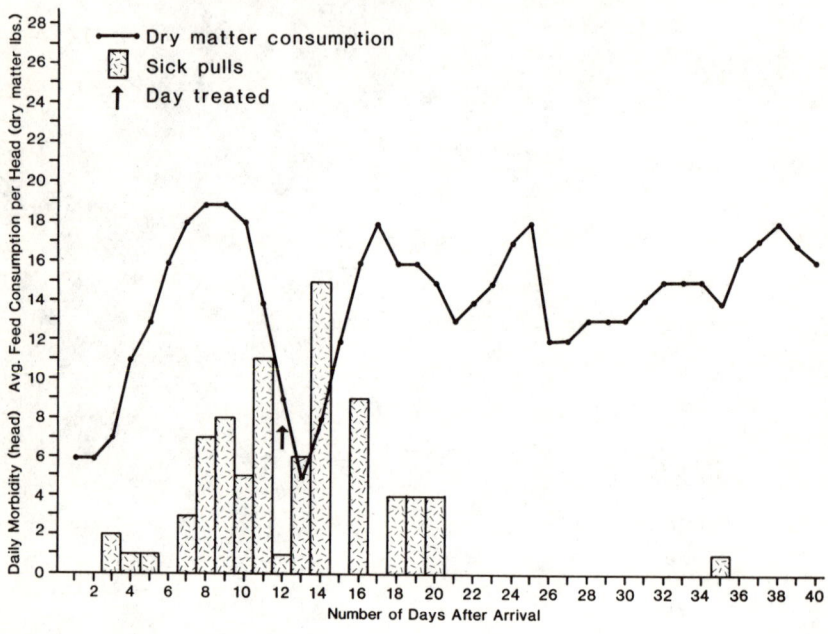

Graph I

**Feed Consumption, Daily Morbidity, and Death Loss
on Newly Received Calves — Lot Number 293**

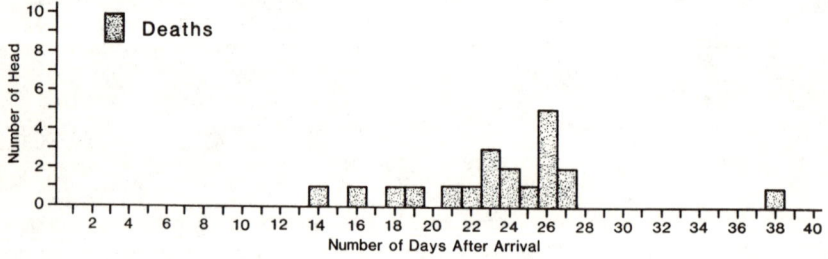

Graph II
Feed Consumption, Daily Morbidity, and Death Loss
on Newly Received Calves — Lot Number 294

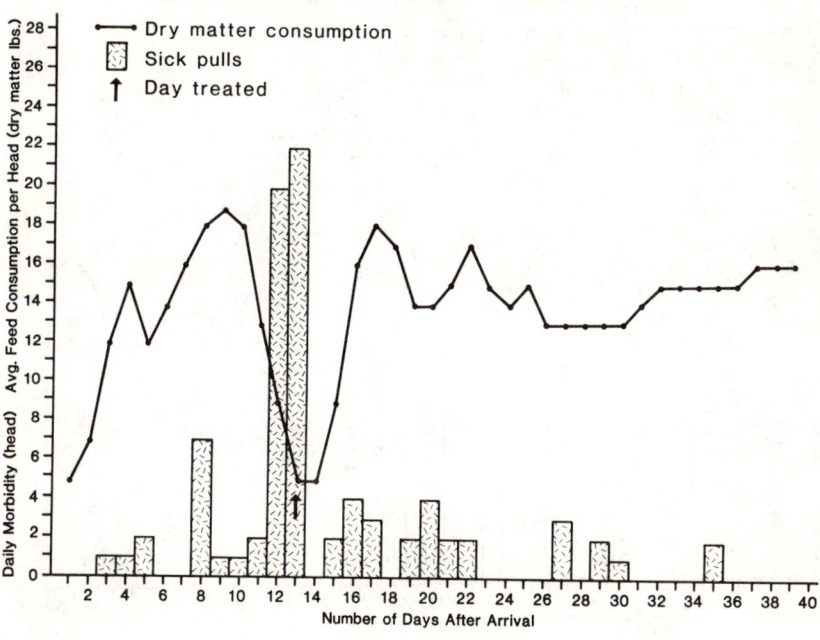

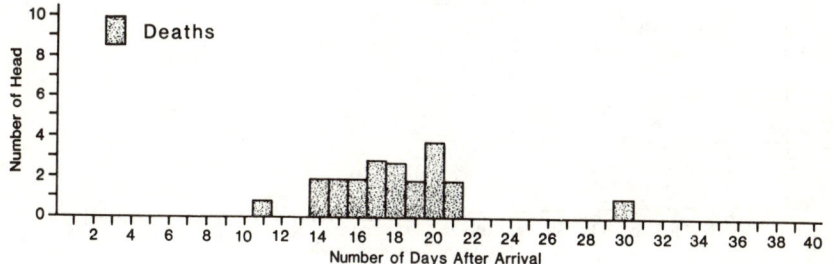

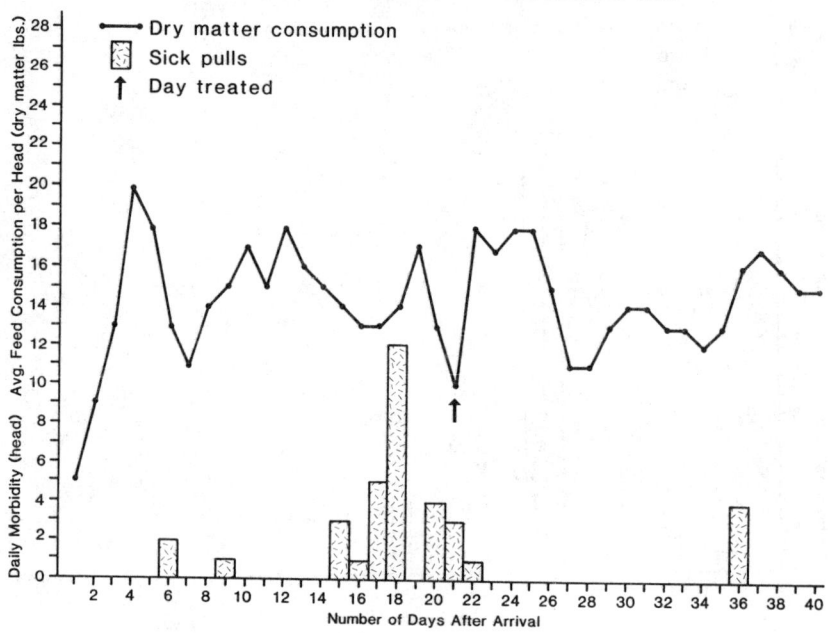

Graph III
Feed Consumption, Daily Morbidity, and Death Loss
on Newly Received Calves — Lot Number 303

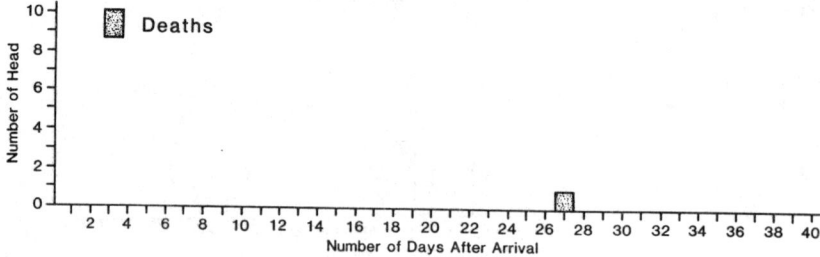

Graph IV
Feed Consumption, Daily Morbidity, and Death Loss
on Newly Received Calves — Lot Number 311

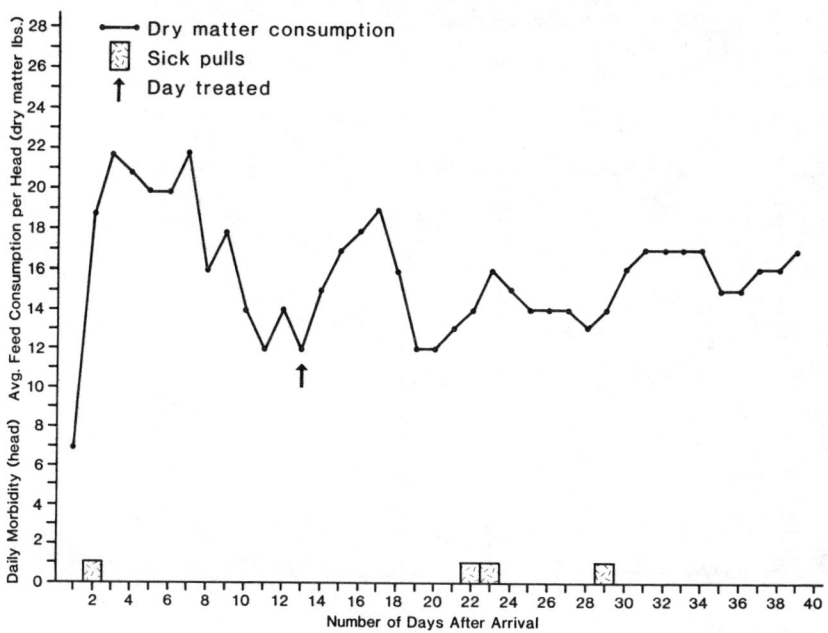

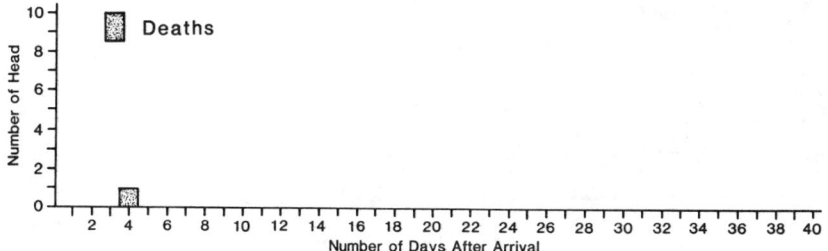

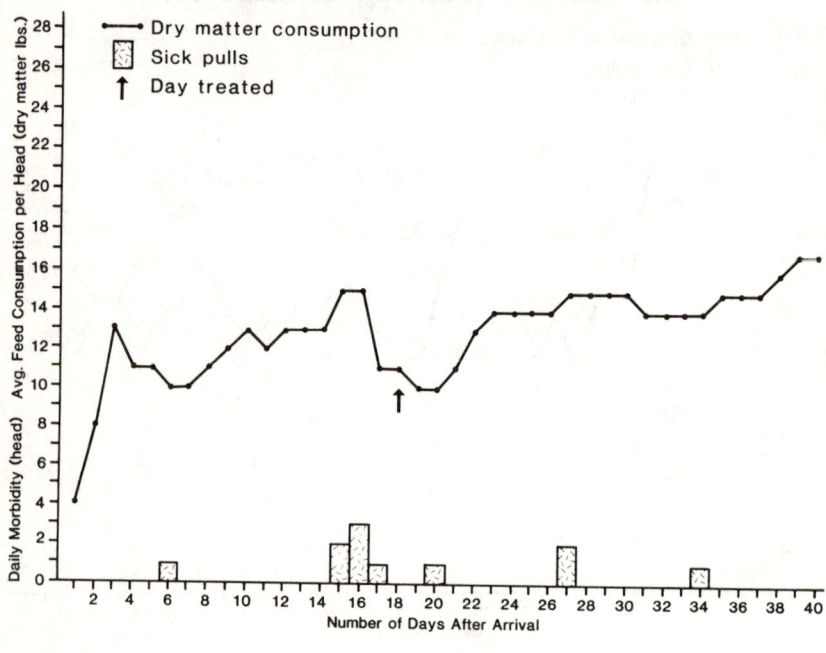

Graph V

**Feed Consumption, Daily Morbidity, and Death Loss
on Newly Received Calves — Lot Number 315**

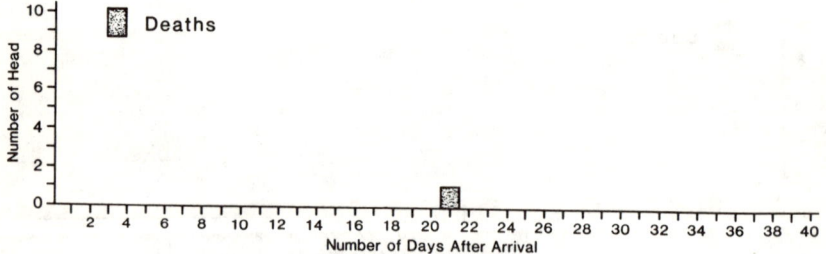

Graph VI
Feed Consumption, Daily Morbidity, and Death Loss
on Newly Received Calves — Lot Number 909

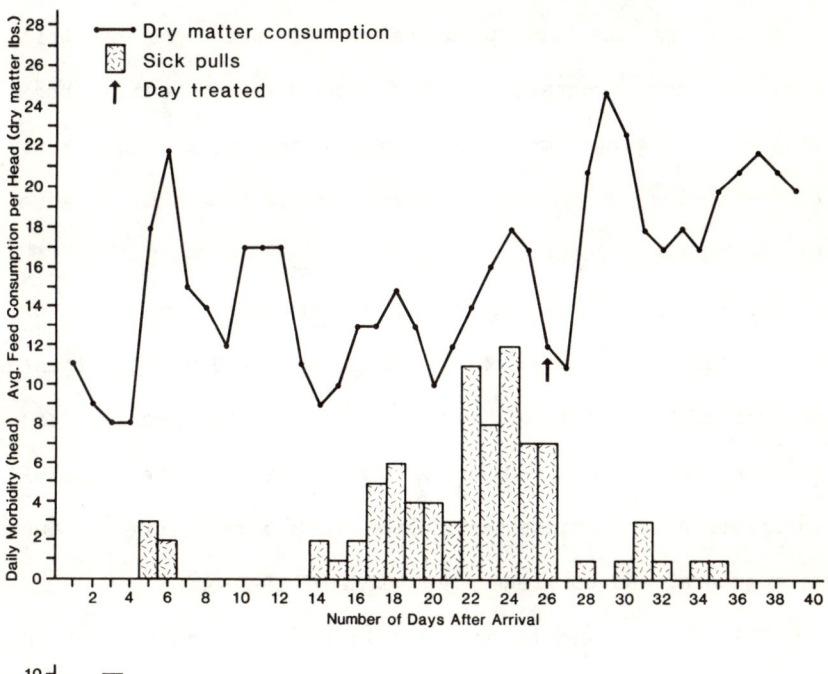

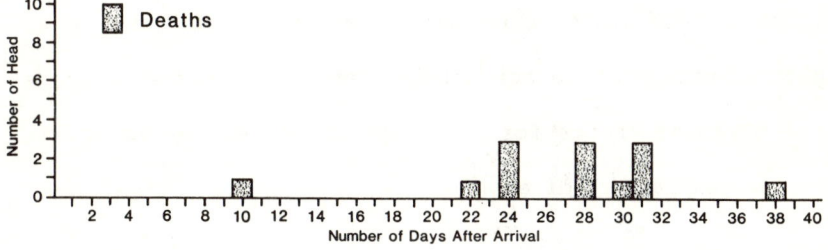

Working Together, Sharing Knowledge

C. W. McMillan

Assistant Secretary for Marketing and Inspection Services
U.S. Department of Agriculture
Washington, D.C. 20250

Introduction

It is my distinct pleasure to be with you on this occasion. My congratulations to the sponsors and members of the organizing committee on this excellent program. Your topic—bovine respiratory disease—is of great importance to the cattle industry.

Sharing information such as this is the very heart of agriculture. The organic act creating the U.S. Department of Agriculture set as our mission "...to acquire and diffuse among the people of the United States useful information on subjects connected with agriculture in the most general and comprehensive sense of the word."

USDA has long had an active role in animal health. I am proud of our many achievements in that field, and I am pleased with what we are doing today. Let me just trace a few of these things for you—especially as they relate to bovine respiratory disease.

Observations

Annual losses from bovine respiratory disease are estimated in excess of $500 million. Reference to the term "bovine respiratory disease" usually includes the word "complex." This appears to be rightly so since a variety of causative agents are implicated--alone and in concert.

There are a number of vaccines available for dealing with causative agents associated with pneumonia. In some cases, their value may be questionable. Some are labeled only as an aid in preventing respiratory diseases. The causative agents we hear most about include: *Pasteurella* sp., infectious bovine rhinotracheitis virus, parainfluenza virus type III, bovine viral diarrhea virus, *Mycoplasma* sp., and one or two others. Probably there are more such agents not yet identified or implicated in the so-called respiratory disease complex.

Stress

We often hear the word "stress" associated with respiratory disease, and there is no doubt that so-called stress does play a role in precipitating outbreaks. We are all familiar with stress associated with adverse weather or transporting over long distances.

Recent research showed the number of isolations of *Pasteurella hemolytica* type 1, which is now widely incriminated in bovine respiratory disease, to be low among cattle on the farm. When cattle were moved to auction barns, however, the number of isolations increased. When cattle were moved again approximately 1,000 miles to a feedyard, the number of isolations increased dramatically.

The very words "shipping fever" imply that respiratory diseases are commonly associated with cattle shipments. One of the aims of USDA's experimental cattle car is to reduce stress and risk of disease when shipping cattle long distances by rail. This palace on wheels, on lease from the Ortner Freight Car Company, is 91 feet long and equipped with an on-board feeding and watering system. As many of you know, the first shipment of cattle using this car took place earlier this year--traveling from Knoxville, Tennessee, to Amarillo, Texas. The next shipment, later this month, will follow the same route.

Also making the trip will be a modified aluminum highway cattle trailer, built by the Wilson Livestock Trailer Company of Sioux City, Iowa. This trailer, with its own feeding and watering facilities, will travel piggyback on a flatcar. For comparison, another load of cattle will travel to Amarillo by standard cattle trailer. Later, the modified trailer and a standard trailer will both make a road trip to Texas. Lemmy Wilson Livestock, Inc. of

Newport, Tennessee, is shipping the cattle.   The Burlington Northern, Chessie System and Norfolk and Southern Railroads will haul the cattle.   Other cooperators include the Metalex Corporation, the National Cattlemen's Association, Ralston Purina Company, the Texas Agricultural Experiment Station and five agencies of USDA.   In my view, this experimental car project, initiated in 1977, is an excellent example of industry and government working together to accomplish something worthwhile.   I might mention that Ringling Brothers-Barnum & Bailey Circus has expressed keen interest in this experimental cattle car project. Apparently they have their own special problems shipping animals over long distances.

I am reminded of an event described by historian T. Harry Williams in his biography of Huey P. Long. Sometime back in the 1930's, the circus was in Texas, about to depart for Louisiana.   Huey, who was then governor of Louisiana, became alarmed when he learned that the circus would open in Baton Rouge on the very same day LSU would play an important football game.   LSU football was something special to Huey; so taking the phone, he called John Ringling and asked him to postpone the circus' arrival by one day. Ringling declined, explaining his tight travel schedule and related problems.   But Huey had other ideas.

He told Ringling, "We have livestock laws in this state. Have you ever tried to dip a lion, a tiger or an elephant, Mr. Ringling?" LSU played that Saturday without a circus distraction. Huey's example was not exactly one of cooperation with industry, but times have changed.

USDA's Office of Transportation, working with the Statistical Reporting Service, has compiled some tables summarizing cattle shipments for a five-year period. They cover incoming shipments of feeder cattle and calves to nine states which feed more than 80 percent of the nation's fed cattle. More than half of the cattle shipped to Texas traveled 1,000 miles or more.

I have talked a little about transportation as it relates to stress and respiratory disease. But researchers are also concerned with the effects of nutrition and diet, in combination with transportation, as they relate to stress and respiratory disease. Studies are underway to better understand so-called stress and unknown factors which may result in stress. Current and future work includes evaluating the influences of post-transit diets, pre-shipment management, and other management practices and factors affecting feed consumption of stressed calves—all aimed at developing regimens that will be most beneficial to animals during and after transport.

Cooperation in Research

I note that the Regional Technical Committee for NC-107, Bovine Respiratory Diseases, is one of our Symposium sponsors along with the Texas Agricultural Experiment Station and Texas A&M University's College of Veterinary Medicine. This example of cooperative regional research brings together the scientific talents of State Agricultural Experiment Stations, USDA, and other institutions and government agencies. Through team effort, problems too costly in manpower and funds for a single Experiment Station to attack can be resolved.

Over the past five years, USDA's Cooperative State Research Service has awarded grants totaling more than $5.5 million for research specifically on bovine respiratory disease. Currently, more than a dozen such projects are underway at various universities. Within the same time frame, USDA's Agricultural Research Service spent an additional $3.5 million on bovine respiratory disease reseach. So we have various disciplinary approaches being taken to identify causes and develop control measures to prevent the respiratory disease complex. Of course, much of the research on respiratory diseases of other animal species can be applied to cattle.

Breakthroughs

Recently we have seen major scientific breakthroughs which will permit new approaches to this disease complex. New technology such as recombinant DNA and monoclonal antibody technology is being used. These, along with other emerging technologies, will permit us to better understand diseases in general. These revolutionary approaches should offer even greater understanding of disease processes and host reactions—including susceptability and resistance. Entirely new approaches for diagnosis, control, prevention and treatment of diseases should become a reality within five to ten years. This same new technology should impact favorably on production and management practices.

Interferons have created a lot of excitement lately, offering thousands of possible uses. For regulatory purposes, however, a question had to be settled about who would control their uses. Quite recently the APHIS administrator, Bert Hawkins, and I met with Edward Brandt, an assistant secretary with the Department of Health and Human Services. We agreed that interferons would be treated as drugs under FDA regulatory control. On the other hand, veterinary biologics would remain under USDA control.

Many of you who saw the advent of antibiotics witnessed what was, at that time, a miracle. Information developed within the past few years, augmented by current and future research findings, could put us into a whole new ball game in dealing with animal as well as human disease. But every new advance is not without its problems.

Residues

In recent years, we have faced growing concerns about the problem of drug and chemical residues in the meat supply due, in part, to use of drugs for treatment or prevention of respiratory diseases. Efforts to combat this problem are coordinated by USDA's Food Safety and Inspection Service. Contrary to some published criticisms, the Department has had great success in residue prevention and control, due in large part to the equally committed efforts of industry. We believe it is best to deal with these chemicals prudently and cautiously, using the best information science can provide. This means we do *not* test for every possible compound that may be in the food supply. That would be impractical and costly--potentially adding up to $500 billion each year if every carcass were analyzed for every compound used in agriculture. What we do instead is implement a program combining regulatory and nonregulatory initiatives, aiming for the best of both worlds.

In the regulatory area, USDA uses valid, well-founded procedures to identify those residues most likely to occur in meat and poultry and those considered hazardous to humans.   On the basis of our monitoring data, which we continually evaluate, we adjust the sampling rate for specific compounds and animal species.   In this way, we can best choose how and where to allocate the resources we have available, still allowing the program to evolve and meet changing needs.   It is this kind of flexibility that allowed us to expand the number of compounds that can be monitored from 46 in 1977 to approximately 60 in 1983.   By year's end, we expect to add some one-half dozen more.

The nonregulatory aspects of the program include exploratory surveillance efforts, which enable the Department to see where residue problems exist and whether regulatory efforts are needed.   They also include the Residue Avoidance Program--a grass-roots strategy that aims to build residue prevention into every stage of food animal production.

Monitoring, combined with education on prevention, is the most effective way of dealing with residue problems. Experience bears this out, and bears out as well the impracticality of trying to catch each violative shipment.

USDA has entered into cooperative agreements with industry to encourage residue avoidance. Under these agreements, when company-conducted testing suggests that a residue problem may be present, the firm informs USDA so that appropriate, joint preventive actions can be taken.

The Residue Avoidance Program also includes a cooperative effort with USDA's Extension Service. We transferred $1.5 million to Extension for 35 projects which are carried out by Land Grant colleges in 31 states. Many of these projects include educational components which enable findings to be passed along to producers.

Of course, we also have a mission to protect consumers from violative residues and other hazards in foreign meat and poultry. Our import inspection program centers on two activities--the review of foreign inspection programs, including the determination of their eligibility for exporting to the United States, and the inspection of foreign products at ports of entry in the United States. These activities ensure that foreign systems impose inspection requirements "equal to" all provisions of this country's federal meat and poultry laws and regulations.

Rewards of Partnership

We can all be proud of these achievements in public and animal health. Our success in providing sound programs is due, in large measure, to a magnificent partnership over the years--the Department of Agriculture, Land Grant colleges and universities, Experiment Stations, the Extension system, the producers and all the agriculture-related industries. Regardless of the criticisms that have been laid at the door of one or the other of these partners, the most important point is: the partnership works!

Science has provided both fundamental and applied research to serve the producer. A dynamic educational system and the related Extension system have produced people ready and able to use this knowledge. And a free agricultural industry has produced abundant livestock and poultry--providing wholesome animal protein for American consumers as well as people overseas. In the United States, we spend only 16 percent of our personal consumption expenditures on food. In the United Kingdom, that expenditure is 23 percent; in Italy, it is 34 percent; and in less-developed countries, it may exceed 60 percent. In far too many countries, percentages hardly matter. Simply getting food is a constant problem.

The Bureau of Animal Industry (BAI)

A century ago, animal agriculture was controlled more by traditions of the past and local conditions than by scientific knowledge. Since the establishment of the Department of Agriculture, scientific advances have dramatically changed the picture. We can find many landmarks along the road we have traveled. Let me cite one in particular, one prompted in large measure by a bovine respiratory disease outbreak.

Almost 100 years ago, in 1884, Congress established the Bureau of Animal Industry, the first agency of the Department of Agriculture. For the first time, the federal government was mandated to tackle major animal disease problems, which then threatened to shut off American livestock exports. Great Britain and other countries were refusing our shipments because of bovine pleuropneumonia.

Under the leadership of Dr. D. E. Salmon, the BAI immediately took dramatic steps. It began a campaign to eradicate bovine pleuropneumonia. It established USDA's first Experiment Station. And it developed the basic principles that, to this day, are the foundation of cooperative state-federal animal health programs.

As Assistant Secretary, responsible for regulatory affairs, I have the privilege of carrying on the traditions of the animal health programs begun by the BAI. Regulatory programs are administered by APHIS, FSIS and the Packers and Stockyards Administration. My colleagues in ARS and

CSRS share in the traditions which were embodied in the historic research initiated by BAI.   My friends in state animal health agencies share traditions that began when the BAI made its first cooperative agreements, enabling state and USDA inspectors to work effectively for common goals. Thanks to the vision, leadership, scientific knowledge (and a lot of hard work) that Dr. D. E. Salmon brought to the BAI, bovine pleuropneumonia was eradicated in just eight years.

We might note here that this disease still plagues many areas of the world.   Just this past year, it appeared in Portugal.   A significant number of herds had to be depopulated to bring the outbreak under control and hopefully eradicate it.   The disease also crops up frequently in southern France.   But the Portuguese blamed Spain, not France, for their outbreak. These continuing troubles in Europe suggest that Dr. Salmon's eradication policy was quite sound.

BAI also initiated the research and the strategies that eradicated Texas fever from the United States--one of the most monumental and historic struggles against an animal disease in modern times.   Defeating the disease we know as bovine piroplasmosis required hard, basic research--first to identify the causative agent, *Babesia bigemia,* a blood parasite, then to demonstrate that it was spread by ticks, and finally to learn the life cycle of ticks and how they might be eradicated.

The groundwork was completed in only ten years. Eradication, which meant rigid quarantines and the dipping of cattle again and again, took 40 years of persistent determination.

Significantly, the research on cattle fever lead to understanding of the mosquito's role in spreading yellow fever and malaria. This, in turn, led to our completing the Panama Canal after the French had given up.

In the "point-with-pride" department, I could mention many more recent achievements, such as the eradication of screwworms and hog cholera. And, of course, this same period has seen outstanding advances in genetics, breeding, feed utilization, transportation, handling, housing, processing, and all other aspects of animal agriculture.

National Animal Disease Surveillance System

Today the USDA has cooperative agreements with the states and industries to eradicate or control a number of diseases that can best be handled on a national basis. Very little data is available, however, on many other diseases (including the bovine respiratory disease complex) that can best be handled by individual herd owners. This is a serious omission, for this information is needed by many.

I believe we can gain a lot from a national animal disease surveillance system—one designed to give statistically reliable information. The cost of animal diseases to consumers, to producers and to the country as a whole has been estimated at between $4 and $6 billion annually, but no one can be certain.

If we can establish such a system, if we can generate valid, consistently reliable field data about animal disease nationwide, we will form the basis for analysis never before available in any country:

1. We will have sound economic grounds for the programs we propose.

2. Producers will have reliable information on which to base their management practices. They will know when and where to take preventive or remedial measures.

3. Research agencies and institutions can determine what projects are most needed and they can justify them to the public or to the legislators or boards that appropriate the funds.

This month in Ohio and Tennessee, we begin developing and testing procedures which will build the nationwide system we need. These pilot projects will continue for one year. More will follow. It will take time, but we expect to see a nationwide animal disease surveillance system in place by 1989.

Conclusion

Any USDA project is, or should be, squarely in the public interest. Few, if any, of our projects could ever succeed without public support. To gain and maintain that support, we seek and welcome opportunities such as this to give an accounting.

The Basis of Immune Protection and Immunopathologic Disease Accompanying Virus Infections

Michael B. A. Oldstone, M.D.

Department of Immunology
Scripps Clinic and Research Foundation
10666 Torrey Pines Road
La Jolla, California 92037

Spread of Virus Infection

Virus may spread to infected cells by one of three routes. By the first one, infectious virus carried in fluids comes in contact with permissive cells. Protection against this spread of infection relies on humoral effectors, primarily antibody and complement, either alone or acting in concert. The second way virus infection can spread from one cell to another is via contiguous cytoplasmic bridges. Protection against this spread depends on three factors. Virus-specific structural or nonstructural unique antigens must be expressed on the cell surface. Cytotoxic lymphocytes and/or antibody primed to these antigens must be raised and able to bind and interact. Finally, after antibody and/or cytotoxic lymphocyte binding, effector molecules are brought to play, the infected cells' membranes must be perturbed and disrupted to allow lysis to occur. Since viral-coded antigens are expressed on the cell's surface prior to the forming and release of newly manufactured and infectious virus, the host immune system can effectively remove factories that would ordinarily form more infectious virus. The third modality of viral spread is again by cell-to-cell but without viral release to external fluids. In this instance, viral genetic information is incorporated into host genetic material and passed along with normal cell division and growth. In this instance, the immune surveillance system would be unable to function appropriately until such "vertically transmittable infected cells" express foreign antigens on their surfaces. Of course, in most instances they do, as in "tumor-associated viral antigens."

Humoral Immune System

The host's immune response is segregated, for convenience, into humoral, cellular and combined humoral-cellular categories (Figure 1). The humoral system consists primarily of antibody and complement (C'). Antibody attaches to antigen that stimulates its production through its Fab'2 binding site. The result is a conformational change in the antibody's Fc portion, modifying it for binding to C'1, the first component of C'. Thereafter, each component of the C' system is activated sequentially in an autocatalytic manner.   The interaction of the various components of the C' system have been reviewed (1,2) and are shown schematically in Figures 2 and 3.   Recently the molecular mechanism by which cells of human origin, infected with any one of several RNA or DNA viruses, are lysed by specific antiviral antibody and complement have been uncovered (3).   The infected cell itself, in the absence of antibody, activates C' via the alternative pathway.   Despite the activation of C' components and their binding to the cells' surfaces, lysis does not occur until specific antiviral antibodies are added.   The reason that lysis does not occur in the absence of antibody is because there is an insufficient buildup of C'3b-like molecules on the cell's surface.   However, upon the addition of specific antiviral antibodies, more C'3b binding sites are uncovered and membrane-bound C'3b is protected so as to preclude inactivation by its inactivating enzymes C'3b INA and B1H (4,5).   Recent evidence indicates that this mechanism of exclusive alternative C'-pathway-activation and antibody cooperation in lysis of human cells (from several origins and infected with a wide variety of human RNA and DNA viruses) has been extended by Gorman to the study of distemper virus infection of animal cells (6).   Clearly, more data collection is needed to know whether similar principles apply to other animal virus-induced diseases. However, this activation of the alternative C' pathway by virus-infected cells appears to have a commonalty with other microbial agents as shown by recent observations with both bacteria and parasites.

Complement alone, in the absence of antibody, can be activated on incubation with certain viruses (7). In the best-studied system, human complement when incubated with any one of several retroviruses, is activated, binds to the infected virion and succeeds in inactivating the virus. Of interest is that other animal C' sources are not as effective (7,8).

Cell-Mediated Immune System

The major cellular immune component is thymus-derived (T) lymphocytes. Nonspecific cellular activity is supplied mainly by macrophages, granulocytes and natural killer (NK) cells. Evidence indicates that recognition of virus-infected cells by cytotoxic T lymphocytes requires not only virus antigen specificity but also matching of the major histocompatibility complex of the two cell types (9). Current evidence indicates that the portion of the histocompatibility complex associated with cytotoxic T cell recognition and lysis of virus-infected cells in the mouse maps to the D and/or K region of the H-2 and to the corresponding A, B and C portions of the human HLA complex. Evidence indicates that, at least with some virus infections, the lytic process may favor a preference for one of the two or three haplotypes. Among the other components of cellular immunity, interest in NK cells has focused on the finding that they are active early in infection prior to the induction of cytotoxic T cells. Thus, NK cells may be important early in infection. However, NK cells lack a degree of specificity in killing targets that cytotoxic T lymphocytes possess as they kill both infected and uninfected cells. Recent evidence indicates that NK cells can be activated to kill targets by viral glycoproteins either free in the fluid phase or expressed on the cell surface. Activation and killing occurs within two hours of exposure and by an interferon-independent mechanism (10,11). At a later time, after one cycle of virus replication, NK cells can be activated via a different mechanism (the classic NK cell activation) that has an absolute dependence on interferon production (10). Cytotoxic lymphcytes (T lymphocytes, NK cells), macrophages and granulocytes can be attracted to an area of tissue injury by chemotactic factors released by lymphoid cells themselves or by injured target cells.

Ordinarily, this process involves cellular release of proteolytic enzymes that cleave nearby C' components, specifically C'5, resulting in the formation of the C'5a chemotactic peptide (Figure 1). C'3 and C'4 cleaved proteins are now believed to release little, if any, chemotactic factors (12).

Combined Humoral-Cellular Immune System

Humoral and cell-mediated mechanisms may also combine to kill virus-infected cells. For example, in antibody-dependent cell-mediated killing (ADCC), specific antibody binds to antigen on the cell's surface. Subsequently a killer (K) cell binds via the antibody's Fc fragment and the result is lysis of the target cell (13). There are reports of cytophilic macrophages killing cells, presumably by a mechanism that resembles K-cell-induced injury.

Immunopathologic-Mediated Disease Associated with Virus Infection

The mechanisms resulting in clearing of virus or virus-infected tissues are identical to those responsible for inducing immunopathologic disease. Indeed, infection by a virus offers many opportunities for development of immunologically-mediated disease. The virus as a replicating agent offers many macromolecular antigens that elicit a host immune response. Tissue injury in both acute and chronic viral infections is associated with the interaction of the immune response against the virus or the cell infected by the virus. The severity of injury is directly related to the degree of immune responsiveness and the ability of the immune reactants to reach and interact with the target tissue or cell. It is likely that immune reactions against viruses or virus-infected cells are basically the same during acute and chronic or persistent infections. With acute infection, the immune system determines the balance between recovery (immunity) or death. With persistent or chronic infections, the time scale is lengthened and the interactions between the immune system and the infecting microbe often lead to chronic disease.

Immunologically-mediated tissue injury during virus infection basically follows one or both of two pathways (Figure 1). In the first pathway, components of the immune system react against either specific antigens found uniquely on cells or tissues or against neoantigens expressed on the cell's surface. In this instance, immune components react specifically against those antigens that cause their induction or against the complex of those antigens with the host's histocompatibility antigens in the

case of cytotoxic T-derived lymphocytes.   In addition,
virus-induced specific antibodies may also react with
normal self-components. This phenomenon, termed "molecular
mimicry," is believed due to the sharing of antigenic
determinants between a viral polypeptide and the
self-antigen.   Recently my colleagues and I have
demonstrated such an occurrence with either measles virus
phosphoprotein polypeptides or herpes simplex virus
glycoprotein and normal cytoskeleton component (14). The
second pathway by which immune reagents can cause damage
occurs by deposition of virus antigen-antibody immune
complexes (Figure 4). In this instance, antibodies combine
with their corresponding antigens or with self-antigens
that share common antigenic sites, in the blood or other
body fluids, to form complexes that may become trapped by
basement membranes where they cause injury, usually by
activating inflammatory mediators.   This pathway of
immune-response injury occurs frequently in naturally and
experimentally-induced animal diseases as well as in
naturally-occurring virus infections of man. The study of
animals with either the natural or induced infections
provided much of the information for understanding
virus-induced immune complex disease (15,16). Immune
complexes commonly develop after exposure to foreign

antigens. Thus, hosts infected by any of a wide variety of
DNA and RNA viruses mount immune responses in which
antibodies to these agents combine with the corresponding
viral antigen to form immune complexes.   In this respect,
immune complex formation probably represents a natural host
mechanism for clearing infecting microbes.   However, when
virus infection is continuous, constant viral antigen
stimulation results in a continuing load of immune
complexes.   Any disability that impedes their clearance may
enable these complexes to deposit in tissues, potentially
causing immune complex disease.   The events leading to
immune complex formation in disease are clear. Recently it
has been shown that the degree of immune complex formation
is under the control of host immune response genes
controlling the responsiveness of the antibody (17).

Conclusions

The relationship between virus infection and immune
response leading to immunity and/or tissue injury was noted
nearly 200 years ago by Jenner (18).   Advances in the
understanding of immune response and its manipulation have
led to, and are leading to, the control of many infectious
diseases. Similarly, our understanding of the tissue injury
produced by virus infection and/or the immune response
responding against virus-infected cells is known. The tasks

in the future are the uncovering and manipulation of genes regulating immune responses toward various virus determinants and learning how to modify responses in both the controlling of virus diseases and ablation of immunopathologic-mediated injury.

Figure 1. A cartoon of the generation of immune reactants and their involvement in causing injury during virus infection. K cells: killer cells involved in antibody-dependent cell-mediated killing (ADCC); NK cells: "natural killer cells"; T cells: thymus-derived lymphocytes.

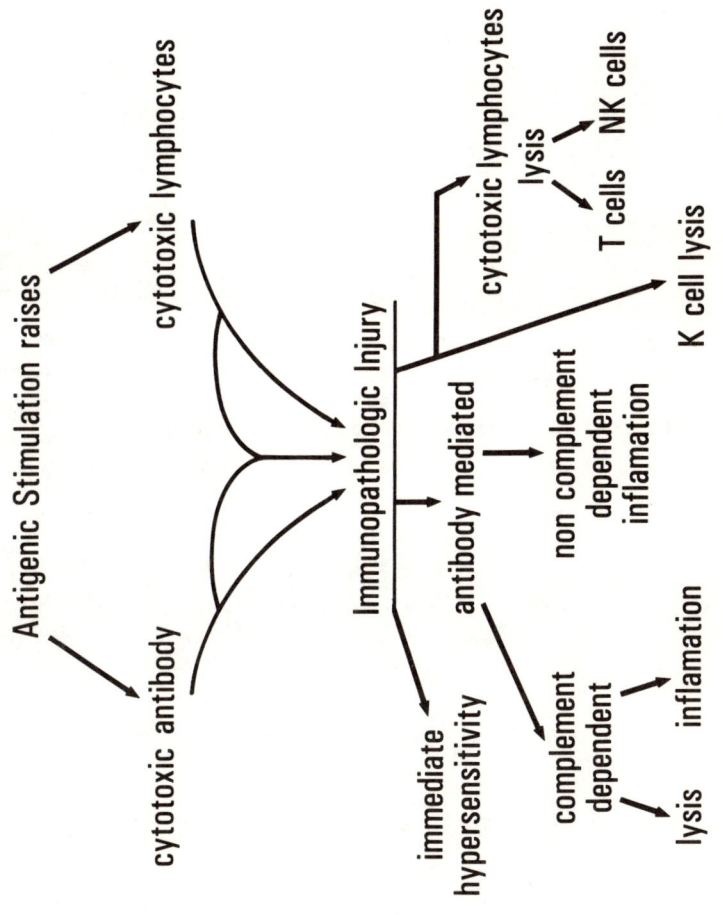

Figure 2.   A cartoon of the classical complement (C'1, C'4, and C'2) and alternative complement (P, B, D, B1H, C'3b INA) pathways and the biological effect of their activated products in immunopathologic-mediated injury.

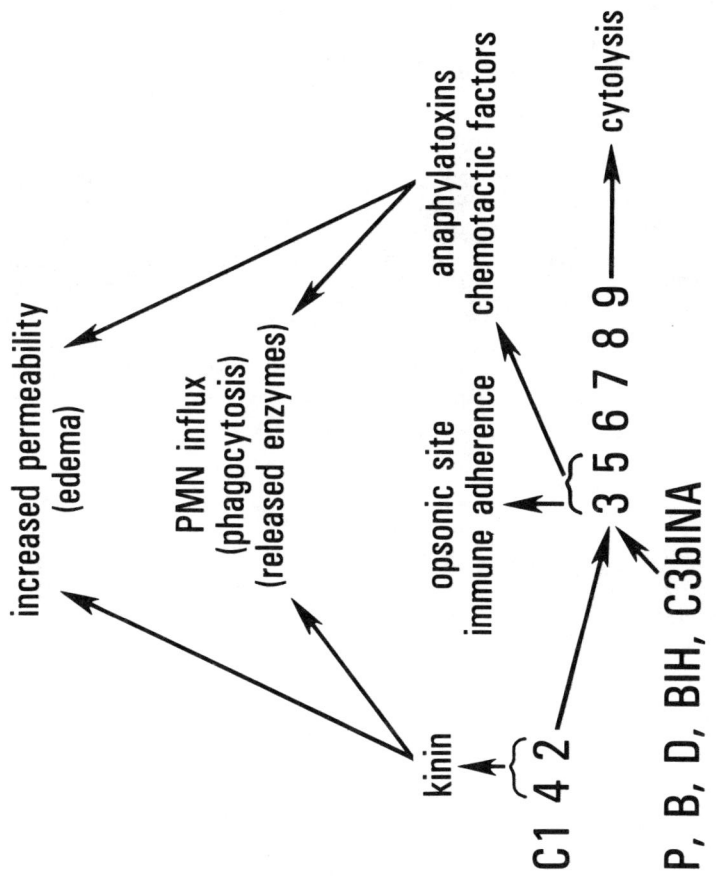

Figure 3. A cartoon of the complement pathways with details of the alternative pathway in the feedback loop. The alternative pathway/amplification system is shown in heavier lettering. By convention, major cleavage products of complement proteins are designated "b" and minor "a"; a subscript bar indicates an active enzyme. In this diagram,⌁ indicates a proteoloytic cleavage. On the surface of activating particles or cells, C'3b escapes from regulation in the positive feedback within the enclosed box.

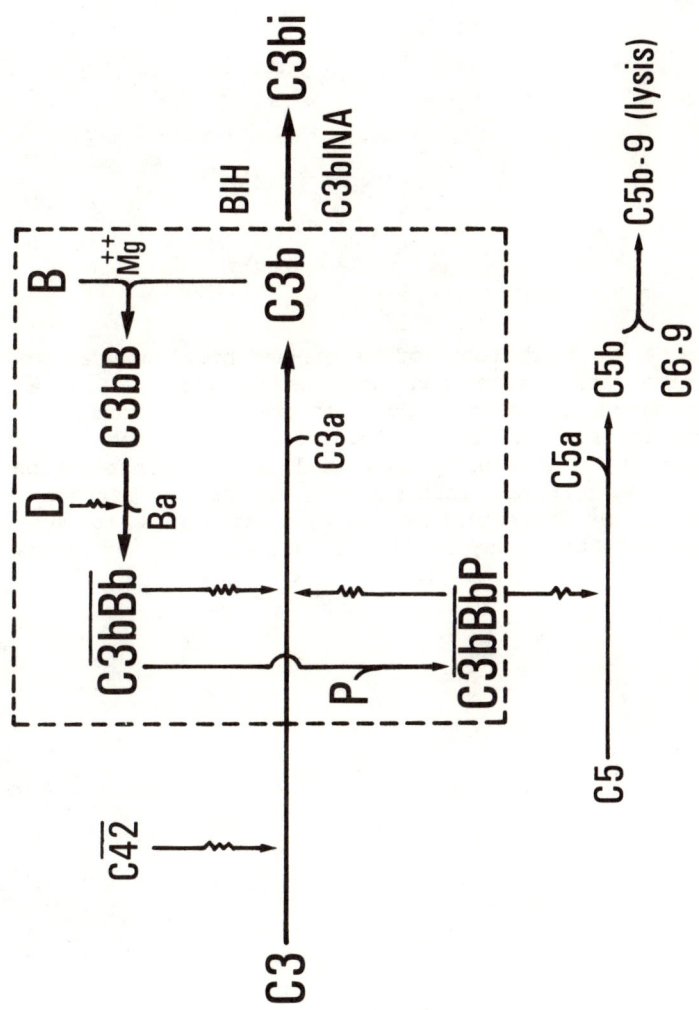

Figure 4. A cartoon of virus-antibody immune complex formation and deposition in target tissues. Note the formation of virus-antibody complexes which occur by the direct interaction of antibodies with virion or viral antigens in the fluid phase and by the interaction of antibody with viral antigens on the cell's surface. In addition, by "molecular mimicry," antibodies to specific viral determinants may react with normal cell components.

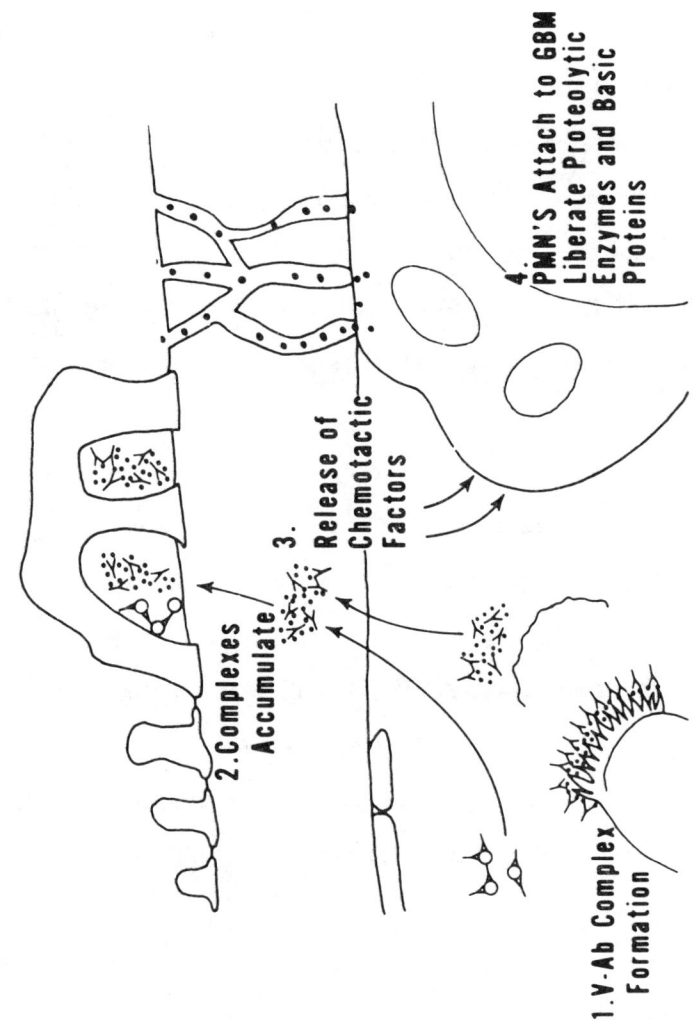

2. Complexes
   Accumulate

3. Release of
   Chemotactic
   Factors

4. PMN'S Attach to GBM
   Liberate Proteolytic
   Enzymes and Basic
   Proteins

1. V-Ab Complex
   Formation

References

1.   Cooper NR:The complement system, in Fudenberg HH, Stites DP, Caldwell JV (ed):Basic and Clinical Immunology, ed. 3. Palo Alto, California, Lang Medical Publishers, 1980, pp. 83-95.

2.   Muller-Eberhard HJ, Schreiber RD:Molecular biology and chemistry of the alternative pathway of complement. Adv Immunol 29:1-53, 1980.

3.   Sissons JGP, Oldstone MBA:Antibody-mediated destruction of virus-infected cells.   Adv Immunol 29:209-260, 1980.

4.   Sissons JGP, Oldstone MBA, Schreiber RD:Antibody independent activation of the alternative complement pathway by measles virus-infected cells. Proc Nat Acad Sci USA 77: 559-562, 1980.

5.   Sissons JGP, Schreiber RD, Perrin LH, Cooper NR, Muller-Eberhard HJ, Oldstone MBA:Lysis of measles virus-infected cells by the purified cytolytic alternative complement pathway and antibody.   J Exp Med 150:445-454, 1979.

6.   Gorman NT, Lachmann PJ:*In vitro* modulation of viral cell surface glycoproteins by antiviral antibody in the presence of complement. Clin Exp Immunol 50:507-514, 1982.

7.   Cooper   NR,   Welsh,   RM   Jr.:Antibody   and complement-dependent viral neutralization, in Miescher P, Muller-Eberhard   HJ   (eds):   Springer   Seminars   in Immunopathology, vol. 2, no. 3.   New York, Springer-Verlag, 1979, pp. 285-310.

8.   Welsh RM Jr., Cooper NR, Jensen FC, Oldstone MBA:Human   serum   lyses   RNA   tumor   viruses.   Nature 257:612-614, 1975.

9.   Zinkernagel RM, Doherty PC:MHC-restricted cytotoxic T cells: studies on the biological role of polymorphic major   transplantation   antigens   determining   T   cell restriction, specificity, function and responsiveness.   Adv Immunol 27:52-177, 1979.

10.   Casali P, Sissons JGP, Buchmeier MJ, Oldstone MBA:*In vitro* generation of human cytotoxic lymphocytes by virus.   Viral   glycoproteins   induce   nonspecific cell-mediated cytotoxicity without release of interferon. J Exp Med 154:840-855, 1981.

11.   Casali P, Oldstone MBA:Mechanisms of killing of measles   virus-infected   cells   by   human   lymphocytes: interferon-associated   and   unassociated   cell-mediated cytotoxicity.   Cell Immunol 70:330-344, 1982.

12.   Hugli TE:The structural basis for anaphylatoxin and chemotactic functions of C3a and C5a, in Critical Reviews

in Immunology I, No. 4.   Boca Raton, Florida, GRC Press
Review, 1981, pp. 321-366.

13.   Perlmann P, Cerottini JC:Cytotoxic lymphocytes, in
Sela M (ed):   The Antigens, vol. 5.   New York, Academic
Press, 1979, pp. 173-281.

14.   Fujinami RS, Oldstone MBA, Wroblewska Z, Frankel
ME, Koprowski H:Molecular mimicry in virus infection:
cross-reaction of measles virus phosphoprotein or of herpes
simplex virus protein with human intermediate filaments.
Proc Natl Acad Sci USA, in press, 1983.

15.   Oldstone MBA:Virus neutralization and virus-induced
immune complex disease: virus-antibody union resulting in
immunoprotection or immunologic injury--2 different sides
of the same coin, in Melnick JL (ed):   Progress in Medical
Virology, vol. 19, Basel, S. Karger, 1975, pp. 84-119.

16.   Oldstone MBA, Buchmeier MJ, Doyle MV, Tishon
A:virus-induced immune complex disease: specific antiviral
antibody and Clq binding material in the circulation during
persistent lymphocytic choriomeningitis virus infection.   J
Immunol 124:831-838, 1980.

17.   Oldstone MBA, Tishon A, Buchmeier MJ:Virus-induced
immune complex disease: genetic control of Clq binding
complexes in the circulation of mice persistently infected
with lymphocytic choriomeningitis virus.   J Immunol
130:912-918, 1983.

18.   Jenner E:An inquiry into the causes and effects of the variolae vaccinae, a disease discovered in some western countries of England, particularly Gloucestershire, and known by the name of cowpox.   1798.   Reprinted by Cassell, London, 1896.

Acknowledgments

This is Publication Number 2993-IMM from the Department of Immunology, Scripps Clinic and Research Foundation, La Jolla, California 92037.

This research was supported by U.S.P.H.S. grants AI-09484, AI-07007 and NS-12428.

Humoral and Cell-Mediated Resistance Mechanisms of Cattle

B. N. Wilkie, D.V.M., Ph.D.

Department of Veterinary Microbiology and Immunology
Ontario Veterinary College
University of Guelph
Guelph, Ontario, Canada N1G 2W1

Introduction

Knowledge of resistance mechanisms within relatively compartmentalized locations such as the respiratory system has evolved progressively following early veterinary recognition of mucosal antibody in relation to mucosal infection (1). While investigation of the relationship between systemic and mucosal resistance mechanisms and of surface resistance systems in general has been intense (2), practical exploitation of the accumulating knowledge for the benefit of veterinary preventive medicine has been difficult because of incomplete understanding. Bovine respiratory disease is of unquestioned economic importance but of uncertain etiology and pathogenesis. Serious evaluation of bovine mucosal resistance mechanisms has occurred only superficially during the present decade and the majority of commercial vaccines have been produced without benefit of a strong scientific base knowledge of the relevant agents, their virulence mechanisms and of crucial host defense systems. The efficacy of contemporary control measures for bovine respiratory disease is in question (3) and it is likely that effective techniques will follow only from precise understanding of host-parasite interactions in the bovine respiratory system. Critical analysis will be necessary in order to determine key manipulable resistance factors, essential microbial virulence mechanisms and appropriate methods of exploiting this information to the economic advantage of the producer. Specific investigation of individual disease-producing agents will be necessary since important differences occur between potential bovine respiratory tract pathogens in major aspects of their interaction with the host. Although generalizations may be made on mechanisms of resistance in the bovine respiratory system, these may need to be heavily modified for individual pathogens.

Observations

The general scheme of host-parasite interaction is illustrated in Figure 1 together with the most important currently recognized mediators of specific (immunological) and nonspecific host resistance. The inventory of resistance mechanisms available differs between surface and subsurface locations as well as between sites at different levels of the respiratory system so that accurate consideration must be given to the most relevant mechanism and site of resistance to any given agent. Objectives which center upon prevention of infection may have more stringent requirements for effective surface resistance while resistance to agents which have already penetrated respiratory system surfaces may be more easily obtained. Similarly, persistent surface infection especially of the more external respiratory epithelia may be difficult to control while colonization of epithelia located more deeply may be more readily preventable.

The respiratory system, in common with other externally-opening organ systems and in contrast to the closed body compartments, cannot accumulate mediators of specific or nonspecific resistance so that effective resistance may be restricted to periods of active local response or of transfer of mediators from systemic to local respiratory compartments. Since the duration of availability of mediators may be restricted, attempts to induce respiratory system resistance must be based upon timing of the prophylactic inducer in relationship to expected challenge. In addition, anamnesis of resistance may be the most relevant characteristic since actual effectors of resistance may not be present on the surface at the time of challenge. Whatever the scheme of resistance-induction that may be suggested by systematic laboratory investigation, it must be evaluated critically under field conditions since the complexities of the microbiological, nutritional and stressful influences upon the host are such that procedures devised in less intricate circumstances may prove invalid in actual use.

Resistance to Respiratory Infection

Immunologically-specific as well as nonspecific resistance mechanisms mediating protection of the respiratory system have been described in several species and a composite impression has emerged (4-7) against which resistance mechanisms of the bovine respiratory system may be studied. The general mechanisms of nonspecific and specific respiratory resistance are illustrated in Table 1 and Figures 1 and 2.

Nonspecific Resistance Mechanisms. Agents of relatively low virulence or of subvirulent dose may be adequately controlled as a result of nonspecific mechanisms operating within the upper and lower respiratory tract. Clearance of particles from the respiratory system is mediated by ciliary action above the alveoli which elevates material within fluid secretions to be swallowed or expectorated and by phagocytosis in the alveolus especially by lung macrophages. The site of particle deposition is a function of particle size, the larger particles (>10μ m) impinging upon nasal mucosa while smaller particles (0.5 - 3μ m) may reach the lung (8,9). Bovine lung clearance of *Pasteurella haemolytica* may reach 90 percent or more of the delivered dose by four hours post-inoculation (10) and bacterial clearance is impaired at seven days post-infection with PI-3 virus. Both PI-3 virus and bovine herpesvirus 1 (BHV-1) have been shown to enhance susceptibility to pneumonic pasteurellosis induced by *P. haemolytica* given by aerosol at discrete time intervals of three-ten days for PI-3 and greater than four days for BHV-1 (11,12). *Mycoplasma bovis* and bovine virus diarrhea virus (BVDV) failed to impair clearance of *P. haemolytica* in one reported experiment (13). In contrast to these findings, Corstvet (14) observed pneumonia in cattle challenged with a relatively low dose of *P. haemolytica* while actively infected with BVDV although animals not infected with the virus remained healthy. Investigation of viral and bacterial synergism in lung clearance using laboratory mice has strongly suggested that impaired clearance relates to defective alveolar macrophage bacterial killing (15). Limited studies of viral bacterial synergism in bovine pneumonia are inconclusive on the mechanisms involved.

While *in vitro* BHV-1-virus infection of bovine lung macrophages impaired cell function in antibody-dependent cell-mediated cytotoxicity (ADCC), this effect was not observed in macrophages infected *in vivo* (16).

In vitro infection of bovine alveolar macrophages with PI-3 virus has actually been shown to enhance cell resistance to cytotoxicity induced by *P. haemolytica* (17). Apparently resistance was associated with increased size of the macrophage due to syncitia induced by the virus. Detrimental effects of virus infection of macrophages *in vivo* may result from immune response to viral antigen with subsequent injury to cells expressing this antigen (18), an effect which would not occur spontaneously *in vitro*. Similarly, calves given *Corynebacterium parvum (Propionobacter acnes)* intravenously one week before sequential infection at an interval of one week with PI-3 and *P. haemolytica* had significantly enhanced lung clearance of *P. haemolytica* (19). Alveolar macrophage size was correlated significantly with enhanced bacterial clearance, an effect which was most likely attributable to nonspecific activation of macrophages by *C. parvum* which is known to enhance host resistance to a variety of microbial pathogens as well as to tumors (19).

The alveolar macrophage, the most numerous cell type in bovine lung lavage fluids (20) may well be the principal mediator of nonspecific resistance in the lung. *P. haemolytica* has been shown to produce a potent cytotoxin which is active against ruminant leukocytes, including alveolar macrophages, both impairing phagocytosis and killing the leucocyte (21,22,23). Cytotoxin-neutralizing antibody has been shown to correlate positively with resistance to pneumonic pasteurellosis in feedlot cattle (24). In addition, *P. haemolytica* has been shown to inhibit production of leukocyte chemotactic factors, an important component of nonspecific resistance, by bovine alveolar macrophages (25). The observed dose relatedness of *P. haemolytica*-induced bovine pneumonia (26) as well as the increase of *P. haemolytica* nasal colony counts in shipped calves judged to be unhealthy (27) suggests that in nonimmune cattle nonspecific respiratory system resistance is overcome by increasing numbers of *P. haemolytica* entering the lung with inspired air (28).

Macrophage-rich bovine pulmonary alveolar washing cells inhibit replication of BHV-1 virus in bovine tracheal organ cultures, an effect which is enhanced by soluble factors, including interferon, released from mitogen-activated bovine lymphocytes (29). These results suggest that interferon, or other lymphokines which are known to activate macrophages, may enhance macrophage-mediated nonspecific resistance to respiratory viruses, however, related *in vivo* and *in vitro* studies are inconclusive since results both support (30,31) and refute (32,33) a positive role for interferon in relation to resistance to BHV-1.

Nasal secretions of calves have been shown to contain an unidentified soluble factor which nonspecifically induces resistance to PI-3 virus infection (34,35). This is particularly effective in young calves and for virus strains having low neuraminidase content (36). Leukocytes in bovine nasal secretions have been studied only minimally (37) and apparently not at all in the context of nonspecific resistance in spite of the apparent importance of the site in colonization, infection and shedding of bacterial and viral pathogens (38,39).

Bovine lung lavage cell natural killer (NK) or spontaneous cell-mediated cytotoxicity has been reported against virus-infected and tumor cell targets (40). Cytotoxicity occurred against PI-3 virus but not against BHV-1-infected cells which were observed to be somewhat more resistant to NK cytotoxicity than were uninfected cells (40). The same effector cells mediated antibody-dependent cell-mediated cytotoxicity (ADCC) against both PI-3 virus and BHV-1-infected target cells (40). Natural cytotoxicity for PI-3-virus-infected cells was previously detected in association with bovine lung macrophages obtained from gnotobiotic calves (41).

Nonspecific resistance mechanisms operating in the bovine respiratory tract may well include nonspecific opsonization by IgG and IgM or complement as has been reported in other species (42) and the contribution of lysozyme, lactoferrin or other antibacterial substances as described in other species (43) may also be significant in cattle but are presently undescribed. The resistance afforded by macrophage, and likely also neutrophil function, is apparently substantial. This component may prove amenable to extrinsic regulation to enhance microbial killing (17,19). Alteration of bovine alveolar macrophage function to assist nonspecific resistance to infection and disease may also provide conditions within the lung more conducive to immunologically-specific resistance since in the bovine lung resident macrophages are reported to be inhibitory of lymphocyte mitogenic responses (44). A systematic search should therefore be undertaken to identify methods effective in enhancing bovine nonspecific respiratory resistance to infection.

Immunologically-Specific Resistance Mechanisms. Products of specific antibody or cell-mediated immune response are complementary to preexisting nonspecific resistance and clearance mechanisms. A relatively large body of information pertaining to respiratory immune response has accumulated from studies of several animal species so that the following general concepts have emerged (4-7):

1. The respiratory system is relatively compartmentalized from blood and blood-derived immune response, particularly in the upper areas but less so in the lung.

2. The respiratory system is itself compartmentalized immunologically into upper, middle and lower areas with apparent functional differences occurring by area.

3. Both antibody and cell-mediated immune responses occur within the respiratory system.

4. Surface respiratory system immune mediators can be induced by surface or by parenteral immunization and surface mediators are better correlated with resistance than are serum mediators. Respiratory immune response varies qualitatively and quantitatively in relation to route and method of its initiation.

5. Mechanisms of immunologically-mediated respiratory resistance are similar to those operating in other sites and are subject to the same limitations imposed by immunoglobulin isotype-related function as well as availability of immunoglobulin and cells.

6. Presence of respiratory surface immune mediators is transient in the absence of ongoing stimulation by antigen.

7. Memory can be established and measured in relation to surface immunization of the respiratory system.

Antibody-Mediated Immune Response.   Immune response in the bovine respiratory system has been studied only minimally but sufficient information is available to substantially confirm the generalizations given above. Regional differences exist in secreted immunoglobulin isotypes (20,45) with the ratio of IgA:IgG favoring IgA in nasal secretions (0.43± 0.27) approaching unity in lung lavage fluids (1.09± 1.3) and strongly favoring IgG in serum (185± 134) (20).   In the majority of individual animals, IgA predominates in lung washings (20,46) over IgG which is in slightly lower concentration. Lung lavage fluids and nasal secretions may contain IgM in very low concentrations as reflected by average ratios of IgA.IgM which are respectively 9.29 and 6.96 while the ratio in serum is 0.112 (20).   Others have failed to detect IgM in nasal secretions or in lung-washing fluids (45,46).

The presence of complement components in secretions of the bovine respiratory system has not actually been confirmed but by extrapolation from other species it seems likely that a functional complement system should exist, at least in alveolar fluids (47).   Complement is important in opsonization of bacteria for phagocytosis by lung macrophages and in lung clearance of bacteria in mice and rabbits (42).   Bovine alveolar macrophages have receptors for rabbit immunoglobulin G Fc (94 percent) and less frequently (39 percent) for C_3 b (48) both of which function in opsonization *in vitro.* Serum heated to destroy complement activity had reduced ability to opsonize *P. haemolytica* for phagocytosis by bovine alveolar macrophages (49).

Purified bovine lung-washing IgG, which was predominantly IgG1, and IgA did not opsonize *P. haemolytica in vitro* whether or not the immunoglobulin came from nonimmunized or immunized conventional calves (46,50). Similarly, whole reconstituted bovine lung lavage fluids failed to opsonize and impaired *in vitro* alveolar macrophage phagocytosis of *P. haemolytica* but not of *Yersinia enterocolitica.* Blocking occurred particularly with "normal" lung fluids or with fluids of calves previously exposed to killed *P. haemolytica* by intrabronchial infusion (51). Lung fluids obtained from calves immunized by subcutaneous injection of killed adjuvanted *P. haemolytica* rarely impaired phagocytosis in contrast to fluids from animals exposed to the bacterium by the respiratory route. The opposing effects occurred in spite of similar bacterial agglutinating antibody activity in opsonizing and phagocytosis inhibiting lung fluids. Although immunoglobulin isotypes were not fractionated from the lung fluids used in these experiments, the authors speculated that the observed phagocytosis inhibitory effect may have been due to a preponderance of antibody in the IgA class following respiratory immunization. This isotype is nonopsonizing (52) and may block phagocytosis (51). It is known that respiratory immunization of calves with killed *Mycoplasma bovis* induces production of lung-washing IgA-associated antibody as well as IgG while parenteral immunization favors antibody of the IgG isotype including IgG1 and IgG2 (53). Both IgG1 and IgG2 can fix bovine complement (54) and may therefore induce bacteriolysis or virolysis. Opsonization for phagocytosis by fresh macrophages and neutrophils occurs with IgG2 but not with IgG1 (54) but, since both isotypes occur in bovine lung lavage fluids (53), enhanced phagocytosis of microorganisms may occur in that site with beneficial or adverse consequences. Since phagocytic uptake of *P. haemolytica* leads to macrophage killing (21) parenteral immunization with this organism may be detrimental if the immunogen fails to induce cytotoxin-neutralizing antibody. Surface immunization with propensity to induce nonopsonizing IgA antibody may be less detrimental and beneficial if toxin neutralization occurs. For organisms which do not possess macrophage-injuring ability, or which do not survive within phagocytic cells, induction of respiratory IgG antibody by parenteral immunization may be advantageous. Caution must be exercised however since it is not yet firmly established that IgG isotypes, in contrast to IgA, do opsonize in the lung. Macrophage Fc receptors (55) and opsonization (54) have been recorded *in vitro* but others (56) could demonstrate phagocytic uptake of bacteria only by bovine lung macrophages *in situ* and not by macrophages cultured with antigen-specific IgG or IgA obtained from lung fluids.

Secreted immunoglobulin may arise by secretion from plasma cells immediately beneath the epithelium of the respiratory system or from tissue fluids by transudation. Neonatal calves have much higher concentrations of IgM and IgG1 in nasal secretions than do older animals in which IgA is present in higher concentration (57).   These changes likely reflect early secretion of colostrum-derived Ig into respiratory secretions and a gradual increase of endogenous epithelium-associated production of IgA.   Passive transfer of colostral Ig to nasal secretions of lambs has been formally demonstrated (58).   In small airways-associated lymphoid cells of normal calves, IgA producers predominate but with development of pneumonia the proportion of IgG1-producing cells increases (59). Physiologically-delayed onset of respiratory immunoglobulin synthesis may be important in predisposition to neonatal respiratory disease by analogy with the calf intestine in which local antibody production is also delayed (60).

Specialized bronchial-associated lymphoid tissue (BALT) with membranous antigen-absorbing overlying epithelium has been extensively studied in several species but not in cattle (6).   BALT, and the intestinal analogue GALT, are precursors of IgA-producing lymphocytes which migrate preferentially and interactively to mucosal sites thus providing the possibility of dissemination of mucosal resistance from an exposure at only one mucosal organ system.   It appears likely that IgA secreted in the bovine respiratory tract may be the product of BALT-derived precursors.   Knowledge of this aspect of respiratory immunology may influence development of methods for vaccination by local administration of antigen if an advantage can be shown to follow antigen uptake by BALT or a functionally-equivalent structure.

Induction of antibody within bovine respiratory tract secretions can be accomplished by local or parenteral administration of antigen (34,37,53,61). Antibody readily appears in lung-washing fluids following parenteral immunization but induction of nasal-secretion antibody apparently requires more rigorous immunization with adjuvanted or replicating agents (53). In parenterally immunized calves, lung washings contain antibody only transiently (61) and without apparent relationship to serum antibody titre (53,61). Lung washings of calves immunized parenterally with killed *M. bovis* contained protective antibody associated with IgG while intratracheal or intratracheal and intramuscular immunization resulted in IgA-related activity but this was minor relative to coexisting IgG antibody (53). In these experiments, resistance to respiratory challenge was related to lung antibody and was independent of serum antibody titres. Similarly, the best correlate of resistance in calves challenged with *P. haemolytica* was nasal antibody present after exposure to the live organism (62) and nasal antibody was found to be associated with reduced nasal *P. haemolytica* colony counts (63). Nasal antibody was not increased in calves immunized subcutaneously with adjuvanted killed *P. haemolytica* (61). Following intramuscular vaccination with attenuated BHV-1 virus, two of four cattle had nasal antibody only in association with IgG while intranasal vaccination resulted in more virus-neutralizing IgA than IgG at 14 days and the reverse by 28 days after vaccination (37). Serum antibody was detected at fourteen days after intramuscular vaccination and at higher titer than after intranasal vaccination which resulted in detectable antibody by day 21. Anamnesis was induced by both routes since serum antibody increased by five days after challenge to a higher titer than in controls which did not produce detectable antibody until day 12 (37). Both nasal and serum antibody occurred in calves vaccinated intranasally or intramuscularly with modified live PI-3 virus vaccines (64-66) although nasal vaccination produced higher nasal antibody titres.

Although memory response has been demonstrated within the respiratory secretions of laboratory animals after local (67-69) or local and parenteral immunization (70), it is not clear if this potential exists in cattle and if so how it may best be generated. Since specific antibody in lung fluids has been shown to inhibit antigen uptake in rabbits and to increase antigen catabolism within the lung (71,72), it is conceivable that preexisting lung antibody may impair further specific immune response.   This is suggested, but not confirmed, by studies involving immunization and challenge of calves with *P. haemolytica* (61).

Cell-Mediated Immune Response (CMI). CMI occurs within the lung of several species and is partially compartmentalized from parenteral CMI as is true for antibody-mediated respiratory immune response (73). Compartmentalization can be eroded by rigorous immunization. The alveolar macrophage is responsive to lymphokines secreted from antigen-stimulated immune T lymphocytes (9) and can be activated for enhanced killing of intracellular parasites (73).

Limited information is available concerning CMI within populations of bovine respiratory system cells. Calf nasal leucocytes were found to contain macrophages (44 percent), lymphocytes (41 percent) and neutrophils (15 percent) which were able to inhibit replication of BHV-1 virus *in vitro,* after immunization with modified live virus vaccine. Calf lung-washing lymphocytes were able to produce macrophage migration inhibition factor when cultured with antigens of

Micropolyspora faeni (74); however, populations of calf lung-washing cells did not respond to lymphocyte mitogens or to specific antigen (44) in the presence of alveolar macrophages which were markedly inhibitory for all bovine lymphocyte responses. Alveolar washing cells, partially depleted of macrophages by carbonyl iron treatment, formed rosettes with sheep erythrocytes (SRBC) (2.3± 1.1 percent), and with antibody and complement-coated SRBC indicating a preponderance of B lymphocytes (20). On the basis of binding to *Helix pomatia* lectin, the majority of lymphocytes in another study were found to be T cells (75). Cell-mediated immunity can be induced by respiratory infection or vaccination with BHV-1 or PI-3 virus as measured by peripheral blood lymphocyte blastogenesis, viral plaque reduction, generation of macrophage-migration inhibition factor or of delayed skin hypersensitivity (37,76-80). Similar studies of respiratory system cells are not reported.

Mitogen-stimulated bovine peripheral blood lymphocyte supernatants did not enhance bovine alveolar macrophage ability to phagocytize *P. haemolytica* or to resist bacterial cytotoxin (51) and actually inhibited phagocytosis. Peripheral blood lymphocytes of BHV-1-immunized calves did not diminish BHV-1 production when cultured together with virus-infected calf tracheal organ cultures; however, supernatants of BHV-1-stimulated immune bovine lymphocytes added to normal calf lung lavage cells did significantly reduce virus production (29). Interferon, a product of antigen-activated lymphocytes, has inhibited BHV-1 production in some studies of bovine tracheal organ cultures (81) but not in others (33).

Clearly, pertinent information on the CMI capability of the bovine respiratory immune system is deficient and should be sought in view of the apparent importance of cell-associated viruses (BHV-1) and macrophage function in production of bovine respiratory disease.

Protective Effect of Bovine Respiratory Immune Response. The protective potential of the respiratory immune system varies by region--there being apparently more effective resistance in the lung than the nose where antibody is more likely to be IgA with attendant limitations in antimicrobial mechanisms possibly enhancing the likelihood of the carrier state (Figure 2). Agents which remain upon the surface of epithelia at any level of the respiratory system are subject to a more restricted inventory of immunological control mechanisms than are those that penetrate and spread beyond the portal of entry. The most pertinent question is, therefore, the effect of immune mediators upon agents prior to their entry to epithelia; however, experiments reported to date are frequently such that this distinction cannot be made. Pragmatically it matters only that the host is made resistant to agents which characteristically induce respiratory disease and it may be academic as to whether the source of resistance is within or outside the respiratory system. However, prevention of infection may be the most important objective so that the disadvantages of persistent foci of infection and serological positivity, common features of BHV-1, PI-3 and *P. haemolytica* infection may be avoided. Surface resistance may be needed to provide this.

Although respiratory protection is generally best correlated with immune mediators within the secretions of the respiratory system (53,62,64,82), advantage does not clearly result from local rather than parenteral administration of modified live PI-3 virus, BHV-1 or live *P. haemolytica* when compared in terms of induced protection against homologous respiratory challenge (14,37,66,82,83) or the advantage is slight (56). Parenteral vaccination with BHV-1-modified live virus may result in fewer post-vaccinal clinical signs (82) than respiratory vaccination although with greater risk of inducing abortion (84). Parenteral vaccination with formalin-killed *P.*

haemolytica, however, failed to protect calves and was associated with more severe reaction to homologous respiratory challenge (85). While the exact pathogenesis of this response has not been elucidated, it is thought to be due to inappropriate specificity of immune response for surface antigens rather than cytotoxin or other virulence factors induced as well as possibly inappropriate class bias (IgG opsonins in excess of virulence-neutralizing IgG or IgA) of lung antibody. Similar antigen given locally does not induce adverse reaction but fails to protect against challenge.

Clearance of BHV-1 from the nose of aerosol-immunized calves was more rapid (10^9 PFU in less than one hour, 10^6 PFU in less than five minutes) than in nonimmunized controls (10^9 PFU in less than four hours, 10^6 PFU in less than one hour) and reinfection persisted for only 24 hours by comparison with twelve days (38). BHV-1 viral shedding ceases as sensitized T lymphocytes (CMI) are detected and begins again under the influence of dexamethasone treatment even though virus-neutralizing antibody titers are high in serum (76). Shedding again stops as CMI is detected. It is thought that CMI is crucial in resistance to BHV-1 but NK activity and ADCC may also contribute (40,48,80,86).

Vaccination with live *P. haemolytica* by aerosol or by subcutaneous injection induced resistance to homologous challenge by direct injection into the lung. Protection was associated with enhanced phagocytosis of the bacterium *in vivo* and reduced extent of pneumonic lesions and resulted in no mortality (14,56). Subcutaneous vaccination resulted in more intact intracellular bacteria than did aerosol vaccination. Vaccination with killed *M. bovis* also induced enhanced lung clearance in relation to protection of calves (53).

Conclusion

The incentive is great to provide effective preventive methods for bovine respiratory disease. Systematic analysis of the cause and pathogenesis of economically important conditions may provide targets for prophylaxis which can utilize developing knowledge of microbial genetics, functional interaction of specific and nonspecific resistance mechanisms, immunogenetics and hybridoma technology. Available knowledge is slight and fragmentary and new studies must be designed with strict concern for real economic benefit to the producer from any instituted preventive measures. Future studies may benefit from the recognition that specific immune response functions to enhance host resistance by improving preexisting nonspecific resistance mechanisms. Attention may profitably be turned toward direct enhancement of nonspecific resistance as well as the more traditional attempts to stimulate immune response. The latter clearly carries the potential for inadvertent induction of adverse reaction if inappropriate antigens or immune mediators are involved. Attention should also be given to bovine genetics and immunogenetics in relation to specific and nonspecific resistance as well as to husbandry systems that may optimize intrinsic ability to remain healthy.

Novel immunomodulating materials including synthetic thymic hormone peptides, interleukin 1, interleukin 2 and interferon may find a place in prevention of bovine respiratory disease as may synthetic immunogen-carrier-adjuvant molecules. The immediate challenge is to provide the foundation knowledge of bovine respiratory host-parasite interaction upon which these promising new methods may be based.

Table 1. Nonspecific resistence mechanisms of the respiratory system

Cell Mediated	Humoral
Particle deposition and clearance by cilia, sneeze, cough	Complement-mediated opsonization and microbial lysis
Phagocytosis by resident alveolar macrophages and by neutrophils chemotactically attracted to upper and lower airways	Interferon inhibition of intracellular pathogens
Natural cytotoxicity by surface leucocytes	Macrophage activation by lymphocyte products, microorganisms or particulate matter
	Lysozyme and lactoferrin-mediated antibacterial systems
	Nonspecific viral inhibitors
	Pulmonary surfactant enhancement of bacterial phagocytosis and killing
	Protease inhibitors

Figure 1. Immunologically-Specific   and   Nonspecific
Mechanisms of   Host   Resistance to Microbial
Infection

The largest circle represents host surface epithelium, the
smaller a host cell and the smallest the cell nucleus.
⬢Microbial pathogen.
●Microbial   antigen,   microbial-induced   antigen   or
altered host antigen expressed on the cell surface.

Mediators of nonspecific resistance are symbolized in the
lower sections of the figure:
MO, macrophage
PMN, neutrophil
C', complement
Ifn, interferon
Mucus, mucus secretions
Lysin, microbial lysing substances
Lysozyme, lysozyme
NK, natural killer cell
K, killer cell

Mediators   of   immunologically-specific   resistance   are
symbolized in the upper sections of the figure:
K, killer cell
CMI, cell-mediated immunity
Ab, antibody
C', complement

Numerals and arrows indicate stages in the interaction of
parasite and host:

1. Release of pathogen from original host

2. Surface attachment and penetration

3. Movement within interstitial or other internal body
fluids

4. Infection of host cell

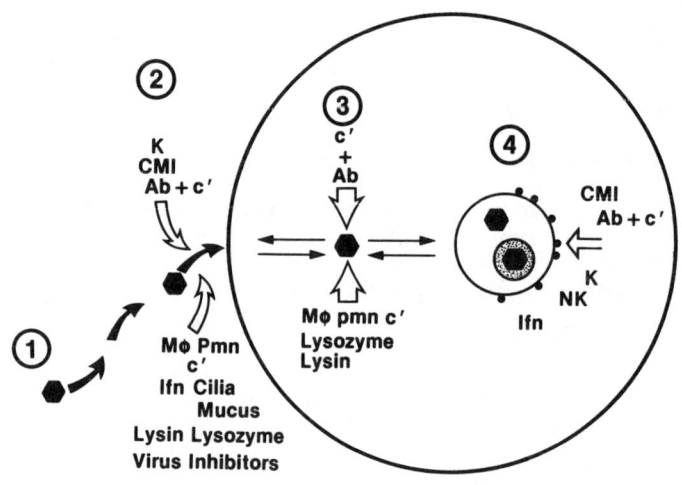

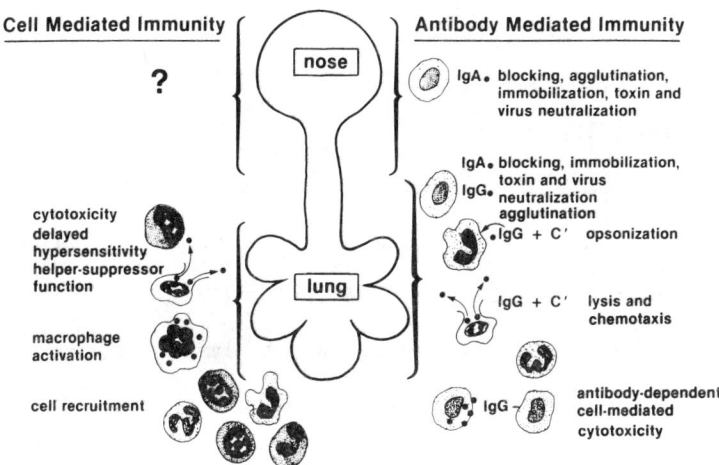

Figure 2.   Respiratory   Antibody   and   Cell-Mediated
            Resistance Mechanisms.

? Function undescribed in this location.
O Microbial pathogen.
C' Complement

References

1.   Pierce AE:Specific antibodies at mucosal surfaces. Vet Rev and Annotat 5:17-36, 1959.

2.   Bienenstock J, Befus AD:Mucosal immunology. Immunology 41:249-270, 1980.

3.   Martin SW:Vaccination: is it effective in preventing respiratory disease or influencing weight gains in feedlot calves? Can Vet J 24:10-19, 1983.

4.   Wilkie BN:Respiratory tract immune response to microbial pathogens. J Am Vet Med Assoc 181:1074-1079, 1982.

5.   Newhouse M, Sanchis J, Bienenstock J:Lung defense mechanisms. N Engl J Med 295:990-997, 1045-1052, 1976.

6.   McDermott MR, Befus AD, Bienenstock J:The structural basis for immunity in the respiratory tract, in Richter GW, Epstein MA (eds): Int Rev Exp Path, New York, Academic Press, 1981.

7.   Green GM, Jakab GJ, Low RB, Davis GS:Defense mechanisms of the respiratory membrane. Am Rev Resp Dis 115:479-514, 1977.

8.   Kaltreider HB, Caldwell JZ, Adam E:The fate and consequence of an organic particulate antigen instilled into bronchoalveolar spaces of normal canine lungs. Am Rev Resp Dis 116:267-280, 1977.

9.   Kaltreider HB, Turner FN, Salmon SE:Expression of immune mechanisms in the lung.   Am Rev Resp Dis 113:347-379, 1976.

10.   Lopez A, Thomson RG, Savan M:The pulmonary clearance of *Pasteurella haemolytica* in calves infected with bovine parainfluenza-3 virus.   Can J Comp Med 40:385-391, 1976.

11.   Jericho KWF, Daniel CLeQ, Langford EV:Respiratory disease in calves produced with aerosols of parainfluenza-3 virus and *Pasteurella haemolytica*. Can J Comp Med 46:293-301, 1982.

12.   Jericho KWF, Langford EV:Pneumonia in calves produced with aerosols of bovine herpesvirus 1 and *Pasteurella haemolytica*. Can J Comp Med 42:269-277, 1978.

13.   Lopez A, Maxie MG, Savan M, Ruhnke HL, Thomson RG, Barnum DA, Geissinger MD:The pulmonary clearance of *Pasteurella haemolytica* in calves infected with bovine virus diarrhea or *Mycoplasma bovis*. Can J Comp Med 46:302-306, 1982.

14.   Corstvet RE, Panciera RJ, Newman P:Vaccination of calves with *Pasteurella multocida* and *Pasteurella haemolytica*. Proc Am Assoc Vet Lab Diag 21:67-90, 1978.

15.   Jakab GJ, Green GM:Defect in intracellular killing of *Staphylococcus aureus* within alveolar macrophages in

Sendai virus-infected murine lungs. J Clin Invest 57:1533-1539, 1976.

16. Forman AJ, Babiuk LA, Baldwin F, Friend SCE:Effect of infectious bovine rhinotracheitis virus infection of calves on cell populations recovered by lung lavage. Am J Vet Res 43:1174-1179, 1982.

17. Angulo AB:Parainfluenza-3 virus infection of bovine alveolar macrophages, in Butler JE (ed): The Ruminant Immune System. New York, Plenum, 1981.

18. Jakab GJ:Mechanisms of virus-induced bacterial superinfections of the lung. Clinics in Chest Med 2:59-66, 1981.

19. Al-Izzi SA, Maxie MG, Savan M:The pulmonary clearance of *Pasteurella haemolytica* in calves given *Corynebacterium parvum* and infected with parainfluenza-3 virus. Can J Comp Med 46:85-90, 1982.

20. Wilkie BN, Markham RJF:Broncheoalveolar washing cells and immunoglobulins of clinically normal calves. Am J Vet Res 42:241-243, 1981.

21. Markham RJF, Wilkie BN:Interaction between *Pasteurella haemolytica* and bovine alveolar macrophages: cytotoxic effect on macrophages and impaired phagocytosis. Am J Vet Res 41:18-22, 1980.

22.   Shewen PE, Wilkie BN:Cytotoxin of *Pasteurella haemolytica* acting on bovine leucocytes. Infect Immun 35:91-94, 1982.

23.   Shewen PE, Wilkie BN:*Pasteurella haemolytica* cytotoxin: production by recognized serotypes and neutralization by type-specific rabbit antisera. Am J Vet Res 44:715-719, 1983.

24.   Shewen PE, Wilkie BN:*Pasteurella haemolytica* cytotoxin neutralizing activity in sera from Ontario beef cattle. Can J Comp Med 47:497-498, 1983.

25.   Markham RJF, Ramnaraine MLR, Muscoplatt CC:Cytotoxic effect of *Pasteurella haemolytica* on bovine polymorphonuclear leukocytes and impaired production of chemotactic factors by *Pasteurella haemolytica*-infected alveolar macrophages. Am J Vet Res 43:285-288, 1982.

26.   Yates WDG, Jericho KWF, Doige CE:Effect of bacterial dose on pneumonia induced by aerosol exposure of calves to herpesvirus-1 and *Pasteurella haemolytica*. Am J Vet Res 44:238-243, 1983.

27.   Thomson RG, Chander S, Savan M, Fox ML:Investigation of factors of probable significance in the pathogenesis of pneumonic pasteurellosis in cattle. Can J Comp Med 39:194-207, 1975.

28.   Grey CL, Thomson RG:*Pasteurella haemolytica* in the tracheal air of calves. Can J Comp Med 35:121-128, 1971.

29.   Bouffard A, Derbyshire JB, Wilkie BN:Effects of lymphocytes and bronchoalveolar washing cells on the replication of bovine herpesvirus type 1 in tracheal organ cultures. Vet Microbiol 7:241-251, 1982.

30.   Todd JD, Volerec FJ, Paton IM:Interferon in nasal secretions and sera of calves after intranasal administration of avirulent infectious bovine rhinotracheitic virus: association of interferon in nasal secretions with early resistance to challenge with virulent virus. Infect Immun 5:699-706, 1972.

31.   Smorodintsev AA:The production and effect of interferon on organ cultures of calf trachea. BrJ Exp Pathol 49:511-515, 1968.

32.   Savan M, Angulo AB, Derbyshire JB:Interferon, antibody responses and protection induced by an intranasal infectious bovine rhinotracheitis vaccine. Can Vet J 20:207-210, 1979.

33.   Bouffard A, Derbyshire JB:Effects of some components of the humoral immune response on the replication of bovine herpesvirus type 1 in tracheal organ cultures. Vet Microbiol 6:129-141, 1981.

34.   Morein B:Immunity against parainfluenza-3 virus in cattle; immunoglobulins in serum and nasal secretions after subcutaneous and nasal vaccination. 2. Immun-Forsch 144:63-74, 1972.

35.   Smith WD, Wells PW, Burrells C, Dawson AML:Immunoglobulins, antibodies and inhibitors of parainfluenza-3 virus in respiratory secretions of sheep. Arch Virol 49:329-337, 1975.

36.   Bergman R, Moreno-Lopez J, Mollerberg L, Morein B:Parainfluenza-3 virus: difference in capacity of neuraminidase-weak and strong strains to infect young calves and to elicit cellular immune response. Res Vet Sci 25:193-199, 1978.

37.   Gerber JD, Marron AE, Kucera CJ:Local and systemic cellular and antibody immune responses of cattle to infectious bovine rhinotracheitis virus vaccines administered intranasally or intramuscularly. Am J Vet Res 39:753-760, 1978.

38.   Lupton HW, Reed DE:Clearance and shedding of infectious bovine rhinotracheitis virus from nasal mucosa of immune and nonimmune calves. Am J Vet Res 41:117-119, 1980.

39.   Pass DA, Thomson RG:Wide distribution of *Pasteurella haemolytica* type 1 over the nasal mucosa of cattle.   Can J Comp Med 35:181-185, 1971.

40. Campos M, Rossi CR, Lawman MJP:Natural cell-mediated cytotoxicity of bovine mononuclear cells against virus-infected cells. Infect Immun 36:1054-1059, 1982.

41. Probert M, Stott EJ, Thomas LH:Interactions between calf alveolar macrophages and parainfluenza-3 virus. Infect Immun 15:576-585, 1977.

42. Guckian JC, Christensen GD, Fine DP:The role of opsonins in recovery from experimental pneumococcal pneumonia. J Inf Dis 142:175-190, 1980.

43. Turner-Warwick M:Clinical aspects of protective immunity of the respiratory tract. Thorax 30:601-611, 1975.

44. Bendixen PH, Shewen PE, Wilkie BN:Inhibition of the blastogenic response of peripheral blood mononuclear cells to mitogen and antigen by bovine pulomonary macrophages and their culture supernatants. Res Vet Sci 31:272-277, 1981.

45. Duncan JR, Wilkie BN, Hiestand F, Winter AJ:The serum and secretory immunoglobulins of cattle: characterization and quantitation. J Immunol 108:965-976, 1972.

46. Walker RD, Corstvet RE, Lessley BA, Panciera RJ:Study of bovine pulmonary response to *Pasteurella haemolytica:* specificity of immunoglobulins isolated from the bovine lung. Am J Vet Res 41:1015-1023, 1980.

47.   Reynolds HJ, Thompson RE:Pulmonary host defenses. I. Analysis of protein and lipids in bronchial secretions and antibody responses following vaccination with *Pseudomonas aeruginosa.* J Immunol 111:358-368, 1973.

48.   Forman AJ, Babiuk LA:Effects of infectious bovine rhinotracheitis virus infection on bovine alveolar macrophage functions.   Infect Immun 35:1041-1047, 1982.

49.   Maheswaran SK, Berggren KA, Simonson RR, Ward GE, Muscoplatt CC:Kinetics of interaction and fate of *Pasteurella haemolytica* in bovine alveolar macrophages.   Infect Immun 30:254-262, 1980.

50.   Walker RD, Corstvet RE, Panciera RJ:Study of bovine pulmonary response to *Pasteurella haemolytica:* pulmonary macrophage response.   Am J Vet Res 41:1008-1014, 1980.

51.   Markham RJF, Wilkie BN:Influence of bronchoalveolar washing supernatants and stimulated lymphocyte supernatants on uptake of *Pasteurella haemolytica* by cultured bovine alveolar macrophages.   Am J Vet Res 41:443-446, 1980.

52.   Corbeil LB, Schurig GG, Duncan JR, Wilkie BN, Winter AJ:Immunity in the female bovine reproductive tract based on the response to *"Campylobacter fetus,"* in Butler JE (ed):   The Ruminant Immune System. New York, Plenum, 1981.

53.   Howard CJ, Gourlay RN, Taylor G:Immunity to *Mycoplasma bovis* infections of the respiratory tract of calves. Res Vet Sci 28:242-249, 1980.

54. McGuire TC, Musoke AJ:Biologic activities of bovine IgG subclasses, in Butler JE (ed): The Ruminant Immune System. New York, Plenum, 1981.

55. Rossi CR, Kiesel GK:Bovine immunoglobulin G subclass receptor sites on bovine macrophages. Am J Vet Res 38:1023-1025, 1977.

56. Newman PR, Corstvet RE, Panciera RJ:Distribution of *Pasteurella haemolytica* and *Pasteurella multocida* in the bovine lung following vaccination and challenge exposure as an indicator of lung resistance. Am J Vet Res 43:417-422, 1982.

57. Morgan K, Bradley P, Bourne FJ:The immune system of the bovine respiratory tract. Proceedings of the Seminar on Respiratory Diseases of Cattle, Commission of the European Community, Edinburgh, 1977.

58. Wells PW, Dawson A, Smith WD, Smith BSW:Transfer of IgG from plasma to nasal secretions in newborn lambs. Vet Rec 97:455, 1975.

59. Allan EM, Pirie HM, Selman IE, Wiseman A:Immunoglobulin containing cells in the bronchopulmonary system of non-pneumonic and pneumonic calves. Res Vet Sci 26:349-355, 1979.

60. Husband AJ:Ontogeny of the gut associated immune system, in Butler JE (ed): The Ruminant Immune System. New York, Plenum, 1981.

61.   Wilkie BN, Markham RJF:Sequential titration of bovine lung and serum antibodies after parenteral or pulmonary inoculation with *Pasteurella haemolytica*. Am J Vet Res 40:1690-1693, 1979.

62.   Friend SCE, Wilkie BN, Thomson RG, Barnun DA:Bovine pneumonic pasteurellosis: experimental induction in vaccinated and nonvaccinated calves. Can J Comp Med 41:77-83, 1977.

63.   Duncan JR, Thomson RG:Preliminary observations on the effect of specific immunity on nasal bacterial flora. Can J Comp Med 34:90-93, 1970.

64.   Frank GH, Marshall RG:Relationship of serum and nasal secretion-neutralizing antibodies in protection of calves against parainfluenza-3 virus. Am J Vet Res 32:1707-1713, 1971.

65.   Marshall RG, Frank GH:Neutralizing antibody in serum and nasal secretions of calves exposed to parainfluenza-3 virus. Am J Vet Res 32:1699-1706, 1071.

66.   McKercher DG, Sarto JK, Franti CE, Wada EM, Crenshaw GL:Response of calves to parainfluenza-3 vaccines administered nasally or parenterally.   Am J Vet Res 33:721-730, 1972.

67.   Kasturi K, Hannoun C:Immune responses to influenza virus in rabbits after local immunization. I.   Local and

systemic humoral response.   Ann Microbiol (Inst Pasteur) 128:97-117, 1977.

68.   Kasturi K, Hannoun C:Immune responses to influenza virus in rabbits after local immunization.   II. Local and systemic cell mediated response.   Ann Microbiol (Inst Pasteur) 128:349-364, 1977.

69.   Markham RJF, Wilkie BN:Local adjuvants.   The influence of sodiumdodecylbenzenesulphonate on immunization with aerosolized antigen.   Experientia 35:414-416, 1979.

70.   Thomas WR, Holt PG, Keast D:Local and systemic immune response of mice after intratracheal and intravenous inoculations of sheep erythrocytes.   Int Arch Allergy Appl Immunol 46:487-489, 1976.

71.   Braley JF, Dawson CA, Moore VL:Immunologic block against antigen absorption from isolated perfused rabbit lungs.   J Immunol 121:926-929, 1978.

72.   Thrall RS, Peterson LB, Linehan JH, Abramoff P, Moore VL:The effect of immunization on the uptake of intratracheally administered antigen.   Clin Immunol Immunopath 10:136-147, 1978.

73.   Truitt GL, Mackaness GB:Cell-mediated resistance to aerogenic infection of the lung.   Am Rev Resp Dis 104:829-843, 1971.

74.   Wilkie   BN:Experimental   hypersensitivity pneumonitis. Humoral and cell-mediated immune response of cattle to *Micropolyspora faeni* and clinical response to aerosol   challenge.   Int   Archs   Allerg   Appl   Immunol 50:359-373, 1976.

75.   LeJan C, Johansson C:Characterization of bovine lymphocytes from blood, lung and trachea, in Butler JE (ed): The Ruminant Immune System. New York, Plenum, 1981.

76.   Davies DH, Carmichael LE:Role of cell-mediated immunity in the recovery of cattle from primary and recurrent infections with infectious bovine rhinotracheitis virus.   Infect Immun 8:510-518, 1973.

77.   Hoglund B, Moreno-Lopez J, Morein B:Components of parainfluenza-3 virus, SLP-strain reacting in assays of cell-mediated immunity in cattle.   Arch Virol 53:323-333, 1977.

78.   Johnson K, Morein B:*In vitro* stimulation of bovine circulating lymphocytes by parainfluenza type 3 virus.   Res Vet Sci 22:83-85, 1977.

79.   Morein B, Moreno-Lopez J:Skin hypersensitivity to parainfluenza-3 virus in cattle.   Zbl Vet Med 20:540-546, 1973.

80.   Rouse BT, Babiuk LA:Host defense mechanisms against infectious bovine rhinotracheitis virus II.   Inhibition of

viral plaque formation by immune peripheral blood lymphocytes. Cell Immunol 17:43-56, 1975.

81.   Fulton RW, Root SK:Antiviral activity in interferon-treated bovine tracheal organ cultures. Infect Immun 21:672-673, 1978.

82.   Frank GH, Marshall RG, Smith PC:Clinical and immunologic responses of cattle to infectious bovine rhinotracheitis virus after infection by viral aerosol or intramuscular inoculation. Am J Vet Res 38:1497-1502, 1977.

83.   McKercher DG, Crenshaw GL:Comparative efficacy of intranasally and parenterally administered infectious bovine rhinotracheitis vaccines. J Am Vet Med Assoc 159:1362-1369, 1971.

84.   Kucera CJ, White RG, Beckenhauer WH:Evaluation of the safety and efficacy of an intranasal vaccine containing a temperature-sensitive strain of infectious bovine rhinotracheitis virus. Am J Vet Res 39:607-610, 1978.

85.   Wilkie BN, Markham RJF, Shewen PE:Response of calves to lung challenge exposure with *Pasteurella haemolytica* after parenteral or pulmonary immunization. Am J Vet Res 41:1773-1778, 1980.

86.   Rouse BT, Wardley RC, Babiuk LA:The role of antibody dependent cytotoxicity in recovery from herpesvirus infections. Cell Immunol 22:182-186, 1976.

Immunosuppression and Immunomodulation in Bovine Respiratory Disease

James A. Roth, D.V.M., Ph.D.

Department of Veterinary Microbiology and Preventive Medicine
College of Veterinary Medicine
Iowa State University
Ames, Iowa 50011

Introduction

The bovine respiratory disease complex (BRD) has been extensively investigated in recent years and is the subject of numerous scientific reports. In spite of these efforts, the pathogenesis and etiology of BRD is still incompletely understood. Respiratory disease ("shipping fever") is particularly prevalent after animals have been weaned, transported and placed in a feedlot. The economically important clinical signs, lesions, and death loss in shipping fever can usually be attributed to bacterial pneumonia, but efforts to reproduce these lesions by challenging normal cattle with bacterial agents alone are typically unsuccessful. The bacteria which are most frequently isolated from the lower respiratory tract of affected cattle are also commonly found in the nasopharyngeal area of normal animals. These observations have led to the concept that BRD has a multifactorial etiology involving a complex interaction between stressors and viruses predisposing to bacterial infection and fulminant disease (1).

The purpose of this report is to review the evidence that stressors, viruses and bacteria associated with BRD impair host defense mechanisms, to characterize the nature of the impairments and to discuss the potential for immunomodulators to reduce the losses associated with BRD.

Observations

Immunosuppression by Stress

There is ample evidence that environmental, physical or psychological stress can lead to increased susceptibility to disease and that the increased susceptibility is at least partially due to alterations in immune function (2,3). A general response of the body to stress is the release of ACTH from the anterior pituitary gland which stimulates the adrenal cortex to increase the synthesis and secretion of cortisol (hydrocortisone). Many (but probably not all) of the effects of stress on the immune system are due to the actions of plasma cortisol. The effects of glucocorticoids in general on the bovine immune system and the role for cortisol as a mediator of stress-associated immunosuppression in cattle have recently been reviewed (4,5). Therefore, only a brief summary of the immunosuppressive effects of cortisol on the bovine immune system will be presented here.

Several stressors which are sometimes associated with introduction of cattle to a feedlot have been proven to result in increased plasma cortisol levels. Some of these conditions are castration and dehorning (6), weaning (7,8), handling (7), forced exercise (9), acute pain (10), and transportation (6-8,11,12). There is evidence that high plasma cortisol concentrations affect several aspects of host defense. Primary antibody responses that develop in the presence of high plasma cortisol concentrations are inhibited (8,13). The effects of cortisol on cell-mediated immunity is more difficult to assess. ACTH administration to cattle will inhibit lymphocyte blastogenic responsiveness to the mitogens phytohemagglutinin (PHA) and concanavalin A (Con A) (14). While this cannot be considered a direct measure of cell-mediated immunity, it does indicate that increased cortisol *in vivo* has an effect on lymphocyte function or distribution.

Increased plasma cortisol also impairs certain aspects of neutrophil function. Perhaps the most important effect is to inhibit the immigration of neutrophils into the tissues at sites of inflammation (15). This is a result of the action of cortisol to reduce the "stickiness" of the neutrophil plasma membrane so that it cannot efficiently adhere to endothelial cells and leave the vasculature by diapedesis.   In addition to inhibiting neutrophil accumulation in the tissues, cortisol also inhibits the activity of the hydrogen peroxide-halide-myeloperoxidase anti-bacterial system (probably by inhibiting degranulation) and increases the rate of random migration of neutrophils (14).   These effects may be due to an inhibition of microtubule function with the neutrophil. Increased plasma cortisol due to ACTH administration in cattle does not measurably impair the ability of neutrophils to ingest *Staphylococcus aureus,* generate the burst of oxidative metabolism or mediate antibody-dependent cell-mediated cytotoxicity (14). Dexamethasone, a more potent glucocorticoid does inhibit these activities of bovine neutrophils at pharmacologic dosages (16).   It is possible that cortisol also affects these functions, but in a more subtle fashion which is beyond the limits of sensitivity of the assay systems employed.

The effects of glucocorticoids on macrophage function in the bovine has apparently not been studied.   In other species the macrophage is generally sensitive to glucocorticoids and has reduced phagocytic and bactericidal capabilities (17,18).

The effects of glucocorticoids on the eventual immune response to an antigen capable of replication can be quite different from the effects on the response to a nonviable antigen. When modified live IBR virus was administered to cattle with high plasma cortisol concentrations (due to ACTH administration) the primary antibody response, lymphocyte blastogenic response to IBR antigen, and serum interferon concentration were higher in the ACTH-treated cattle than the controls (Kaeberle and Roth, unpublished observations.) These results are probably explained by the observation that administration of hydrocortisone at the time of IBR-virus inoculation causes a higher and more persistent viremia in spite of a higher and more prolonged serum interferon response (19,20). The suppression of host defense mechanisms (probably phagocytic cell activity) by glucocorticoids early in virus infection apparently facilitated viral replication so that when glucocorticoid concentrations returned to normal the treated animals had a greater antigenic stimulus and produced a stronger immune response.   Recrudescence of the IBR virus with dexamethasone has also resulted in enhancement of the *in vitro* lymphocyte blastogenic response to IBR antigen (21,22).

Immunosuppression by Viruses and Mycoplasmas

The viruses associated with the bovine respiratory disease complex usually do not produce severe lesions and clinical signs when inoculated into normal cattle. Their real importance in BRD is probably due to their detrimental effect on pulmonary defense mechanisms which facilitates secondary infection by bacteria. There are several types of evidence commonly cited to suggest that respiratory viruses are immunosuppressive:

1. Epidemiologic investigation may reveal that infection with, or serologic conversion to, a particular virus is associated with a higher incidence of bacterial pneumonia.

2. Inoculation of experimental animals with a virus may facilitate lung colonization by a subsequent bacterial challenge.

3. Viral infection in the animal may result in defects in host defense mechanisms evaluated by *in vitro* procedures, or

4. Incubation of a virus with lymphocytes or phagocytes *in vitro* may alter cellular functions.

The results of these types of experimental approaches to the question of viral-induced immunosuppression do not always correlate with each other. Each has advantages and disadvantages, with individual investigators finding some types of evidence more convincing than other types.

Parainfluenza-3   Virus.   Previous   infection   with parainfluenza-3 (PI-3) virus has been shown to predispose the lung to fulminant infection after aerosol exposure to *P. multocida* (23,24) or *P. hemolytica* (25-27).   Lopez *et al.* (28) have reported that PI-3 infection impairs the pulmonary clearance of *P. hemolytica,* while other authors were not successful in demonstrating impairment of pulmonary clearance in PI-3-infected calves (29,30). Infection with PI-3 virus will destroy ciliary activity in bovine tracheal ring cultures *in vitro* (31).   The PI-3 virus is capable of replicating in bovine alveolar macrophages *in vitro* (32,33) and has been shown to inhibit phagosome-lysosome fusion in macrophages, an important event in macrophage microbicidal activity (34). *In vitro* infection with PI-3 virus has also been shown to inhibit alveolar macrophage cytotoxic activity (32).   The PI-3 virus may also be immunosuppressive through an effect on lymphocytes.   Pospisil *et al.* (35) have reported that experimental PI-3 virus infection in calves resulted in a depression of *in vitro* lymphocyte blastogenic responsiveness to PHA.   The effects of PI-3 virus infection on a humoral or cell-mediated immune response or on neutrophil function has apparently not been investigated.

Infectious   Bovine   Rhinotracheitis.   Infection   with   the   IBR virus (bovine herpesvirus 1) results in an extensive loss of cilia from the tracheal epithelium resulting in a reduction in the efficiency of the mucociliary defense mechanism (31,36).   Aerosol   exposure   to   IBR   virus   will reproducibly   facilitate   infection   of   the   lung   by   an otherwise   unsuccessful   challenge   with   *P.   hemolytica* resulting in fibrinous pneumonia similar to field cases of shipping   fever   pneumonia   (37-42).   In   a   series   of experiments, Forman *et al.* (43-45) attempted to determine if IBR   virus   infection   altered   alveolar   macrophage   function sufficiently to explain the increased susceptibility to *P. hemolytica* infection.   They and other investigators found that the IBR virus could replicate in alveolar macrophages (33,45). Infection of alveolar macrophages *in vitro* resulted in   decreased   Fc   receptor-mediated   activity,   decreased phagocytosis, an initial increase followed by a decrease in C3b   receptor   activity,   and   a   rapid   inhibition   of antibody-dependent   cell-mediated   cytotoxicity   by   alveolar macrophages (44).   When they attempted to reproduce these results *in vivo* by evaluating the activity of alveolar macrophages lavaged from infected animals, they found that only a small proportion of the alveolar macrophages became infected   and   their   function   was   not   measurably   altered

(43). They concluded that IBR virus infection *in vivo* does not directly alter alveolar macrophage function sufficiently to explain the increased susceptibility to challenge with *P. hemolytica.* They pointed out that their experimentation did not rule out the possibility of an indirect effect of the IBR virus on alveolar macrophage function.

There are apparently no reports on the effects of IBR virus infection on lymphocyte or neutrophil function in cattle.

Bovine Viral Diarrhea Virus. The BVD virus is capable of producing severe illness and death in susceptible cattle (mucosal disease), but this is a relatively rare event and is probably due to a preexisting problem with the animal's immune system. These severely affected animals usually have a persistent viremia and fail to produce antibody (46). Experimental infection of healthy cattle with BVD virus usually results in a transient febrile response and leukopenia with only mild clinical signs manifested as depression, decreased appetite and perhaps an increased respiratory rate (47). Serologic evidence indicates that it is common for cattle to have been infected with BVD virus without any observable symptoms of disease (47). The importance of the BVD virus in bovine respiratory disease lies in its effects on host defense mechanisms during a mild or inapparent infection resulting in increased susceptibility to bacterial pneumonia. Evidence for immunosuppression by the BVD virus comes from studies on animals fatally affected with mucosal disease and on animals mildly affected by BVD virus after experimental inoculation.   The evidence indicates that mucosal disease is associated with immunosuppression, (46,48,49) but it is difficult to determine if the immune defects were already present in the animal before infection and if the animal was predisposed to mucosal disease, or if they are due directly to the BVD virus. Dexamethasone administration has been shown to immunosuppress calves and convert an otherwise mild infection with BVD virus into the fatal viremic form of mucosal disease (50).   The altered immune function observed in animals severely affected by BVD virus may be nonspecific and secondary to severe illness (46).

There is clinical evidence that a mild infection with BVD virus is capable of impairing host defense mechanisms against bacterial infection and predisposes to bacterial pneumonia.   Some authors have reported an increased incidence of bacterial pneumonia in calves recently infected with or seroconverting to BVD virus (51-53). Experimental infection with virulent BVD virus has also been shown to result in a spontaneous bacteremia in up to 85 percent of animals (54). The bacteremia was presumably of endogenous origin and due to an inhibition of normal clearance mechanisms responsible for removing bacteria from the blood stream.

Just as with IBR and PI-3 virus, experimental infection with BVD virus under the appropriate conditions will facilitate the production of pneumonia by an otherwise nonpathogenic aerosol inoculation of *P. hemolytica* (55) (L.N.D. Potgieter, personal communication, 1983). During experimentation to evaluate the efficacy of using live *P. multocida* or *P. hemolytica* by aerosol exposure as a vaccine, it was observed that calves naturally infected with BVD virus developed pneumonia after the aerosol vaccination procedure. The vaccines produced no gross lung lesions in healthy calves (56). Infection with BVD virus *in vitro* (like IBR and PI-3) will destroy the ciliary activity of tracheal ring cultures (31).

In contrast to the evidence suggesting that BVD virus infection predisposes to bacterial pneumonia, Lopez *et al.* (57) could not demonstrate that infection with BVD virus (or *Mycoplasma bovis*) inhibited pulmonary clearance of *P. hemolytica*. The authors state, "This lack of effect of treatment (BVD or *M. bovis* infection) was largely due to great variation within and between animals of the same experimental groups." Variation of this magnitude renders the assay relatively insensitive for detecting differences between experimental groups. The results of this experiment should not be interpreted as proof that BVD virus and *M. bovis* have no effect on pulmonary clearance of *P. hemolytica* (i.e., there was a failure to reject the null hypothesis rather than an acceptance of the null hypothesis).

The BVD virus has been shown to have specific effects on cells of the immune system. In mucosal disease there is depletion of lymphocytes from lymphoid tissue and necrosis of Peyers patches (58). Even mild infections with BVD virus will result in lymphopenia (59). Some of the effects of BVD virus on lymphocytes may be due to the observation that it can infect and replicate *in vitro* in lymphocytes from immune and nonimmune animals (60).

Lymphocyte blastogenesis has been used by several authors as a measure of the effect of the BVD virus on lymphocyte function with conflicting results. Some authors have reported that experimental infection with BVD virus results in an inhibition of lymphocyte blastogenic responsiveness to mitogens (35,54). These experiments were performed on lymphocytes isolated from the peripheral blood and incubated in fetal bovine serum. Other authors did not find a suppression of lymphocyte blastogenesis in experimentally-infected cattle using isolated lymphocytes in fetal bovine serum (61) or a whole-blood lymphocyte culture technique (62). The reasons for the differing results are not apparent but probably lie in differences in cattle, experimental design or methods used.

Lymphocyte blastogenesis has also been reported to be depressed in animals fatally affected with BVD-MD. Johnson and Muscoplat (49) reported suppressed blastogenesis of lymphocytes to PHA when using either a whole-blood culture method or lymphocytes isolated from whole blood and cultured in the presence of fetal bovine serum. Steck *et al.* (46) reported that in mucosal disease the suppression of lymphocyte blastogenesis was due to a serum factor which was capable of suppressing blastogenesis of normal lymphocytes. Lymphocytes from BVD-MD-affected cattle responded normally to mitogens when washed free of autologous plasma and incubated in fetal bovine serum. They also proposed that the serum suppressive factor was not specific for BVD infection since they found that serum from two cattle severely ill with non-BVD-related problems would suppress blastogenesis by normal lymphocytes.

Even the *in vitro* infection of lymphocytes with BVD virus has produced conflicting results. *In vitro* treatment of lymphocytes with a commercially-prepared modified live vaccine strain of BVD virus has been reported to dramatically inhibit lymphocyte blastogenesis (63). Steck *et al.,* (46) citing unpublished results, stated that "lymphocytes infected by several strains of virulent BVD virus can still be stimulated by PHA and Con A."

Infection with BVD virus has been demonstrated to have some effects on humoral immunity. Two calves severely affected with BVD-MD had a decreased percentage of circulating lymphocytes with detectable surface immunoglobulin (B cells) (48). Other authors reported that experimentally-infected calves with relatively mild disease had no significant change in the percentage of surface immunoglobulin-staining lymphocytes (61). Calves that were fatally affected with BVD-MD failed to produce antibody against the virus and had decreased amounts of circulating IgG1, IgM and IgA (46). These fatally affected cattle produced an antibody response to ferritin (in incomplete Freund's adjuvant) which was comparable to that of normal controls. Brownlie *et al.* (61) reported that calves experimentally infected with BVD had an antibody response to killed *Brucella abortus* which was 50 percent lower than control calves at one week post-inoculation, but this difference was not statistically significant by their analysis (based on the inverse of the agglutination titer; an analysis based on the $\log_2$ of the inverse of the titer may have produced a different level of statistical significance).

The BVD virus may facilitate bacterial pneumonia through its effects on phagocytic cells. It has been reported to infect and replicate in monocytes isolated from peripheral blood (31,60) and in alveolar macrophages (33). Ketelsen et al. (64) have reported that incubation of bovine peripheral blood monocytes with bovine viral diarrhea virus (either Singer or NY-1 strain) caused a decrease in their random locomotion and migration toward a chemotactic lymphokine. In their protocol they incubated virus with ficoll-hypaque-purified mononuclear cells in a virus-to-cell ratio of one or two TCID 50 of virus per 80 mononuclear cells for 30 minutes then washed the cells and evaluated locomotion and chemotaxis in a three-hour assay. It is not clear if the inhibition of locomotion and chemotaxis was due to a direct effect of the virus on the macrophage or due to a soluble mediator produced through an interaction between the virus and the lymphocytes present.

Experimental infection with BVD virus also alters neutrophil function. Infection with either a cytopathic or non-cytopathic BVD virus resulted in a marked impairment of the activity of the myeloperoxidase-hydrogen peroxide-halide antibacterial system of the neutrophil as measured by the iodination reaction (59). Ingestion and oxidative metabolism were normal in these neutrophils. This defect in neutrophil function lasted for about three weeks after infection and was compounded by a neutropenia.

The use of MLV-BVD vaccine has been associated with post-vaccinal cases of BVD-MD (65,66) and with an increased incidence of BRD (67). This suggests that the modified live virus may have retained its immunosuppressive potential. When cattle were injected intranasally and intramuscularly with a vaccine strain of MLV-BVD virus (Singer strain), a suppression of lymphocyte and neutrophil function similar to that produced by field isolates was observed (i.e., a mild lymphopenia and neutropenia, a suppression of lymphocyte blastogenic responsiveness to mitogens, and a suppression of neutrophil iodination) (68). In addition, a suppression of neutrophil-mediated antibody-dependent cell-mediated cytotoxicity (ADCC) was observed. (This was not evaluated in cattle infected with virulent virus.) Neutrophil-mediated ADCC is purportedly important in resistance to herpesvirus infections in cattle (i.e., IBR virus) (69). The suppression of iodination by neutrophils was evident for three-four weeks after MLV-BVD virus administration.

When ACTH was administered to cattle given the MLV-BVD virus in an attempt to crudely mimic vaccination at times of stress, the suppression of neutrophil and lymphocyte function was even more pronounced than in those cattle which received the MLV-BVD virus alone (68). Two of the four animals so treated developed an increased body temperature and respiratory distress. These results indicate that the immunosuppressive effects of cortisol and the BVD virus can be additive.

A very interesting phenomenon associated with BVD virus is tolerance resulting from early *in utero* infection. *In utero* infection may result in fetal death or congenitally-infected neonatal calves which are generally unthrifty and usually do not survive for more than a few months. Coria *et al.* (70) have reported the occurrence of immune tolerance in an adult bull that was persistently infected with BVD virus. Virus was isolated from the peripheral blood of this animal at birth (pre-colostral) and periodiclly for at least 2.5 years. The bull remained in apparently good health during this period and did not produce an antibody response to the virus. The virus isolated from this bull was pathogenic for other cattle. If the apparent immunosuppressive effects of BVD infection discussed above were due to a direct effect of the virus on cell function, one would expect this bull to have impaired host defense mechanisms and to suffer from recurrent infections. The function of the host defense mechanisms in this animal was not reported, but the lack of clinical problems indicate that it was probably near normal. This case suggests that the immunosuppression observed in BVD infection is due to aspects of the host response to the virus rather than to a direct effect of replicating virus. Presumably antibody would not mediate the detrimental effect since animals fatally affected with mucosal disease usually do not produce antibody (46). This hypothesis of course would require further testing.

Respiratory Syncytial Virus. Infection with bovine respiratory syncytial virus (BRSV) has been suggested to predispose to secondary bacterial infection due to damage to ciliated respiratory epithelium (71) and to facilitate secondary infection by other viruses (72). Experimental inoculation with BRSV was found to produce a mild leukopenia (73) and BRSV was shown to be capable of replicating in a small proportion of bovine alveolar macrophages *in vitro* (33). There are apparently no published reports of investigations into the effects of BRSV on lymphocyte or phagocyte function in cattle.

Other Virus. Several other viruses have been associated with the bovine respiratory disease complex (including bovine adenovirus, DN599 herpesvirus [Movar], rhinoviruses, reoviruses and bovine parvovirus) (74,75). This author was not able to find any reports dealing with their immunosuppressive potential.

Mycoplasma Species. The mycoplasmas most frequently associated with bovine respiratory disease are *M. bovis, M. dispar,* and ureaplasmas (76). Uncomplicated infection with these agents usually results in subclinical pneumonia. The mycoplasmas are probably more important in BRD as predisposing factors to secondary bacterial infection than as primary pathogens (76). In one survey of calves which died from pneumonia and were necropsied at a diagnostic laboratory, over 90 percent of the calves from which *Mycoplasma* spp. were isolated also were infected with *Pasteurella* spp. (77). Houghton and Gourlay (78) reported a synergistic effect resulting in a much more severe pneumonia when gnotobiotic calves were infected with both *M. bovis* and *P. hemolytica.*

The mechanisms by which mycoplasmas predispose to secondary infection are not clear, but impairment of selected aspects of host defense by mycoplasmas has been reported. Bennett *et al.* (79) reported that calves tended to have a lower lymphocyte blastogenic response to PHA after infection with *M. bovis* than before infection, suggesting that *M. bovis* infection may result in impairment of lymphocyte function. *M. dispar* has been shown to inhibit ciliary activity in organ cultures of bovine fetal trachea (80). Geary *et al.* (81) reported that *M. bovis* has a toxin which is a complex polysaccharide that is capable of activating complement and increasing vascular permeability. The authors proposed a role for this toxin in *M. bovis*-induced mastitis, but its significance in the pathogenesis of *M. bovis*-induced respiratory disease is not certain.

Lopez *et al.* (57) have reported that *M. bovis* infection did not consistently impair pulmonary clearance of *P. hemolytica.* However, the authors point out that this lack of detection of impaired clearance may be due to the great variability of results between animals treated alike. (For a discussion see the section on BVD virus.)

Simberkoff and Elsbach (82) found that *Mycoplasma hominis* would attach to neutrophils but were not ingested or killed.   They also found that neutrophils coated with mycoplasma had a reduced ability to kill *E. coli*. If the mycoplasmas which infect cattle have similar inhibitory effects on phagocytic cell function, it may be important in allowing secondary infection to occur.

Impairment of Host Defense Mechanisms by Bacteria

The bacteria associated with bovine respiratory disease are frequently found colonizing the nasopharyngeal area of normal cattle, but are not found in the lower respiratory tract.   Apparently the bacterial clearance mechanisms in the lung are efficient enough to prevent colonization in this area when functioning properly. When stress or viral infection impair these clearance mechanisms sufficiently, bacterial colonization of the lungs can occur (83). Bacterial pneumonia in bovine respiratory disease is almost always due to one of only three species of bacteria *(P. hemolytica, P. multocida,* or *H. somnus)*. Apparently the host defense mechanisms of the lung are still functioning well enough, even in the presence of stress and viral infection, to prevent other bacteria from colonizing.   This implies that the BRD bacterial pathogens have special properties which enable them to overcome the moderately-impaired pulmonary defense mechanisms.   The three bacterial species involved have all been found to be capable of inhibiting bovine phagocytic cell activity.

P. hemolytica elaborates a cytotoxin which is toxic for bovine neutrophils (84-86), lymphocytes (86) and macrophages (86-89). The cytotoxin has been variously reported to be greater than 300,000 MW (85) or to be approximately 150,000 MW (88). It is not clear if this discrepancy is due to the existence of two different cytotoxins or to differences in experimental techniques.

The capsule of type A *P. multocida* has been demonstrated to inhibit the ingestion of the organism by bovine neutrophils (90). When the encapsulated bacteria were treated with hyaluronidase to remove the capsule, the decapsulated organisms were ingested normally. This led the authors to suggest that the inhibitory factor was hyaluronic acid (90). Ryu *et al.* (90a) extended this work by removing the capsule from the organism through heat extraction in 2.5 percent NaCl (56° C, 1 hour) and evaluating the effects of the extracted capsule on bovine neutrophil function *in vitro.* The capsular material was found to inhibit the ability of neutrophils to ingest *Staphylococcus aureus* and to iodinate protein through the myeloperoxidase-hydrogen peroxide-halide antibacterial system. It did not affect the oxidative metabolism of the neutrophils. The active material was retained by a 300,000 MW cutoff membrane both before and after treatment with hyaluronidase. Purified hyaluronic acid (human umbilical cord origin) did not affect bovine neutrophil function *in vitro*. It was concluded that the inhibitory substance in the capsule was probably not hyaluronic acid but it may be structurally associated with it. *H. somnus* was also found to have heat-extractable surface material that was capable of inhibiting *S. aureus* ingestion and iodination by bovine neutrophils without affecting neutrophil oxidative metabolism. However, unlike *P. multocida,* the *H. somnus* activity was due to two heat-stable substances with differing molecular weights and effects. The material that inhibited bacterial ingestion was greater than 300,000 MW while the material that suppressed iodination was less than 1,000 MW (R. Hubbard *et al.,* manuscript in preparation). The chemical nature and biologic activities of both the *P. multocida* and *H. somnus* neutrophil inhibitory factors are being further characterized.

Immunomodulation in Bovine Respiratory Disease

Levamisole. Levamisole is a widely-used anthelmintic for cattle which has received a lot of attention as a potential immunomodulator. Levamisole has been shown to have its greatest effect on cells of the immune system which are not functioning properly, with little or no effect on normal cells. The effects of levamisole on the immune system are apparently heavily dependent upon the dosage used, time of administration and condition of the animal (91). Most of the research on levamisole as an immunomodulator has been conducted in species other than cattle. This review will consider only that research which has been conducted in cattle relative to the bovine respiratory disease complex.

In *in vitro* experimentation with bovine cells, levamisole has been shown to increase the lymphocyte blastogenic response to mitogens and specific antigens, to increase immune interferon production by mononuclear cell cultures and to increase macrophage Fc receptor activity (92). *In vivo* experimentation in which levamisole was given to cattle vaccinated with attenuated IBR virus has produced inconsistent results. Irwin *et al.* (93) reported that levamisole (8 milligrams/kilogram, SC) given simultaneously with IBR vaccination (IM) had a moderate inhibitory effect on the subsequent antibody response. They found no effect on the percentage of circulating lymphocytes with detectable surface immunoglobulin. Babiuk and Misra (92) found that levamisole (6 milligrams/kilogram, SC) given at the same time as intranasal vaccination with attenuated IBR virus resulted in a moderate decrease in the antibody response to IBR virus, a decrease in the lymphocyte blastogenic response to IBR antigen and a decrease in direct lymphocyte cytotoxicity for IBR-infected target cells. In a later report, Babiuk and Misra (94) found that an identical dosage of levamisole given at the time of vaccination or seven days later produced an enhanced antibody response to IBR virus. In the earlier report they speculate that the decreased immune responsiveness to IBR virus in the levamisole-treated cattle was due to an effect of levamisole to rapidly increase the immune response to the virus resulting in a reduced amount of antigen available for continued stimulation of the immune response. The reason for the discrepancy between the reports which showed mild suppression of antibody response by levamisole (92,93) and the later report which showed enhancement (94) are not apparent.

Zipprin *et al.* (95) reported that levamisole administration (10 milligrams/kilogram, orally) did not affect neutrophil numbers in normal or shipping-stressed cattle. Saperstein *et al.* (96) evaluated the effects of levamisole on selected parameters in cattle experimentally infected with BVD virus. The cattle were subjected to transportation stress then inoculated with a cytopathic strain of BVD virus 24 hours later. The calves displayed mild clinical signs on day 7 post-inoculation. Beginning on day 7, one-half of the animals were given levamisole

(2.047 milligrams/kilogram, SC) daily for three days.   No difference in severity of infection, virus shedding, speed of recovery or antibody response was detected between levamisole-treated and untreated animals. The total number of lymphocytes in the peripheral blood of levamisole-treated cattle was higher than in the non-levamisole-treated cattle, but this difference also existed before infection.

In an attempt to determine if levamisole was capable of preventing or reversing some of the effects of glucocorticoids on the immune system, levamisole was administered at six different dosage levels to dexamethasone-treated cattle (Roth JA, Kaeberle ML:Failure of levamisole to enhance lymphocyte blastogenesis or neutrofil function in dexamethasone-treated cattle. Am J Vet Res, accepted for publication). Dexamethasone (0.4 milligram/kilogram, IM) and levamisole (0.5, 1.0, 2.0, 4.0 or 8.0 milligrams/kilogram orally) were administered daily for three days.   Another group of animals received the three-day treatment regimen with dexamethasone and a single 6.0 milligrams/kilogram dose of levamisole (the recommended anthelmintic dose) on the first day of dexamethasone administration.   Levamisole had no apparent consistent ability to normalize lymphocyte blastogenic responsiveness (to the mitogens PHA, Con A, or PWM or in a one-way mixed lymphocyte reaction) or to normalize neutrophil function (random migration, nitroblue tetrazolium reduction, iodination or antibody-dependent cell-mediated cytotoxicity) in dexamethasone-treated cattle.

Perhaps the most convincing type of experiments for determining if levamisole may be effective in reducing the losses due to shipping fever are those experiments in which large numbers of cattle arriving at a feedlot are treated with levamisole and the morbidity and mortality in these animals are compared to that in closely matched, co-mingled control animals. In one such experiment involving 1,464 feedlot cattle, a single treatment with levamisole phosphate (8 milligrams/kilogram SC) was associated with a significantly-reduced incidence of shipping fever as compared to the morbidity observed in cattle treated with either thiabendazole (66 milligrams/kilogram orally) or levamisole hydrochloride (8 milligrams/kilogram orally) (97). This beneficial effect was observed only in those animals that became ill between approximately day 8 through 30 after levamisole administration. The two forms of levamisole were administered by different routes; it is not known why one form of levamisole appeared to have an effect while the other did not. Unfortunately, the management practices in the commercial feedlot involved did not allow the observance of disease incidence in a control group which did not receive anthelmintic.

The efficacy of levamisole phosphate in reducing morbidity due to shipping fever was also evaluated in another experiment involving a total of 2,241 cattle in six trials located in different states (98). In each trial 300 to 470 animals were processed and randomly allotted to control or treated groups. The treated group received a single 6 milligrams/kilogram injection (SC) of levamisole phosphate. There was no statistically significant difference in incidence of respiratory disease or in mortality between the two groups. The levamisole-treated group did have an improvement in average daily gain and in feed efficiency, probably due to the removal of worms.

In summary, levamisole has on occasion produced results which could be interpreted to be beneficial to animals affected with or susceptible to shipping fever. More often, negative results have been found. The cumulative results to date are insufficient to recommend the use of levamisole as an effective immunomodulator in bovine respiratory disease.

Thiabendazole. Thiabendazole, like levamisole, is a commonly-used anthelmintic in cattle which has been reported to have immunomodulating properties. At relatively low dosages (2 milligrams/kilogram and 20 milligrams/kilogram) thiabendazole has been observed to enhance immune responsiveness in mice (99,100), while at high dosages (200 milligrams/kilogram, 1,000 milligrams/kilogram, and 2,000 milligrams/kilogram) it has been reported to be immunosuppressive (101). Also like levamisole, the immunomodulating activity of thiabendazole was observed to be the most pronounced in immunosuppressed animals (99).

Thiabendazole was evaluated for its ability to prevent or reverse some of the effects of glucocorticoids on the bovine immune system using a protocol similar to that described above for levamisole (Kaeberle and Roth, submitted for publication). Dexamethasone (0.04 milligram/kilogram, IM) and thiabendazole (0, 1, 3, 6, 12, 25, 50, or 100 milligrams/kilogram, orally) were administered concurrently each day for three consecutive days. Thiabendazole administration in the dosage range from 1.0 to 25.0 milligrams/kilogram was associated with a significant enhancement of lymphocyte blastogenic responsiveness to PHA, Con A, PWM and allogeneic cells in dexamethasone-treated cattle. This immunonormalizing effect was not observed at the 50 or 100 milligrams/kilogram dosage levels or when the thiabendazole treatment was initiated 24 hours prior to dexamethasone administration. Thiabendazole did not produce a consistent significant normalization of any parameter of neutrophil function in dexamethasone-treated cattle (random migration, nitroblue tetrazolium reduction, iodination or antibody-dependent cell-mediated cytotoxicity).

Since thiabendazole had some activity in normalizing lymphocyte blastogenesis in dexamethasone-treated animals, an experiment was undertaken to determine its effect on antibody responses in stressed cattle (Roth et al., submitted for publication). Fifty-one calves were divided into a control group and a thiabendazole-treated group. Animals in both groups were stressed by weaning, castration, placement in a feedlot and injection of antigens (equine ferritin, tetanus toxoid and killed Brucella abortus strain 19) on the day that thiabendazole therapy was started. Thiabendazole administered orally for five consecutive days at a dosage of 20 milligrams/kilogram did not enhance the antibody response to any of the antigens. Thiabendazole treatment did significantly inhibit the antibody response to B. abortus. The reasons for the discrepancy in the effect of thiabendazole on lymphocyte blastogenesis in dexamethasone-treated cattle and the effect on antibody responses in stressed calves are not known. Since Hewlett et al. (101) demonstrated that high dosages of thiabendazole in mice are immunosuppressive, it may be that the five-day treatment period was too long to achieve an immunoenhancing effect.

The sum of the evidence concerning levamisole and thiabendazole is that the dosage, frequency and timing of administration relative to the immunosuppressive event are critical to obtaining immunorestoration. These factors will probably prevent either of these compounds from ever being an effective immunomodulator on a practical basis in bovine respiratory disease. They do serve as useful prototypes in the search for practical immunomodulating compounds.

Another compound which has received some attention as an immunomodulator in cattle is the lipoidal amine CP 20,961 (N,N-dioctadecyl-N'N'-bis[2-hydroxyethyl]   propanediamine) (102).   It has been evaluated in cattle and found to enhance the bactericidal activity of peripheral blood neutrophils after intramuscular administration to yearling cattle.   Further work is needed to determine if this compound will prove to be a clinically-useful immunomodulator.

Summary

In summary, there is ample evidence that impairment of host defense mechanisms by stressors, viruses and/or mycoplasmas are prerequisite for the establishment of bacterial pneumonia in the bovine lung (with a reasonable bacterial challenge). Even when the immune system is impaired by these factors, there is still sufficient pulmonary defense to prevent infection by the majority of bacteria in the bovine environment. The bacteria which can successfully colonize the lung in immunosuppressed cattle are species which have specialized virulence factors that inhibit phagocytic cells. These virulence factors by themselves will not allow the bacteria to colonize the lower respiratory tract unless the pulmonary defense mechanisms have already been impaired. These observations suggest that pulmonary defense mechanisms in normal cattle are quite efficient and a "multiple hit" on these defense mechanisms is necessary for the development of respiratory disease. If man could intervene and reduce the number of "hits" on the defense mechanisms, the incidence of bovine respiratory disease should be decreased. Possible approaches are:

1. reduce the amount of stress on the animals,

2. use immunomodulators to reduce the effects of stress on the immune system,

3. vaccinate to prevent infection by viruses and mycoplasmas,

4. use immunomodulators to reduce the immunosuppressive effects of viruses and mycoplasmas,

5. block the activity of the bacterial virulence factors through pharmacologic or immunologic means, or

6. enhance immunity against the bacterial agents through effective vaccines.

A special problem with vaccination is that there are several viruses and mycoplasma species which are widespread and capable of predisposing to bacterial pneumonia. It may be necessary to induce immunity to a majority of these before a reduction in the incidence of respiratory disease is seen. Similarly with the bacterial agents, an immunosuppressed animal which is immune to two of the common bacterial agents is still susceptible to the third. It will be difficult to induce effective immunity against all three common agents in one animal.

The use of immunomodulators to prevent or reverse the immunosuppression also promises to be complex. Stress and the various viruses, mycoplasma and bacteria probably use a variety of mechanisms to induce immunosuppression. It is unlikely that a single immunomodulator will be effective against this host of immunosuppressive factors. Experimentation on compounds which have been shown to have some immunomodulatory activity indicates that the dosage and time of administration relative to the initiation of immunosuppression are critical for determining the effectiveness of the immunomodulator. Until this problem is overcome, it will limit the clinical usefulness of immunomodulators.

There is currently a great deal of research aimed at producing and characterizing new immunomodulating compounds for eventual use in man. In order to take full advantage of this research and apply it to the bovine respiratory disease problem, the nature of the immunosuppression which occurs in BRD due to stress or infectious disease must be thoroughly characterized. This knowledge would provide a basis for predicting the properties that would be desirable in an immunomodulator for use in stressed or virus-infected cattle.

References

1.   Hoerlein AB, Marsh GL:Studies on the epizootiology of shipping fever in calves.   J Am Vet Med Assoc 131:123-127, 1957.

2.   Kelley KW:Stress and immune function: a bibliographic review. Ann Res Vet 11:445-478, 1980.

3.   Roe CP:A review of the environmental factors influencing calf respiratory disease.   Agricultural Meteorology 26:127-144, 1982.

4.   Roth JA, Kaeberle ML:Effect of glucocorticoids of the bovine immune system.   J Am Vet Med Assoc 180:894-901, 1982.

5.   Roth JA:Cortisol as a mediator of stress-associated immunosuppression in cattle, in Moberg G (ed):   Animal Stress.   Bethesda, Maryland, American Physiological Society, in press, 1984.

6.   Johnston JD, Buckland RB:Response of male Holstein calves from seven sires to four management stresses as measured by plasma corticoid levels. Can J Anim Sci 56:727-732, 1976.

7.   Crookshank HR, Elissalde MH, White RG, *et al.*:Effect of transportation and handling of calves upon blood serum composition.   J Anim Sci 48:430-435, 1979.

8. Gwazdauskas FC, Gross WB, Bib TL, *et al.*:Antibody titers and plasma glucocorticoid concentrations near weaning in steer and heifer calves. Can Vet J 19:150-154, 1978.

9. Arave CW, Walters JL, Lamb RC:Effect of exercise on glucocorticoids and other cellular components of blood. J Dairy Sci 61:1567-1572, 1978.

10. Stephens DB:Stress and its measurement in domestic animals. A review of behavioral and physiological studies under field and laboratory situations. Adv Vet Sci Comp Med 24:179-210, 1980.

11. Simensen E, Laksesvela B, Blom AK, *et al.*:Effects of transportation, a high lactose diet, and ACTH injections on the white blood cell count, serum cortisol, and immunoglobulin G in young calves. Acta Vet Scand 21:278-290, 1980.

12. Shaw, KE, Nichols RE:Plasma 17-hydroxycorticosteroids in calves: the effects of shipping. Am J Vet Res 25:252-253, 1964.

13. May I, Manoiu I, Donta C, *et al.*:Stress und immunitat beim rind. Arch Exp Veterinaemed, Leipzig 33:87-98, 1979.

14. Roth JA, Kaeberle ML, Hsu WH:Effects of ACTH administration on bovine polymorphonuclear leukocyte

function and lymphocyte blastogenesis. Am J Vet Res 43:412-416, 1982.

15. Carlson GP, Kaneko JJ:Influence of prednisolone on intravascular granulocyte kinetics of calves under nonsteady state conditions. Am J Vet Res 37:149-151, 1976.

16. Roth JA, Kaeberle ML:Effects of *in vivo* dexamethasone administration on *in vitro* bovine polymorphonuclear leukocyte function. Infect Immun 33:434-441, 1981.

17. Fauci AS:Immunosuppressive and anti-inflammatory effects of glucocorticoids, in Baxter JD, Rousseau GG (eds): Glucocorticoid Hormone Action. Berlin, Springer Verlag, 1979, pp. 449-465.

18. Parrillo JE, Fauci AS:Mechanisms of glucocorticoid action on immune processes. Ann Rev Pharmacol Toxicol 19:179-201, 1979.

19. Cummins JM, Rosenquist BD:Effect of hydrocortisone on the interferon response of calves infected with infectious bovine rhinotracheitis virus. Am J Vet Res 38:1163-1166, 1977.

20. Cummins JM, Rosenquist BD:Leukocyte changes and interferon production in calves injected with hydrocortisone and infected with infectious bovine rhinotracheitis virus. Am J Vet Res 40:238-240, 1979.

21.   Davies DH, Carmichael LE:Role of cell-mediated immunity in the recovery of cattle from primary and recurrent infections with infectious bovine rhinotracheitis virus. Infect Immun 8:510-518, 1973.

22. Pastoret PO, Babiuk LA, Misra V, *et al.*:Reactivation of temperature-sensitive and non-temperature sensitive infectious bovine rhinotracheitis vaccine virus with dexamethasone. Infect Immun 29:483-488, 1980.

23.   Heddleston KL, Reisinger RC, Watko LP:Studies on the transmission and etiology of bovine shipping fever. Am J Vet Res 23:548-553, 1962.

24.   Hetrick FM, Chang SC, Byrne RJ, *et al.*:The combined effect of *Pasteurella multocida* and myxovirus parainfluenza-3 upon calves. Am J Vet Res 24:939-946, 1963.

25.   Baldwin DE, Marshall RG, Wessman GE:Experimental infection of calves with myxovirus parainfluenza-3 and *Pasteurella haemolytica*. Am J Vet Res 28:1773-1782, 1967.

26.   Trapp AL, Hamdy AH, Gale C, *et al.*:Lesions in calves exposed to agents associated with the shipping fever complex. Am J Vet Res 27:1235-1242, 1966.

27.   Jericho KWF, Darcel CQ, Langford EV:Respiratory disease in calves produced with aerosols of parainfluenza-3 virus and *Pasteurella haemolytica*. Can J Comp Med 46:293-301, 1982.

28. Lopez A, Thomson RG, Savan M:The pulmonary clearance of *Pasteurella hemolytica* in calves infected with bovine parainfluenza-3 virus. Can J Comp Med 40:385-391, 1976.

29. Al-Izzi SA, Maxie MG, Savan M:The pulmonary clearance of *Pasteurella haemolytica* in calves given *Corynebacterium parvum* and infected with parainfluenza-3 virus. Can J Comp Med 46:85-90, 1982.

30. Gilka F, Thomson RG, Savan M:The effect of edema, hydrocortisone acetate, concurrent viral infection and immunization on the clearance of *Pasteurella hemolytica* from the bovine lung. Can J Comp Med 38:251-259, 1974.

31. Rossi CR, Kiesel GK:Susceptibility of bovine macrophage and tracheal-ring cultures to bovine viruses. Am J Vet Res 38:1705-1708, 1977.

32. Probert M, Stott EJ, Thomas CH:Interactions between calf alveolar macrophages and parainfluenza-3 virus. Infect Immun 15:576-585, 1977.

33. Toth TH, Hesse RA:Replication of five bovine respiratory viruses in cultured bovine alveolar macrophages. Arch Virol 75:219-224, 1983.

34. Hesse RA, Toth TE:Effects of bovine parainfluenza-3 virus on phagocytosis and phagosome-lysosome fusion of cultured bovine alveolar macrophages. Am J Vet Res 44:1901-1907, 1983.

35.   Pospisil Z, Machatkova M, Mensik J, *et al.*:Decline in the phytohaemagglutinin responsiveness of lymphocytes from calves infected experimentally with bovine viral diarrhoea-mucosal disease virus and parainfluenza-3 virus. Acta Vet Brno 44:369-375, 1975.

36.   Allen EM, Msolla PM:Scanning electron microscopy of the tracheal epithelium of calves inoculated with bovine herpesvirus I.   Res Vet Sci 29:325-327, 1980.

37.   Jericho KWF, Langford EV:Pneumonia in calves produced with aerosols of bovine herpesvirus I and *Pasteurella haemolytica.* Can J Comp Med 42:269-277, 1978.

38. Jericho KWF:Histological changes in the respiratory tract of calves exposed to aerosols of bovine herpesvirus I and *Pasteurella haemolytica.* J Comp Path 93:73-82, 1983.

39.   Yates WDG:A review of infectious bovine rhinotracheitis, shipping fever pneumonia and viral-bacterial synergism in respiratory disease of cattle. Can J Comp Med 46:225-263, 1982.

40.   Yates WDG, Jericho KWF, Doige CE:Effect of viral dose on experimental pneumonia caused by aerosol exposure of calves to bovine herpesvirus 1 and *Pasteurella haemolytica.* Can J Comp Med 47:57-63, 1983.

41.   Yates WDG, Babiuk LA, Jericho KWF:Viral-bacterial pneumonia in calves: duration of the interaction between

bovine herpesvirus 1 and *Pasteurella haemolytica.* Can J Comp Med 47:257-264, 1983.

42.   Yates WDG,   Jericho   KWF,   Doige   CE:Effect   of bacterial dose on pneumonia induced by aerosol exposure of calves to bovine herpesvirus-1 and *Pasteurella haemolytica.* Am J Vet Res 44:238-243, 1983.

43.   Forman AJ, Babiuk LA, Baldwin F, *et al.*:Effect of infectious bovine rhinotracheitis virus infection of calves on cell populations recovered by lung lavage. Am J Vet Res 43:1174-1179, 1982.

44.   Forman AJ, Babiuk LA:Effect of infectious bovine rhinotracheitis virus infection on bovine alveolar macrophage function.   Infect Immun 35:1041-1047, 1982.

45.   Forman AJ, Babiuk LA, Misra V, *et al.*:Susceptibility of bovine macrophages to infectious bovine rhinotracheitis virus infection.   Infect Immun 35:1048-1057, 1982.

46.   Steck   F,   Lazary   S,   Fey   H,   *et   al.*:Immune responsiveness in cattle fatally affected by bovine virus diarrhea-mucosal disease. Zbl Vet Med B 27:429-445, 1980.

47.   Malmquist WA:Bovine viral diarrhea-mucosal disease: etiology, pathogenesis and applied immunity. J Am Vet Med Assoc 152:763-770, 1968.

48.   Muscoplat CC,   Johnson   DW,Teuscher   E:Surface immunoglobulin of circulating lymphocytes in chronic bovine

diarrhea: abnormalities in cell populations and cell
function. Am J Vet Res 34:1101-1104, 1973.

49.   Johnson DW, Muscoplat CC:Immunologic abnormalities
in calves with chronic bovine viral diarrhea. Am J Vet Res
34:1139-1141, 1973.

50.   Shope RE, Muscoplat CC, Chen AW, et al.:Mechanism of
protection from primary bovine viral diarrhea virus
infection I.   The effects of dexamethasone. Can J Comp Med
40:355-359, 1976.

51.   Reggiardo C:Role of BVD virus in shipping fever of
feedlot   cattle.   Case   studies   and   diagnostic
considerations.   Proc Amer Assn Vet Lab Diag 22:315-320,
1979.

52.   Stott EJ, Thomas LH, Collins AP, et al.:A survey of
virus infections of the respiratory tract of cattle and
their association with disease. J Hyg, Camb 85:257-270,
1980.

53.   Hamoud M, Imrey PB, Woods GT, et al.:An
epidemiologic study of acute respiratory disease in beef
calves after weaning.   Bovine Practice 2:7-11, 1981.

54.   Reggiardo C, Kaeberle ML:Detection of bacteremia in
cattle inoculated with bovine viral diarrhea virus. Am J
Vet Res 42:218-221, 1981.

55.   Corstvet RE, Panciera RJ:Effect of infectious bovine rhinotracheitis virus and bovine virus diarrhea virus on *Pasteurella haemolytica* infection in the bovine lung. Proc Amer Assoc Vet Lab Diag 25:363-368, 1982.

56.   Corstvet RE, Panciera RJ, Newman P:Vaccination of calves with *Pasteurella multocida* and *Pasteurella haemolytica*. Proc Amer Assn Vet Lab Diag 21:67-90, 1978.

57.   Lopez A, Maxie MG, Savan M, *et al.*:The pulmonary clearance of *Pasteurella haemolytica* in calves infected with bovine virus diarrhea or *Mycoplasma bovis*. Can J Comp Med 46:302-306, 1982.

58.   Tyler DE, Ramsey FK:Comparative pathologic, immunologic, and clinical responses produced by selected agents of the bovine mucosal disease-virus diarrhea complex. Am J Vet Res 26:903-913, 1965.

59.   Roth JA, Kaeberle ML, Griffith RW:Effects of bovine viral diarrhea virus infection on bovine polymorphonuclear leukocyte function. Am J Vet Res 42:244-250, 1981.

60.   Truitt RL, Shechmeister IL:The replication of bovine viral diarrhea-mucosal disease virus in bovine leukocytes *in vitro*. Archiv fur die gesamte Virusforschung 42:78-87, 1973.

61.   Brownlie J, Nuttall PA, Stott EJ, *et al.*:Experimental infection of calves with 2 strains of

bovine virus diarrhoea virus: certain immunological reactions. Vet Immunol Immunopathol 1:371-378, 1980.

62. Snider TG, McConnell S, Adams LG, et al.:In vitro and in vivo immune responses in neonatally thymectomized Holstein-Friesian calves exposed to bovine viral diarrhea virus. Comp Immunol Microbiol Infect Dis 4:9-19, 1981.

63. Muscoplat CC, Johnson DW, Stevens JB:Abnormalities of in vitro lymphocyte responses during bovine viral diarrhea virus infection. Am J Vet Res 34:753-755, 1973.

64. Ketelsen AT, Johnson DW, Muscoplat CC:Depression of bovine monocyte chemotactic responses by bovine viral diarrhea virus. Infect Immun 25:565-568, 1979.

65. Peter CP, Tyler DE, Ramsey FK:Characteristics of a condition following vaccination with bovine virus diarrhea vaccine. J Am Vet Med Assoc 150:46-52, 1967.

66. Lambert G:Bovine viral diarrhea: prophylaxis and postvaccinal reactions. J Am Vet Med Assoc 163:874-876, 1973.

67. Martin SW, Meek AH, Davis DG, et al.:Factors associated with mortality in feedlot cattle: the Bruce County beef cattle project. Can J Comp Med 44:1-10, 1980.

68. Roth JA, Kaeberle ML:Suppression of neutrophil and lymphocyte function induced by a vaccinal strain of bovine viral diarrhea virus with and without the administration of ACTH. Am J Vet Res 44:1366-2372, 1983.

69.   Rouse BT, Wardley RG, Babiuk CA:Antibody-dependent cell-mediated cytotoxicity in cows. Comparison of effector cell activity against heterologous erythrocyte and herpesvirus-infected bovine target cells. Infect Immun 13:1433-1441, 1976.

70.   Coria MF, McClurkin AW:Specific immune tolerance in an apparently healthy bull persistently infected with bovine viral diarrhea virus. J Am Vet Med Assoc 172:449-451, 1978.

71.   Bohlender RE, McCune MW, Frey ML:Bovine respiratory syncytial virus infection. Mod Vet Practice 3:613-618, 1982.

72.   Lehmkuhl LD, Gough PM:Investigation of causative agents of bovine respiratory tract disease in a beef cow-calf herd with an early weaning program. Am J Vet Res 38:1717-1720, 1977.

73.   Elazhary MASY, Galina M, Roy RS, et al.:Experimental infection of calves with bovine respiratory syncytial virus (Quebec strain). Can J Comp Med 44:390-395, 1980.

74.   Potgieter LND:Current concepts on the role of viruses in respiratory tract disease of cattle. Bovine Practitioner 12:75-81, 1977.

75.   Weiblen R, Mock RE, Woods GT, et al.:Possible involvement of bovine parvovirus in the respiratory disease

complex.   Proc Third Intl Symp World Assoc Vet Lab Diag,
361-367, 1983.

76.   Stalheim OHV:Mycoplasmal respiratory diseases of
ruminants: a review and update.   J Am Vet Med Assoc
182:403-406, 1983.

77.   Knutsen W, Anson MA, Reed DE:A microbiologic survey
of calf pneumonia. Abstract presented at the North American
Symposium on Bovine Respiratory Disease, Amarillo, Texas,
September 7-9, 1983.

78.   Houghton   SB,   Gourlay   RN:Synergism   between
Mycoplasma bovis and *Pasteurella haemolytica* in calf pneumonia.
Vet Record 113:41-42, 1983.

79.   Bennett RH, Jasper DE:Immunosuppression of humoral
and cell-mediated responses in calves associated with
inoculation of *Mycoplasma bovis.* Am J Vet Res 38:1731-1738,
1977.

80.   Howard CJ, Thomas LH:Inhibition by *Mycoplasma
dispar* of ciliary activity in tracheal organ cultures.
Infect Immun 10:405-408, 1974.

81.   Geary SJ, Tourtellote ME, Cameron JA:Inflammatory
toxin from *Mycoplasma bovis:* isolation and characterization.
Science 212:1032-1033, 1981.

82.   Simberkoff MS, Elsbach P:The interaction *in vitro*
between polymorphonuclear leukocytes and mycoplasma. J Exp
Med 134:1417-1430, 1971.

83.   Frank GH, Smith PC:Prevalence of *Pasteurella haemolytica* in transported calves. Am J Vet Res 44:981-985, 1983.

84. Markham RJF, Ramnaraine MLR, Muscoplat CC:Cytotoxic effect of *Pasteurella haemolytica* on bovine polymorphonuclear leukocytes and impaired production of chemotactic factors by *Pasteurella haemolytica*-infected alveolar macrophages. Am J Vet Res 43:285-288, 1982.

85.   Baluyut CS, Simonson RR, Bemrick WJ, *et al.*:Interaction of *Pasteurella haemolytica* with bovine neutrophils: identification and partial characterization of a cytotoxin. Am J Vet Res 42:1920-1925, 1981.

86.   Shewen PE,Wilkie BN:Cytotoxin of *Pasteurella haemolytica* acting on bovine leukocytes. Infect Immun 35:91-94, 1982.

87.   Maheswaran SK, Berggren KA, Simonson RR, *et al.*:Kinetics of interaction and fate of *Pasteurella hemolytica* in bovine alveolar macrophages. Infect Immun 30:254-262, 1980.

88.   Himmel ME, Yates MD, Lauermann LH, *et al.*:Purification and partial characterization of a macrophage cytotoxin from *Pasteurella haemolytica*. Am J Vet Res 43:764-767, 1982.

89.   Shewen PE, Wilkie BN:*Pasteurella haemolytica*
cytotoxin: production by recognized serotypes and
neutralization by type-specific rabbit antisera. Am J Vet
Res 44:715-719, 1983.

90.   Maheswaran SK, Thies ES:Influence of encapsulation
on   phagocytosis   of   *Pasteurella   multocida*   by   bovine
neutrophils. Infect Immun 26:76-81, 1979.

90a.   Ryo H, Kaeberle ML, Roth JA, *et al*.:Effect of type
A *Pasteurella multocida* fractions on bovine polymorphonuclear
leukocyte functions. Infect Immun 43:(January), 1984.

91.   Brunner CJ, Muscoplat CC:Immunomodulatory effects
of levamisole. J Am Vet Med Assoc 176:1159-1162, 1980.

92.   Babiuk LA, Misra V:Levamisole and bovine immunity:
in vitro and *in vivo* effects on immune responses to
herpesvirus immunization. Can J Microbiol 27:1312-1319,
1981.

93.   Irwin MR, Holmberg CA, Knight HD, *et al*.:Effects of
vaccination against infectious bovine rhinotracheitis and
simultaneous   administration   of   levamisole   on   primary
humoral responses in calves. Am J Vet Res 37:223-226, 1976.

94.   Babiuk LA, Misra V:Effect of levamisole in immune
responses   to   bovine   herpesviurus-1.   Am   J   Vet   Res
43:1349-1354, 1982.

95.   Ziprin RL, Steel EG, Petersen HD, *et al.*:Hematologic study of effects of levamisole on stressed cattle. Am J Vet Res 41:1884-1885, 1980.

96.   Saperstein G,Mohanty SB, Rockemann DD, *et al.*:Effect of levamisole on induced bovine viral diarrhea. J Am Vet Med Assoc 183:425-427, 1983.

97.   Irwin MR, Melendy DR, Hutcheson DP:Reduced morbidity associated with shipping fever pneumonia in levamisole phosphate-treated feedlot cattle. Southwestern Vet 33:45-49, 1980.

98.   Anon.   Tramisol - immunoresponse cattle trials. Product fact sheet no. 11, Cyanimid Technical Service Department, Wayne, New Jersey.

99.   Lundy J, Lovett EJ:Immunomodulation with thiabendazole: a review of immunologic properties and efficacy in combined modality cancer therapy. Cancer Treat Reports 62:1955-1966, 1978.

100.   Lovett EJ, Lundy J:The effect of thiabendazole in a mixed leukocyte culture.   Transplantation 24:93-98, 1977.

101.   Hewlett EL, Hamid OY, Ruffier J, *et al.:In vivo* suppression of delayed hypersensitivity by thiabendazole and diethylcarbamazine.   Immunopharm 3:324-332, 1981.

102.   Woodard LF, Jasman RL, Farrington DO, *et al.*:Enhanced antibody-dependent bactericidal activity of

neutrophils   from   calves   treated   with   a   lipid   amine
immunopotentiator.   Am J Vet Res 44:389-394, 1983.

Physiology of the Bovine Lung

N. E. Robinson, B.Vet.Med., M.R.C.V.S., Ph.D.

Departments of Physiology and Large Animal Clinical Sciences
College of Veterinary Medicine
Michigan State University
East Lansing, Michigan 48824

R. F. Slocombe, B.V.Sc., M.S., Ph.D.

Department of Pathology
College of Veterinary Medicine
Michigan State University
East Lansing, Michigan 48824

F. J. Derksen, D.V.M., Ph.D.

Department of Large Animal Clinical Sciences
College of Veterinary Medicine
Michigan State University
East Lansing, Michigan 48824

Introduction

Although respiratory diseases of cattle are of great economic importance and there have been numerous studies of lung pathology and of the infectious agents causing lung disease, the physiology of the bovine lung has been neglected. This is strange since all infectious agents produce their clinical signs by altering lung function. An understanding of the mechanisms whereby infectious agents affect lung function may lead to new methods for prevention and treatment of lung disease and a better understanding of how lung disease affects the economic viability of an animal.

A complete review of all aspects of lung physiology is beyond the scope of this paper. We will instead focus upon the unique aspects of bovine lung physiology and those which we believe make cattle susceptible to respiratory problems. We will also review available data on changes in lung function in two types of bovine respiratory disease to demonstrate that functional measurements can indicate the pathogenesis of respiratory disease.

Observations

Anatomy of the Bovine Lung

For its size, the cow has a small lung, yet its resting oxygen consumption is similar to mammals of equal size (1). Alveoli of cattle have few communications with their neighbors because there is paucity of interalveolar pores of Kohn (2) and because interlobular septa completely subdivide the lung into irregularly polyhedral secondary lobules (3). These secondary lobules which contain 30-50 primary lobules are clearly visible on the surface of the lung.

The bronchial anatomy and lobation of cattle lungs is different from many other species. Like other species, cattle have four lobes (cranial, middle, caudal and accessory) on the right side, and two lobes (cranial and caudal) on the left side. However, the bronchus of the right cranial lobe arises directly from the trachea anterior to the carina at approximately the most dependent part of the trachea. Because of the location of the bronchial opening of the right cranial lobe, there may be drainage of secretions into the bronchus tending to make the right cranial lobe susceptible to infections.

The pulmonary arteries of cattle are well-supplied with smooth muscle (4). All mammals have muscular pulmonary arteries at birth but in most species the amount of muscle decreases as the animal matures. The relatively thick muscular layer of cattle pulmonary arteries is thought to contribute to vascular hyperreactivity to many stimuli that cause little response in vessels of other species. The vigorous response to hypoxia, for example, leads to pulmonary hypertension and right heart failure in cattle pastured at altitude (5) and hypoxia may also be the cause of the very high pulmonary arterial pressures we have observed in calves with chronic lung diseases.

Review of Normal Lung Function

The lung's major function, gas exchange, is accomplished by bringing together air and blood in the peripheral gas-exchange portion of the lung. The overall aim is to produce an alveolar oxygen tension of 90-100 torr sufficient to saturate hemoglobin passing through pulmonary capillaries. Delivery of air depends on the respiratory muscles generating sufficient force to overcome both the elastic recoil of the lung and the frictional resistance of the airways. The elastic properties of the lungs are reflected in measurements of lung compliance while the resistive properties of airways are indicated by measurements of pulmonary resistance. Lung diseases generally decrease compliance and/or increase resistance, both of which increase the work of breathing and require additional energy use by respiratory muscles.

Delivery of blood to the lung is determined by the work of the heart and the flow resistance of pulmonary vessels. Because the total cardiac output passes through the lungs, constriction of pulmonary vessels by hypoxia for example increases the work of the right heart and elevates pulmonary arterial pressure.

Ideally air and blood reach the gas-exchange region in a ratio of 0.8 which is optimal for maintenance of a normal alveolar oxygen tension. Even in healthy cattle lungs there is probably some mismatching of ventilation and blood flow (6), but in disease, mismatching is accentuated and gas exchange is severely impaired (7). Hypoxemia occurs particularly when regions of the lung receive blood flow but too little ventilation as a result of atelectasis, consolidation or airway obstruction.

Ventilation

The maximal oxygen consumption which can be achieved by cattle during exercise is less than one-third of that which can be achieved by a horse of similar size.   The cow reaches maximal oxygen consumption at a speed of 4 m/sec whereas a horse must go 10 m/sec (8).   This limited maximal oxygen consumption which is reflected in the relatively small alveolar surface area available for diffusion (9) means that cattle must utilize anaerobic metabolism with its resultant metabolic acidosis when herded or when severely stressed. Metabolic acidosis has been reported to suppress bacterial clearance from the lung (10).

Of the total ventilation entering the lung, only part participates in gas exchange (alveolar ventilation). The remainder ventilates dead space, i.e., the trachea and bronchi or poorly perfused regions of lung. Species vary in the combinations of tidal volume and frequency selected to maintain adequate alveolar ventilation.   In calves, 42 percent of the minute ventilation is dead-space ventilation (7,11).   Dead-space ventilation increases with age and by ten and one-half months accounts for 68.5 percent of minute ventilation (12).   Heat stress increases minute ventilation but 79 percent is dead-space ventilation because cattle begin to pant (12).   Cold stress increases metabolic rate with a resulting increase in oxygen requirements. This is met by an increase in alveolar ventilation accomplished by increasing tidal volume and decreasing both respiratory rate and dead-space ventilation (7). These changes in the pattern of ventilation with both heat and cold stress may facilitate the delivery of infections into the respiratory system.

Mechanics of Ventilation

There have been very few studies of the mechanical properties of cattle lungs. Slocombe and co-workers (11) described the static and dynamic properties of neonatal calf lungs. The calf is like other neonates in that it has a compliant thorax and a lung with a relatively low compliance. The low lung compliance is probably due to closure of peripheral airways at relatively high lung volumes. If airways close during tidal breathing, ventilation perfusion mismatching occurs and hypoxemia can result. Another potential consequence of airway closure is atelectasis distal to the point of closure. The compliant thorax of the calf may facilitate the development of atelectasis by failing to support underlying lung tissue which is beginning to collapse.

Calves have small lungs for their body sizes but the functional residual capacity is a relatively large fraction of total lung capacity (11).   This may be necessary to prevent excessive airway closure during tidal breathing.

Measurements of pulmonary resistance are available for calves, but not for adult cattle.   In calves, resistance averages 3.0-5.0 centimeters $H_2O/L/sec$ (7,11,13-15). Autonomic innervation of calf airways is similar to other species.   There is tonic parasympathetic bronchoconstrictor tone in the larger airways so that vagotomy decreases pulmonary resistance and increases the dead-space/tidal volume ratio (11).   Tonic sympathetic tone opposes vagal tone.   Blockade of beta adrenergic receptors increases pulmonary resistance (16).   There is no information on how autonomic control of airways is affected by disease. Alterations in the reactivity of airways to inhaled stimuli occur in other species following viral and bacterial infection (17,18), intravenous infusion of endotoxin (19), and ozone exposure (20,21) and such alter-actions may play a role in the pathogenesis of bovine respiratory disease.

Matching of Ventilation and Blood Flow

Even in healthy lungs there is some mismatching of ventilation and blood flow (6) so that arterial oxygen tension (PaO_2) is less than alveolar oxygen tension, i.e., there is an alveolar-arterial oxygen difference. Although one group of investigators has reported PaO_2 as high as 94 torr in calves (22), other investigators report PaO_2 between 70 and 80 torr with a considerable alveolar-arterial oxygen difference (7,11,13-16,23). This large difference is probably the result of ventilation perfusion inequalities arising as a result of airway closure during tidal breathing. PaO_2 in adult cattle averages 90-95 torr (12). If adult cattle are like adults of most other large species, the stiff thorax of the adult tends to prevent airway closure during tidal breathing.

During respiratory disease, atelectasis, consolidation and airway obstruction result in regions of lung which are poorly ventilated but continue to receive blood flow. Lungs possess several mechanisms to match ventilation and blood flow. These mechanisms include:

1. collateral ventilation between adjacent regions of lung,

2. interdependence between adjacent regions of lung,

3. hypoxic constriction of pulmonary arteries, and

4. hypocapnic constriction of airways.

The relative importance of each of these mechanisms in different species was recently reviewed (24).

The complete separation of secondary lobules by loose connective tissue prevents collateral ventilation in cattle (25). Following obstruction of an airway, there are no alternate pathways available for ventilation of the obstructed region. Since air cannot enter the obstructed region, coughing is ineffectual in removing any mucus which may be causing the obstruction. Alveoli distal to the obstruction become hypoxemic and atelectasis develops. Hypoxia suppresses macrophage function (26) which may allow infections to persist.

Interdependence is a term used to describe the mechanical interactions of adjacent regions of lung (27). When a region of lung inflates or deflates out-of-phase with the rest of the lung, such as occurs with complete or partial airway obstruction, additional stresses are applied to the region distal to the obstruction so as to cause it to inflate homogeneously with the remainder of the lung. Because all regions of a lobe are interconnected, nonhomogeneous inflation or deflation of a region is prevented by the tethering action of surrounding lung parenchyma. In cattle, the loose interlobular connective tissue allows adjacent lobules to act more independently than in other species (28). It is well accepted that the extensive interlobular connective tissue of cattle (28) and pig lungs (29) results in almost no interdependence between adjacent lobules in excised lungs at low lung volumes. With the thorax intact, interdependence between adjacent regions of lung is increased but there is still less interdependence in lobulated than nonlobulated lungs (e.g., dog) (30,31). This limited interdependence of cattle lungs may be another factor making cattle susceptible to atelectasis and regional alveolar hypoxia following airway obstruction. It should be noted that lung-thorax interdependence cannot restore ventilation to a region of cattle lung supplied by a completely obstructed airway because cattle lack interlobular collateral pathways. Lung-thorax interdependence can only attempt to maintain ventilation in the face of incomplete airway obstruction.

Because of the lack of collateral ventilation, regions of lung supplied by obstructed airways cannot function as gas exchangers. It is therefore appropriate to reduce the blood flow to these regions and redirect blood to the better ventilated regions of lung. The pulmonary arteries of cattle constrict vigorously in response to hypoxia (32,33) and this may facilitate the redirection of blood flow away from poorly ventilated regions (34). The adequacy of this mechanism in maintaining normal ventilation/perfusion matching does not appear to be very good (35). The experiments on redistribution of blood flow in response to graded hypoxia have been performed in species with a meager hypoxic vascular response (i.e., dog, cat and sheep) (36-38). There are no data from cattle with a vigorous hypoxic response to determine if these species are better able to redistribute blood flow away from hypoxic regions of lungs. Evidence from other species suggests that hypoxic pulmonary vasoconstriction reduces blood flow to hypoxic or atelectatic regions of lung particularly if hypoxia or atelectasis is restricted to sublobar regions (39,40). However, the response is inadequate to maintain normal PaO_2 . In acute pneumonia (41) and allergic lung disease (42), the hypoxic constrictor response appears to be overridden probably by mediators of inflammation. Blood flow to diseased portions of lung is not reduced and hypoxemia results.

Constriction of airways in response to hypocapnia (43) has been suggested as a mechanism to reduce ventilation to poorly perfused regions of lung (44). The effectiveness of this mechanism is unknown.

Distribution of Lesions of Pneumonia

It is generally thought that the preferential distribution of pneumonic lesions in the anteroventral regions of the lung is because the orientation of these regions in the gravitational field results in fluid accumulation. Other possible causes include:

1. limited defense mechanisms in these regions,

2. regional variations in mechanics of ventilation which cause preferential inhalation of microorganisms, and

3. regional differences in interdependence.

We are unaware of information on regional variations in defense mechanisms. One study on distribution of ventilation (6) showed that the ventral regions of the lung received less ventilation than dorsal regions suggesting that microorganisms would not be preferentially inhaled into these regions. This same study showed a higher ventilation/perfusion ratio in ventral regions than in dorsal regions. This should result in a higher alveolar oxygen tension in ventral than dorsal regions and therefore regional suppression of macrophage function by hypoxia is not a likely cause of the typical distribution of pneumonic lesions.

We have considered regional variation in interdependence as a cause of the typical distribution of pneumonic lesions (28). In isolated lung preparations, lobules in regions where pneumonia commonly occurs had less interdependence with the rest of the lung than lobules in the caudal and dorsal regions of the caudal lobe where pneumonia seldom occurs. The lack of interdependence could be explained by the limited area of interface with the rest of the lung. It was thus tempting to speculate that following injury to the lung, it is more difficult to maintain ventilation to regions with little interdependence. Alveolar hypoxia ensues, suppressing macrophage function and allowing bacterial proliferation. However, we could not show similar regional differences in interdependence in anesthetized intact calves. It is possible that our failure to measure regional differences was due to anesthesia and the use of positive-pressure ventilation. In spontaneously breathing pigs, Zidulka and co-workers (45) showed that interdependence was greatest in lung regions closest to the diaphragm. It is still possible therefore that the typical distribution of pneumonic lesions results from regional mechanical factors and not just because fluids run downhill.

Lung Function in Infectious Bovine Respiratory Disease

There are no reports in the literature of changes in lung function in cattle with spontaneously-occurring disease. We are aware of only two studies in which lung function has been studied during the onset of infectious bovine respiratory disease. Kiorpes and co-workers (14) studied calves inoculated with infectious bovine rhinotracheitis and more recently Slocombe (7) studied calves which were inoculated intratracheally with *Pasteurella haemolytica.* The two studies provide an interesting comparison of two functionally-distinct types of respiratory disease.

Infectious bovine rhinotracheitis (IBR) produced changes in respiratory function compatible with obstruction of the upper airway and trachea (Figures 1 and 2). Pulmonary resistance increased from a baseline value of 3.1 centimeters $H_2O/L/sec$ to 5.3 centimeters $H_2O/L/sec$ ten days after inoculation. Pulmonary resistance is determined to a large extent by the resistance of the upper airway, trachea and bronchi. An increase in pulmonary resistance can be caused by either obstruction of these large airways or by diffuse obstruction of peripheral airways. In the case of airway obstruction distal to the carina, an increase in pulmonary resistance is usually accompanied by a decrease in dynamic compliance because the obstruction causes inequalities in regional time constants. Calves infected with IBR had no change in dynamic compliance suggesting airway obstruction was restricted to the upper airway and trachea. This was confirmed by the investigators' observation that lesions were restricted to the upper airways and that calves with the greatest increase in resistance had the most extensive airway lesions. Infected calves also developed an increase in functional residual capacity and arterial carbon dioxide tension, both classical signs of airway obstruction. The increase in functional residual capacity was probably due to the prolongation of the time required for passive exhalation. The increase in $PaCO_2$ resulted from an increase in metabolic rate unaccompanied by the required increase in alveolar ventilation. Fever and increased work of breathing probably caused increased metabolism while airway obstruction limited the increase in alveolar ventilation.

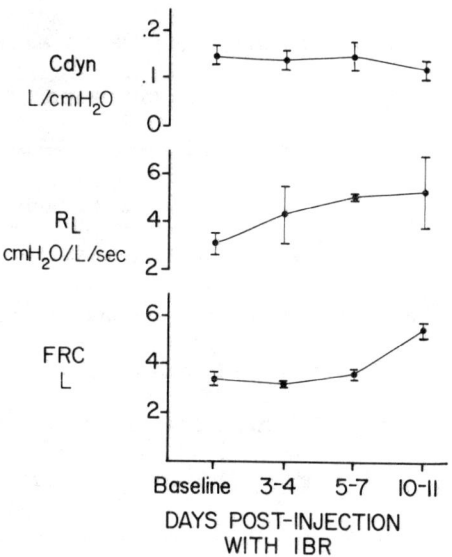

Figure 1.   Dynamic compliance (Cdyn), pulmonary resistance (RL), and functional residual capacity (FRC) in calves infected with infectious bovine rhinotracheitis (from data in reference 13).

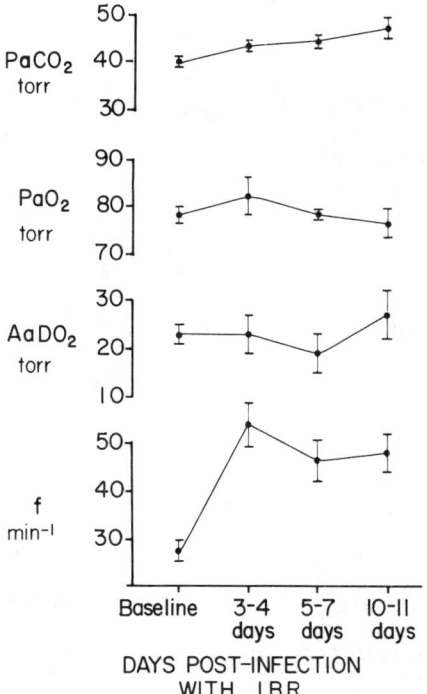

Figure 2.   Arterial carbon dioxide tension (PaCO$_2$), oxygen tension   (PaO$_2$),   alveolar-arterial   oxygen difference (AaDO$_2$), and respiratory   rate (f) in calves infected with infectious bovine rhinotracheitis (from data in reference 13).

There was no physiological evidence of lung damage in calves infected with IBR, dynamic compliance and PaO_2 being unchanged following exposure. These physiological findings were confirmed by necropsy which showed lesions only in large airways.

In contrast to IBR, which presents functionally as an obstruction of large airways, pasteurellosis is a disease of lung parenchyma (Figures 3 and 4). Following intratracheal inoculation of *Pasteurella haemolytica*, PaO_2 decreased significantly by two hours. The decrease was not due to alveolar hypoventilation because $PaCO_2$ remained constant but was the result of an increased alveolar-arterial oxygen difference indicating ventilation perfusion mismatching. Over the next ten hours, hypoxemia became more severe. Further evidence of damage to the lung parenchyma was a decrease in dynamic compliance occurring three-six hours after inoculation. This decrease in compliance was unaccompanied by an increase in pulmonary resistance and therefore indicates either stiffening of the lung by exudates, edema or fibrosis or diffuse obstruction of peripheral airways. Twelve hours after inoculation there was an increase in pulmonary resistance which resulted in hypoventilation (increased $PaCO_2$).

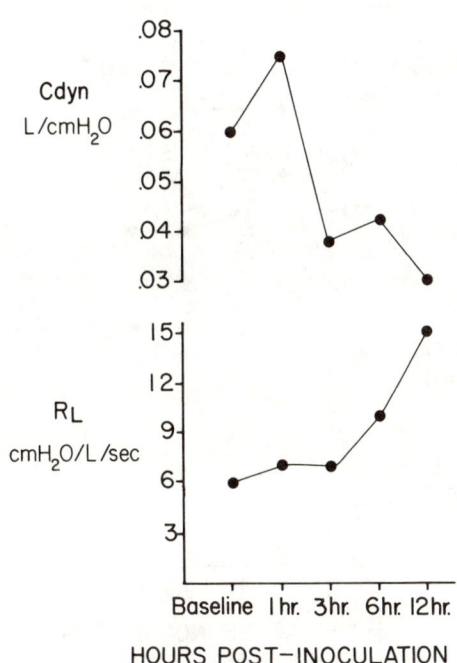

Figure 3.   Dynamic   compliance   (Cdyn)   and   pulmonary
resistance(RL) in calves infected with *Pasteurella haemolytica*
(from data in reference 7).

The sequence of functional changes following *Pasteurella*

challenge, i.e., hypoxemia, decreased compliance, increased

resistance and hypoventilation is compatible with a disease

process beginning in the lung parenchyma and extending into

the peripheral airways.   This was confirmed at necropsy

when disease was limited to alveoli and bronchioles.

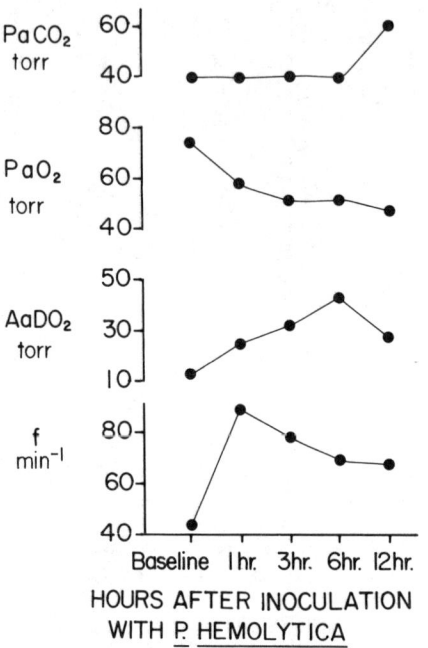

Figure 4. Arterial carbon dioxide tension (PaCO$_2$), oxygen tension (PaO$_2$), alveolar-arterial oxygen difference (AaDO$_2$), and respiratory rate (f) in calves infected with *Pasteurella haemolytica* (from data in reference 7).

One of the interesting observations in both IBR- and *Pasteurella*-infected calves was tachypnea which developed one hour after inoculation with *Pasteurella* and was present three-four days after IBR inoculation. Tachypnea was not in response to hypoxemia or hypercapnia because blood gas tensions were not abnormal when tachypnea occurred. By the time PaO_2 decreased in calves with pasteurellosis, tachypnea abated. In IBR-infected calves, tachypnea may have been in response to fever but body temperature was not elevated in *Pasteurella*-infected calves in which tachypnea was most severe. The tachypnea which occurs in response to allergic (46,47) and toxic (48) lung disease can be abolished by vagal blockade suggesting it results from stimulation of intrapulmonary receptors with vagal afferents. Perhaps infectious agents also stimulate intrapulmonary receptors either directly or by modifying their response to other stimuli such as stretching, edema accumulation or chemical mediators.

The tachypnea of calves with pasteurellosis occurred with no decrease in tidal volume resulting in a large increase in minute ventilation. Alveolar ventilation was unchanged and most of the extra ventilation was dead-space ventilation. This dead-space ventilation could not be explained by the combination of increased frequency and a fixed anatomic dead space. It therefore had to result from ventilation of poorly perfused regions of lung such as would result if much of the pulmonary blood flow was directed away from normal regions toward *Pasteurella*-infected regions of lung.

There are no data available on changes in lung perfusion following challenge by infectious agents. We anticipate a large increase in pulmonary artery pressure when cattle become hypoxemic because of the vigorous vascular constriction in response to hypoxia. Mediators of inflammation may override the vasoconstriction, however, and increase blood flow to the pneumonic areas of lung such as occurs in dogs with streptococcal pneumonia (41). We have measured pulmonary artery pressure in a calf with chronic pneumonia. Pulmonary arterial pressure equaled systemic pressure. When the calf was ventilated and hypoxemia was relieved, pulmonary arterial pressure decreased to normal levels. If pulmonary artery constriction occurs with lung disease, the work load of the right heart will be greatly increased.

Conclusion

There is a vast need for information on basic lung physiology of adult cattle and how and why lung function is altered by disease. Cattle may be particularly prone to lung injury because they have small lungs with little reserve, no collateral ventilation and limited interlobular interdependence. The hyperreactive vasculature may confer an advantage in matching ventilation and blood flow but also may lead to large increases in right ventricular work when animals are hypoxic as a result of lung disease.

Calves, like all newborns, have a compliant thorax which may make them prone to the development of atelectasis. Closure of airways at high lung volumes may also make calves more susceptible to the effects of any agent which can potentially cause airway obstruction.

Only recently have physiological measurements been used to study the pathogenesis of bovine lung disease. The functional changes are consistent with observed lesions. What was so surprising in the case of pasteurellosis was the extremely rapid onset of functional changes.

Acknowledgment

This study was supported in part by a grant from U.S. Department of Agriculture and by Michigan Agricultural Experiment Station.

References

1.   Tenney SM, Remmers JE:Comparative quantitative morphology of the mammalian lung: diffusing area. Nature 197:554-56, 1963.

2.   Mariassy AT, Plopper CG, Dungworth DL:Characteristics of bovine lung as observed by scanning electron microscopy. Ant Rec 183:13-26, 1975.

3.   McLaughlin RF, Tyler WS, Canada RO:A study of the subgross pulmonary anatomy in various mammals. Am J Anat 108:149-165, 1961.

4.   Tucker A, McMurtry IF, Reeves JT, Alexander AF, Will DH, Grover RF:Lung vascular smooth muscle as a determinant of pulmonary hypertension at high altitude. Am J Physiol 228:762-767, 1975.

5.   Alexander AF, Will DH, Grover RF, Reeves JT:Pulmonary hypertension and right venticular hypertrophy in cattle at high altitude. Am J Vet Res 21:199-204, 1960.

6.   Ruiz AV, Bisgard GE, Tyson IB, Grover RF, Will JA:Regional lung function in calves during acute and chronic pulmonary hypertension. J Appl Physiol 37:384-391, 1974.

7.   Slocombe RF:Interactions of cold stress and *Pasteurella hemolytica* in the pathogenesis of pneumonic pasteurellosis of calves. Ph.D. thesis, Michigan State University, 1982.

8.   Taylor CR, Maloiy GMO, Weibel ER, Langman VA, Kamau JMZ, Secherman HJ, Heglund NC:Design of the mammalian respiratory system. III.   Scaling maximum aerobic capacity to body mass: wild and domestic mammals. Resp Physiol 44:25-37, 1980.

9.   Gehr P, Mwangi DK, Ammann A, Malory GMO, Taylor CR, Weibel EW:Design of the mammalian respiratory system. V. Scaling morphometric pulmonary diffusing capacity to body mass: wild and domestic mammals. Resp Physiol 44:61-68, 1981.

10.   Thomson RG, Gilka F:A brief review of pulmonary clearance of bacterial aerosols emphasizing aspects of particular relevance to veterinary medicine.   Can Vet J 15:99-107, 1974.

11.   Slocombe RF, Robinson NE, Derksen FJ:Effect of vagotomy on respiratory mechanics and gas exchange in the neonatal calf. Am J Vet Res 43:1168-1171, 1982.

12.   Hales JRS, Findlay JD:Respiration of the ox: normal values and the effects of exposure to hot environments. Resp Physiol 4:333-352, 1968.

13.   Kiorpes AL, Bisgard GE, Manohar M:Pulmonary function values in healthy Holstein-Friesian calves.   Am J Vet Res 39:773-778, 1978.

14.   Kiorpes AL, Bisgard GE, Manohar M, Hernandez A:Pathophysiologic studies of infectious bovine rhinotracheitis in the Holstein-Fresian calf. Am J Vet Res 39:779-783, 1978.

15.   Slocombe RF, Robinson NE:Histamine H_1, H_2 receptor effects on mechanics of ventilation and gas exchange in neonatal calves. Am J Vet Res 42:764-769, 1981.

16.   Kotlikoff MI, Slocombe RF, Robinson NE:Influence of β-adrenergic antagonism on the response of bovine neonatal lungs to intravenous histamine. Am J Vet Res 43:984-988, 1982.

17.   Empey DW, Laitinen LA, Jacobs L, Gold WM, Nadel JA:Mechanisms of bronchial hyperreactivity in normal subjects after uppper respiratory tract infection. Am Rev Respir Dis 113:131-139, 1976.

18.   Dixon M, Jackson DM, Richards IM:The effect of a respiratory tract infection on histamine-induced changes in lung mechanics and irritant receptor discharge in dogs. Am Rev Respir Dis 120:843-848, 1979.

19.   Hutchison AA, Hinson JM, Jr., Brigham KL, Snapper JR:Effect of endotoxin on airway responsiveness to aerosol histamine in sheep. J Appl Physiol: Respirat Environ Exercise Physiol 54:1463-1468, 1983.

20.   Lee LY, Bleecker ER, Nadel JA:Effect of ozone on bronchomotor response to inhaled histamine aerosol in dogs. J Appl Physiol: Respirat Environ Exercise Physiol 43:626-631, 1977.

21.   Gordon T, Amdur MO:Effect of ozone on respiratory response of guinea pigs to histamine. J Toxicol Environ Health 6:185-195, 1980.

22.   Donawick WJ, Baue AE:Blood gases, acid-base balance and alveolar-arterial oxygen gradient in calves. Am J Vet Res 29:561-567, 1968.

23.   Slocombe RF, Latter W, Derksen FJ, Robinson NE:Pulmonary response of neonatal calves to intravenous and aerosol bradykinin. Am J Vet Res 43:2023-2027, 1982.

24. Robinson NE:Some functional consequences of species differences in lung anatomy. Adv Vet Sci Comp Med 26:1-33, 1982.

25. VanAllen CM, Lindskog GE, Richter HG:Collateral respiration: transfer of air collaterally between pulmonary lobules. J Clin Invest 10:559-590, 1931.

26. Green GM, Kass EH:Factors influencing the clearance of bacteria by the lung. J Clin Invest 43:769-776, 1964.

27. Mead J, Takashima T, Leith D:Stress distribution in lungs: a model of pulmonary elasticity. J Appl Physiol 28:596-608, 1970.

28. Robinson NE, Ingersoll R, Slocombe RF, Olson LE:Regional interdependence in calf lungs. Submitted to J Appl Physiol.

29. Sylvester JT, Menkes HA, Stitik F:Lung volume and interdependence in the pig. J Appl Physiol 38:395-401, 1975.

30. Menkes HA, Lindsay D, Wood L, Muir A, Macklem PT:Interdependence of lung units in intact dog lungs. J Appl Physiol 32:681-686, 1972.

31. Robinson NE:Lobar variations in collateral ventilation in intact dog lungs. Amer Rev Respir Dis 124:68-71, 1981.

32.   Grover RF, Reeves JT, Will DH, Blount SG: Pulmonary vasoconstriction in steers at high altitude.   J Appl Physiol 18:567-574, 1963.

33.   Kuida H, Brown AM, Thorne JL, Lange RL, Hecht H:Pulmonary vascular response to acute hypoxia in normal, unanesthetized calves. Am J Physiol 203:391-396, 1962.

34.   Euler SV, Liljestrand G:Observations on the pulmonary arterial blood pressure in the cat. Act Physiol Scand 12:301-320, 1947.

35.   Grant BJB, Davies EE, Jones H, Hughes JMB:Local regulation   of   pulmonary   blood   flow   and ventilation-perfusion ratios in the coatimundi.   J Appl Physiol 40:216-228, 1976.

36.   Barer GR, Howard P, Shaw JW:Changes in the pulmonary   circulation   after   bronchial   occlusion   in anesthetized dogs and cats.   J Physiol Lond. 211:139-155, 1970.

37.   Rahn H, Bahnson HT:Effect of unilateral hypoxia on gas exchange and calculated pulmonary blood flow in each lung. J Appl Physiol 6:105-112, 1953.

38.   Robinson SM, Cadwallader JA, Hill P McN:Regional alveolar gas composition and lung function in sheep.   Resp Physiol 37:239-254, 1979.

39.   Enjeti S, O'Neill JT, Terry PB, Menkes HA, Traystman RJ:Sublobar atelectasis and regional pulmonary blood flow. J Appl Physiol Respir Environ Exercise Physiol 47:1245-1250, 1979.

40.   Metcalfe JF, Wagner PD, West JB:Effect of large bronchial obstruction on gas exchange in the dog.   Am Rev Resp Dis 117:85-95, 1978.

41.   Light RB, Mink SN, Wood LDH:Pathophysiology of gas exchange and pulmonary perfusion in pneumococcal lobar pneumonia in dogs.   J Appl Physiol Respirat Environ Exercise Physiol 50:524-530, 1981.

42.   Wanner A, Friedman M, Baier H:Study of the pulmonary circulation in a canine asthma model. Am Rev Resp Dis 115:241-250, 1977.

43.   Nisell OI:The action of oxygen and carbon dioxide on the bronchioles and vessels of isolated perfused lungs. Acta Physiol Scand 21:5-62, 1950.

44.   Severinghaus JW, Swenson EW, Finley JN, Lategola MT, Williams J:Unilateral hypoventilation produced in dogs by occluding one pulmonary artery. J Appl Physiol 16:53-60, 1961.

45.   Zidulka A, Sylvester JT, Nadler S, Anthonisen NR:Lung interdependence and lung-chest wall interaction of sublobar and lobar units in pigs.   J Appl Physiol Respirat Environ Exercise Physiol 46:8-13,1979.

46. Cotton DJ, Bleeker ER, Fischer SP, Graf PD, Gold WM, Nadel JA:Rapid shallow breathing after *Ascaris suum* antigen inhalation: role of vagus nerves. J Appl Physiol Respirat Environ Exercise Physiol 42:101-106, 1977.

47. Derksen FJ, Robinson NE, Slocombe RF:Ovalbumin-induced lung disease in the pony: role of vagal mechanisms. J Appl Physiol Respirat Environ Exercise Physiol 53:719-725, 1982.

48. Derksen FJ, Robinson NE, Slocombe RF, Hill RE:Three methylindole-induced pulmonary toxicosis in the horse. Am J Vet Res 43:603-607, 1982.

Viral-Bacterial Interactions in Respiratory Tract Infections: A Review of the Mechanisms of Virus-Induced Suppression of Pulmonary Antibacterial Defenses

George J. Jakab, Ph.D.

Department of Environmental Health Sciences
John Hopkins School of Hygiene and Public Health
John Hopkins University
Baltimore, Maryland 21205

Introduction

Although it was once thought that bacterial infection was merely a function of the virulence of the microbe, it is now known that other pathogens can alter host resistance (1). With regard to viral-bacterial interactions in pulmonary infections, three important factors must be considered: the role of the virus, the role of the bacterium and the immune status of the host. The fact that no one bacterial species is responsible for all human cases of post-influenzal bacterial pneumonia indicates that there is a general impairment of pulmonary antibacterial defenses after viral infection (2-4). The fact that the rate of intrapulmonary killing varies with different bacterial species (5-15) indicates that the superinfecting organisms can themselves play an active role in the dual disease process. Finally, it has been amply demonstrated that the resistance of the host is dependent on a variety of factors which include innate variables such as genetic endowment (16-19) and a multitude of imponderable variables acquired through life experiences which can be considered under the general category of "host factors" (20-24).   All three factors interact and collectively impinge upon the resistance of the host.

Influenza complicated by bacterial pneumonia is probably the best known example of a viral infection that increases the susceptibility of the host to bacterial infections, an example for which there is both clinical and experimental documentation   (2-4,   25,   26).   The   bulk   of   the investigations on the pathogenesis of combined infections have been performed with influenza and parainfluenza viruses and a variety of bacterial pathogens (27,28). This review will summarize those studies which have unraveled some of the mechanisms of the complexities of host-parasite interactions that have given us a more complete understanding of the effects of viral infection on host resistance; specifically, the mechanisms by which virus infections suppress pulmonary antibacterial defenses thus paving the way to bacterial superinfections of the lung.

A unified approach to the current knowledge of the mechanisms   by   which   virus   infections   suppress   host resistance comes from a basic understanding of the antibacterial defenses of the normal lung and the pathogenesis of uncomplicated viral pneumonia. Both subjects have been reviewed recently (29-33), so they will be dealt with here briefly to provide a common basis for the understanding of viral-bacterial interactions in the lungs.

Observations

Pulmonary Antibacterial Defenses

Although bacteria enter the lungs daily by inhalation of small droplets or by aspiration of fluid from the upper respiratory tract, the distal airways and alveoli are normally sterile. This is because the normal lung has the inordinate capacity to inactivate bacteria (29). Bacteria deposited in the lung parenchyma are rapidly engulfed and inactivated by the phagocytic cells of the lungs (34). The rate of intrapulmonary killing greatly exceeds the rate of physical translocation so that in terms of successful resistance against bacterial infections, *in situ* bactericidal mechanisms are more important than transport mechanisms out of the lung.

The resident phagocytes of the lung, the alveolar macrophages, play the pivotal defensive role against bacterial infection (34-37). However, when inflammatory processes are established, the polymorphonuclear leukocytes (PMNs) from the circulation immigrate into the lungs (10,38-47). This leukocytic response brings auxiliary defense capabilities to the lungs and indicates that rather than being wholly dependent on alveolar macrophages, pulmonary antibacterial defense is dependent of a phagocytic system that involves both alveolar macrophages and PMNs (48).

Within one animal model, the rate of intrapulmonary killing varies with different bacterial species (7,8,10). Indeed, with *Pseudomonas aeruginosa* the rate of killing is dependent on the *strain* of the organism (13,15). Microbial virulence factors undoubtedly play a role in the rate of bacterial inactivation in the lungs (49-57). However, the mechanisms by which microbial virulence factors are translated in terms of the rate of intrapulmonary killing of specific bacteria in the lungs is uncertain and may have to be elucidated for each organism. One overall hypothesis which offers an explanation for the differences in the *rate* of intrapulmonary killing among different bacterial species is that certain microbes *proliferate* in the lungs concurrent with bacterial inactivation (58). Since, in the normal lung, bacterial inactivation occurs at a more rapid rate than bacterial proliferation, the *net* effect would be that the bacteria are still killed, albeit at a slower rate than microbes which do not possess the capability to multiply. This hypothesis predicts that, all things being equal, pulmonary resistance against such proliferating organisms can be more easily overcome.   Indeed, with pulmonary virus infections (described below) this appears to be the case.

In addition to the differences in the rate of intrapulmonary bacterial inactivation among the various bacterial species, the overall burden of the number of bacteria of a single species deposited in the lungs also plays a role in the rate of bacterial killing (59).

Environmental manipulations or alterations of the host can modulate pulmonary antibacterial defenses. Conditions known to decrease intrapulmonary killing of bacteria include alveolar hypoxia, pulmonary edema, acidosis, certain pharmacologic agents, stress, inhalation of atmospheric pollutants, pulmonary virus infections and a number of other influences which have been recently reviewed (21).   On the other hand, immune mechanisms enhance the intrapulmonary killing of bacteria (8,60-63). However, as with the rate of intrapulmonary bacterial inactivation described above, immune enhancement of pulmonary bactericidal activity also varies with different bacterial species.   For example, immunization against

Streptococcus pneumoniae or *Staphylococcus aureus* did not enhance the intrapulmonary killing of pneumococci and staphylococci respectively. In contrast, immunization against a specific strain of *Pseudomonas aeruginosa* and *Proteus mirabilis* significantly enhanced the killing of the homologous organism whereas immunization against *Klebsiella pneumoniae* and *Serratia marcescense* was less effective (8). The mechanism(s) for these differences in immune-enhanced bactericidal activity among the different organisms remains to be elucidated.

At the cellular level, the bactericidal armamentarium of the pulmonary phagocytes rapidly inactivates and degrades inhaled and aspirated microorganisms within hours of their entrance into the alveolar region. The ability of the resident macrophage to seek out, ingest and inactivate bacteria results from the integration of a number of complex events. Phagocytes are attracted to bacteria by chemotactic factors. Engulfment is triggered by the attachment of the bacteria to specific immunologic and nonspecific receptors on the macrophage cell membrane. Once ingested, the bacteria are internally isolated in phagosomes. Lysosomes, sequestering microbicidal and degradative enzymes then fuse with the phagosome to form the phagolysosome in which intracellular processing of the

bacteria   occurs.   In   addition   to   lysosomal-killing
mechanisms,   recent   findings   indicate   that   the   alveolar
macrophages are also capable of inactivating organisms by
oxygen-dependent   mechanisms,   such   as   those   involving
peroxide and superoxide, microbicidal compounds of primary
importance in bacterial killing by PMNs.

The mechanism of recruitment of PMNs to the alveoli to
provide auxiliary phagocytic defenses is not completely
understood.   Explanations would include that the alveolar
macrophages secrete chemotactic factors specific for the
recruitment   of   PMNs   (64).   Alternatively,   the   microbes
against which PMNs provide auxiliary phagocytic defenses
are   primarily   Gram-negative   organisms   that   contain
endotoxin.   Endotoxin   is   known   to   activate   complement   of
which   the   C'5   component   has   been   demonstrated   to   be
chemotactic for PMNs (65-68).

Pathogenesis of Uncomplicated Viral Pneumonia

In experimental models of influenza and parainfluenza
virus, the severity and duration of the illness depends on
the infectious dose of virus delivered to the respiratory
tract.   With sublethal infections that cause moderate to
severe pneumonitis, the virus proliferates rapidly in the
lungs, reaching peak titers approximately three to five
days after viral inoculation. Thereafter, pulmonary virus

titers rapidly decline with infectious virus no longer recoverable by days 7 to 9 of the infection.

During the acute stages of the infection, the ciliated epithelial cells of the conducting airways are the principal sites of viral replication. In the affected areas, the ciliated epithelium degenerates and desquamates leaving only a thin layer of basal replacement cells. At this stage, the overall picture consists of spotty but extensive desquamative lesions of the bronchial mucosa. Maximum histopathologic changes occur approximately one week after viral infection. At this time the affected areas of the lung parenchyma are characterized by hyperemia and thickening of the alveolar walls with interstitial infiltration with leukocytes and capillary thrombosis. The alveoli are congested and edematous and contain leukocytic exudates. Concurrently, the luminal side of the affected airways may be partially or completely occluded by the sloughing of degenerated epithelial cells and the influx of inflammatory cells, whereas the peribronchial areas are intensely infiltrated with mononuclear cells.

The virus-induced lesion begins to resolve by the ninth day of the infection, as evidenced by the beginning of repair of the damaged areas of mucosa and the resolution of the consolidation in the lung parenchyma.

Host defenses against the virus infection include interferon (33,69-71) and the specific antiviral immune response (72-75). Interferon concentrations in the lung are usually at their highest levels on approximately the fifth day of infection and then decline as the virus disappears (33,71). Specific antiviral immunoglobulins have been detected in the lungs by the third day of infection (76,77), and by day 8 locally-synthesized antibodies (78) are present in bronchial washings (77); serum antibodies usually appear by day 8 also (71,79). In addition to the humoral immune response, cytotoxic T lymphocytes sensitized to viral antigen also appear in the lungs during the third day of infection. This response peaks at approximately day 7 and thereafter rapidly declines (80-89). Adoptive transfer of such specifically primed T cells to immune-depleted mice has been shown to protect against virus infection (85,88).

Current concepts of antiviral immunity indicate that the host response controls the infection by halting the spread of the virus to extrapulmonary sites and by destroying virus-infected cells. Both humoral and cellular immune responses can participate in the destruction; antibody participates with the aid of complement (90) and T lymphocytes participate through their direct cytotoxic activity (91,92).

Virus-Induced Pulmonary Bactericidal Dysfunction

During the acute phase of the viral infection, the bactericidal mechanisms of the lung become progressively depressed with maximal suppression occurring approximately a week after viral inoculation (93-95).   Thereafter, the antibacterial defenses of the lung become reestablished, being essentially normal by the second week of infection. The extent of the virus-induced suppression of pulmonary bactericidal activity at day 7 is dependent on the amount of virus used for infection (96).   Within the range of sublethal virus inocula that induces a mild-to-severe pneumonia, the virus effect can range from a reduced rate of intrapulmonary bacterial killing to failure of the mechanisms resulting in bacterial proliferation in the lungs with the demise of the host from overwhelming secondary bacterial infection.   With massive lethal doses of the virus, which cause fulminant pneumonitis resulting in viral deaths on the second and third days, intrapulmonary bacterial killing is depressed on the first day after viral infection (93).   The shift in the bactericidal defect from day 7 in the viral infection of intermediate severity to day 1 in the lethal pneumonia presumably reflects the overwhelming viral disease.

Virus-Induced Phagocytic Dysfunctions

The temporal relationship between impaired pulmonary antibacterial defenses and virus-induced anatomic changes led early researchers to stress the importance of the pathologic lesions as the mechanism by which viruses render the lungs more susceptible to bacterial superinfections (97-99).   However, recent studies have questioned the significance of the viral lesion as the *primary* mechanism responsible for pulmonary antibacterial dysfunction (100-103) since bacterial multiplication associated with virus infection of lungs is related to defects in *in situ* bactericidal (phagocytic) mechanisms rather than transport mechanisms of the lung (104).   During the last decade attention has been directed toward functional lesions induced by the virus infection of the biocidal defenses of the lung.

The initial *in vivo* studies related the dysfunction in pulmonary biocidal activity to abnormalities in ingestion and intracellular processing of bacteria by alveolar macrophages (105). In these studies, mice were challenged by aerosol inhalation with staphylococci and the intra- or extracellular location of the bacteria were determined histologically in sections of lungs from virus-infected and noninfected animals.   Shortly after bacterial challenge, a greater percentage of the inhaled staphylococci were extracellularly located in virus-infected lungs indicating an inhibition of the ingestive processes of the macrophage. Thereafter, with time, observable staphylococci disappeared from noninfected lungs reflecting the dissolution of intracellular organisms by the lysosomal degradative enzyme system. In contrast, microcolonies of bacteria were prevalent within macrophages of virus-infected lungs indicating that a defect in the intracellular processing of ingested bacteria was present as well as the defect in phagocytic ingestion (106).

Subsequent studies on the functional activity of alveolar macrophages lavaged from virus-infected lungs during the time of maximum virus-induced suppression of pulmonary bactericidal activity have demonstrated dysfunctions in:

1. immunologic and nonimmunologic membrane receptor binding activity (107,108),

2. immunologic and nonspecific receptor-mediated phagocytic ingestion (107,108),

3. phagosome-lysosome fusion (109),

4. intracellular killing (108,110), and

5. bacterial degradation (111,112).

In addition, alveolar macrophages from virus-infected lungs have abnormally low levels of lysosomal enzymes (113), which undoubtedly also contributes to defects in intracellular processing of microorganisms. These combined observations clearly demonstrate that pulmonary virus infections induce a functional paralysis of the alveolar macrophage phagocytic system.

In contrast to alveolar macrophages, little is known about the effect of viral infection on the phagocytic function of monocytes and PMNs. The most consistently-documented abnormality in peripheral phagocyte function during influenza is impairment of chemotaxis (114-118). What this means in terms of dysfunctions of pulmonary antibacterial defenses during virus pneumonia is uncertain since the virus infection induces a brisk and impressive influx of monocytes and neutrophils into the lungs (119-121).

Experimental animal studies show that peripheral PMN phagocytosis is suppressed at the same time as the dysfunctions observed in the alveolar macrophages, namely, approximately a week after virus infection (122,123). However, clinical observations do not corroborate the experimental data (124,125). One possible explanation for these contrasting results would be that the virus infection in the animals was more severe than that in the clinical situation and, therefore, peripheral phagocyte malfunction is related to the severity of the lung infection. However, this relationship remains to be documented.

To date, the available data demonstrate that virus infection induces a paralysis in lung phagocyte function at a time that coincides with the greatest susceptibility to secondary bacterial pneumonias. The impaired function of the lung phagocytes remains the primary reason most often proposed for the occurrence of bacterial complications after pulmonary virus infection and there is little reason at present to doubt the proposal.

The Involvement of the Antiviral Immune Response in Phagocyte Dysfunction

The growth of virus in the lungs is not immediately accompanied by the transient suppression of pulmonary bactericidal activity (Figure 1). Instead, the impairment of phagocyte function is sometime after peak lung titers of infectious virus are obtained. This temporal relationship suggests that macrophage dysfunction does not result from a direct effect of the virus on the phagocyte (126). Indeed, alveolar macrophages infected with virus *in vitro* inactivate intracellular staphylococci at a rate indistinguishable from noninfected control macrophages (127,128). Insights into the mechanisms by which the virus *induces* the phagocytic defect can be found by examining the dynamic occurrences in the lung during the critical time of the virus infection when pulmonary antibacterial defenses caused by phagocyte dysfunction are maximally suppressed.

The rapid decrease of infectious virus titers occurs concomitantly with the appearance of the antiviral immune response.   These immune mechanisms, consisting of both antiviral antibody and a specific cytotoxic lymphocyte response, are maximal in the lungs at approximately a week after viral infection. An apparent paradoxical association is that during the period of time of decreasing virus titers and increasing immune responsiveness in the lungs, the phagocytic capabilities are maximally suppressed. These simultaneous occurrences indicate that components of the host's antiviral immune response may be involved in producing the phagocytic defect.

Several lines of evidence are emerging that indicate that the immunologic responses of the host play important roles not only in confining respiratory tract infections but also contributing to the pathogenesis of the disease. Leukocyte infiltration of the lungs is known to occur during pulmonary virus infection (119-121).   However, immunodeficient (87,129-131) and immunocompromized mice (132-142) develop much less cellular infiltration and

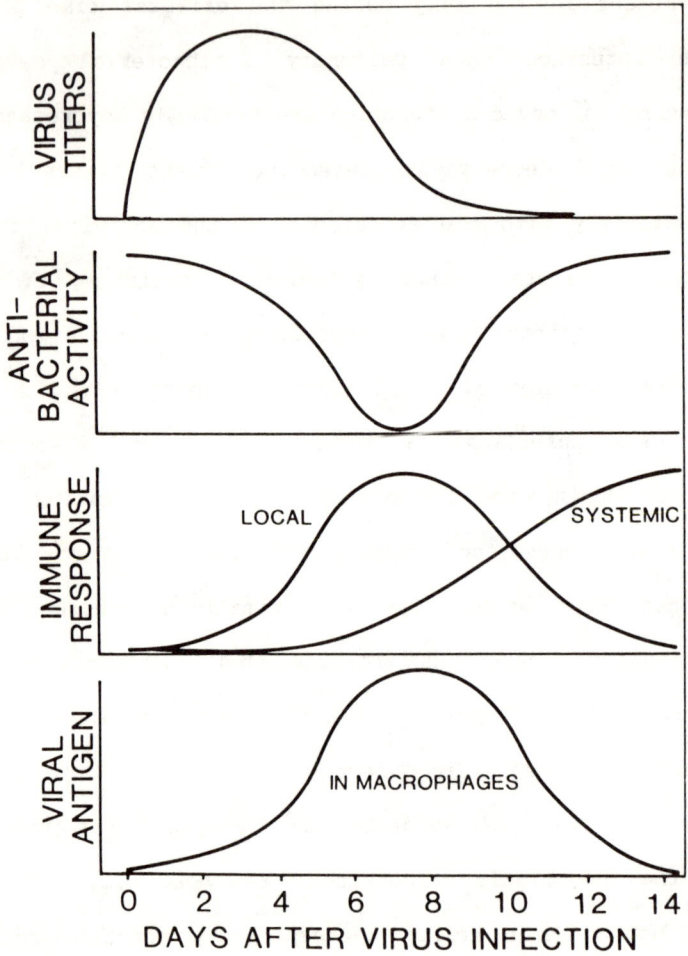

Figure 1.   Diagrammatic summary of the temporal events during virus pneumonia.   Correlation between pulmonary virus titers, virus-induced suppression of pulmonary antibacterial activity, the antiviral immune response and viral antigen in alveolar macrophages.

histopathology than their immunocompetent counterparts.

These correlations between an intact antiviral immune response and increased pathologic alterations of the lung strongly suggest that the immunologic responses of the host contribute to the pathogenesis of the viral pneumonia and, therefore, the antiviral immune responses may also be involved in the virus-induced suppression of pulmonary antibacterial defenses. If this is so, then it can be hypothesized that immunosuppression will ameliorate the phagocytic defect in pulmonary antibacterial defenses and that immune reconstitution would reestablish the dysfunction. Indeed when the hypothesis was tested *in vivo,* the data showed that immunosuppression mitigated the virus-induced pulmonary bactericidal defect (142) whereas passive administration of specific antiserum to immunocompromized animals reestablished the bactericidal dysfunction (143). Furthermore, when the hypothesis was tested at the cellular level it was found that the phagocytic activity of alveolar macrophages lavaged from virus-infected and immunosuppressed animals was largely preserved. However, when in a manner analogous to immune reconstitution *in vivo,* the alveolar macrophages from virus-infected and immunosuppressed animals were incubated with antiviral globulin, the phagocytic defect was reestablished (142).

In vitro studies in which selected antiviral components have been added to alveolar macrophages infected in culture provide additional evidence of immune-enhanced dysfunction of phagocytosis.   Cultured alveolar macrophages infected with virus *in vitro* ingest yeasts and staphylococci normally. However, the treatment of such macrophages with specific antiviral antibody severely inhibits the phagocytic ingestion of both organisms (143,144). In similar studies, the incubation of virus-infected alveolar macrophages with specifically-sensitized lymphocytes also suppressed phagocytosis (143).

The mechanism by which antiviral immune mechanisms participate in the virus-induced derangement of alveolar macrophage phagocytosis remains to be elucidated.   All enveloped RNA viruses (including influenza and parainfluenza) which acquire an outer lipid envelope by budding from the host cell membrane express viral antigen on the cell surface (145-151). Antiviral antibody and specifically-sensitized lymphocytes are known to interact with such virus-infected cells resulting in pertubation of cell function, or even cell death (152-155). Therefore, explanations for the involvement of the antiviral immune mechanisms in the phagocyte derangement would include that the alveolar macrophages become target cells for the antiviral immune response. This is a desirable response because it eliminates virus-bearing cells. It is detrimental to the host because it transiently reduces the phagocytic capacity of the macrophages and thereby the antibacterial defenses of the lung.

That virus-bearing alveolar macrophages become target cells for the antiviral immune response is suggested by the following observations. First, immunofluorescent studies have shown that alveolar macrophages with viral antigen progressively increase to a maximum at approximately a week after infection and thereafter rapidly disappear (156). Second, viral antigen in alveolar macrophages accumulates and disappears in parallel in immunocompromized and immunocompetent animals, suggesting that both sets of phagocytes are equally susceptible to immune injury. However, the phagocytic defect was largely preserved in the immunosuppressed animals in which the antiviral immune response was blunted (142). Third, in culture, the incubation of alveolar macrophages infected *in vitro* with specific antibody resulted in phagocyte dysfunction. In contrast, the treatment of uninfected macrophages with viral antibody had no effect on phagocytosis (144). Thus the antibody appeared to be directed against the viral antigen expressed on the cell surface.

Another immune-mediated mechanism by which phagocytosis is reduced is through the interaction of macrophages with immune complexes (157-160). Such complexes probably form during every infectious process with pulmonary virus infections being no exception (133,161,162). Recently we have documented that influenza virus infections induce immune complexes in the lungs which can be recovered from the acellular portion of lung lavages (163). Early in the infection when the virus proliferates in the lungs, the complexes are in antigen-excess. Then, with the appearance of local antiviral antibody, the virus-induced immune complexes reach equivalence at approximately the seventh to ninth day of infection. Thereafter, with the elimination of infectious virus from the lungs the complexes are in antibody-excess. When cultivated alveolar macrophages are incubated with the virus-induced immune complexes at their equivalence, phagocytic ingestion is severely curtailed. If similar mechanisms are operative in the lungs, then these observations suggest that the alveolar macrophages do not have to be directly affected by the virus, since phagocytic dysfunction could occur simply through the contact of normal macrophages with the immune complexes. Preliminary evidence indicates that PMN phagocytosis may be similarly affected by the virus-induced immune complexes.

Taking this line of thinking one step further, this latter finding may, in part, explain the impairment of peripheral phagocyte function observed in experimental animals (122,123). During the course of viral infection, immune complexes are deposited in the kidneys (164). If these immune complexes reach the kidneys through the circulation, then it might be expected that they would also have the opportunity to interact with peripheral phagocytes which, in turn, may also reduce their phagocytic capabilities. This interpretation, although inviting, remains to be demonstrated.

Immune complexes also induce lung injury (165-168) and therefore may inhibit the phagocytic activities of the alveolar macrophages by mechanisms other than their direct antiphagocytic effect.

Contributing Factors and Other Considerations

The data detailed above demonstrate that virus-induced suppression of pulmonary antibacterial defenses are mediated through defects of the alveolar macrophage phagocytic system and provide strong support that the induction of phagocyte dysfunction is mediated, in part, by the antiviral immune response. However, a number of additional effects are induced during the viral infection which alter the millieu of the lung and undoubtedly also play a role in increasing susceptibility to bacterial superinfection.

First, it has been proposed that as an initial step in bacterial infections, the organisms adhere to the cells of the respiratory tract (169,170). This adherence, in turn, enhances bacterial colonization, which could proceed to bacterial infection and disease (171). Bacteria adhere to cell monolayers infected with virus *in vitro* (172–176), tracheal cells obtained after infection *in vivo* (177,178) and pharyngeal cells from patients with naturally-acquired respiratory illness and from volunteers experimentally infected with influenza virus (179,180). Upper respiratory tract colonization with increased numbers of bacteria may increase the chances of bacterial infection of the lung through either the presence of the microbes in the respiratory tract or, upon aspiration, a bolus containing a larger number of organisms is delivered to the lung.

Second, in the viral lesion in the lung parenchyma, the type 2 alveolar pneumocytes are destroyed. These cells synthesize and secrete surfactant, the level of which is decreased in the consolidated but not in the unconsolidated areas of virus-infected lungs (181,182). Since a component of surfactant is considered to play an important role in the phagocytosis of bacteria by alveolar macrophages

(183-186), its decreased presence may be an additional factor involved in macrophage malfunction. Other extracellular factors believed to have a role in intrapulmonary bacterial killing (187-189) may also be affected by the virus infection. In addition, alveolar macrophages are aerobic cells whose phagocytic capacity is suppressed by hypoxic conditions (190,191); anaerobic conditions brought about by atelectasis and edema would be expected to affect their phagocytic capacity. Altered pulmonary function resulting in reduced ventilatory capacity (192,193) may have a similar effect.

Third, maximal virus-induced inhibition of phagocyte function coincides with the time that the greatest number of alveolar macrophages contain viral antigen (142,156). The source of the antigen is most likely a combination of intracellular viral multiplication and ingestion of cellular debris from the sloughed bronchial epithelium, the site of earlier virus proliferation (33,194). It is known that ingestion of large amounts of material will block subsequent phagocyte function (195). Thus, the lung macrophages that are actively processing ingested cellular debris may have a reduced capacity to ingest additional material (i.e., bacteria). Those affected macrophages that ingest microorganisms, albeit fewer or at a slower rate, may not have the resources to process the additional load intracellularly.

Finally, evidence is accumulating that, in certain instances, the bacterium itself may play a role in diminishing macrophage phagocytosis. *Pasteurella haemolytica* and culture supernatants of the organism are cytotoxic to bovine alveolar macrophages (196,197) and peripheral leukocytes (198,199). This observation would suggest that if the bacteria gained a foothold in the lung through virus-induced macrophage dysfunction, the organism could perpetuate itself through its own toxic mechanism. This added stress on the phagocytic system of the lung may explain the rapid progression and high mortality observed in the natural cattle disease entity of mixed etiology known as "shipping fever," which is caused by bovine respiratory viruses in combination with bacteria of the genus *Pasteurella* (200). Thus, the veterinary data suggest that in some cases the superinfecting bacteria may also play an active role in the progression of the disease instead of merely passively multiplying in the lungs due to paralysis of the lung's phagocytes brought about by the virus infection. Evidence is accumulating that other organisms have similar toxic effects on phagocytes (201,202).

That the bacterial species is important in the *progression* of the disease is also demonstrated by the *rate* of intrapulmonary proliferation of various bacteria in virus-infected lungs. For example, over a four-hour period after bacterial challenge, viable staphylococci only doubled their numbers (106). When the challenge organism was *Proteus mirabilis,* five times as many viable bacteria were recovered (61) and, in the case of *Pseudomonas aeruginosa,* the animals were moribund from overwhelming bacterial pneumonia at four hours after challenge with the organism (Jakab, unpublished observations). The hierarchy of the magnitude of bacterial multiplication of these three organisms in virus-infected lungs reflects their rates of intrapulmonary survival in nonvirus-infected lungs (8). Differential suppression of pulmonary antibacterial defenses by the virus may be one of the mechanisms which determines the selection of a pathogen in bacterial superinfections (203).

The Role of Antiviral and Antibacterial Immunity

The magnitude of the virus-induced suppression of pulmonary bactericidal mechanisms is related to the disease-inducing potential of the virus (96,204). Specific antiviral immunity prevents viral infection and thereby the ensuing decrease in pulmonary antibacterial defenses (205).

Specific antiviral immunity, however, does not preclude infection with a heterologous virus, which would again increase host susceptibility to secondary bacterial complications. This contention is supported by the experimental observation that mice recovered from parainfluenza with influenza virus (206). As with the initial infection, pulmonary antibacterial defenses were again suppressed seven days after the second virus infection.

The efficacy of antibacterial immunity in preventing bacterial superinfections appears to depend on the organism. Active and passive immunization with *Proteus mirabilis* prevents the proliferation of the homologous organism in virus-infected lungs (61). In contrast, when the immunizing and challenge organism was *Staphylococcus aureus,* neither immunization procedure protected the animals from the virus-induced bactericidal defect (27). The reason for these divergent effects of specific bacterial immunity between the two organisms is unknown; however, the results again point out the importance of the bacteria in viral-bacterial interactions in the lungs.

To prevent virus-associated bacterial superinfections, strategies for immunization should consider the fact that the viral infection induces a general impairment of pulmonary antibacterial defenses. This is amply demonstrated by the observation that even one of the most innocuous bacterial species *(Serratia marcescens)* will proliferate in the lungs of animals with experimental influenza (Jakab, unpublished observations) and that in the case of human influenza no one bacterial species is responsible for all cases of post-influenzal bacterial pneumonia. Loosli (3,4) suggested that the prevalence of a specific superinfecting microbe during influenza epidemics depended on the presence of the bacteria in the community at the time of the virus infection. Thus, the picture emerges that a multitude of bacteria are capable of superinfecting a lung predisposed by infection with a single virus (207-214). Therefore, it would appear that immunization against the virus may be more targeted in terms of protection against bacterial superinfections than immunization against a multitude of bacteria. The *caveat,* however, remains that each case has to be considered independently.

Discussion and Summary

This review has dealt primarily with influenza and parainfluenza virus infections of the rodent lung as a model to elucidate the mechanisms by which virus infections predispose to secondary bacterial pneumonias. Since the healthy lung parenchyma is sterile and the lung has the inordinate capacity to inactivate large numbers of inhaled or aspirated bacteria, the approach has stressed the antibacterial defenses of the lung and the mechanisms of suppression by virus infection which, in turn, paves the way to secondary bacterial superinfections.

The bulk of the reviewed literature has dealt with *in vivo* studies. Other studies used the *"semi-in vitro"* approach of harvesting alveolar macrophages from virus-infected animals and examining phagocytic activity *in vitro* which allows virus-macrophage interactions to take place in the intact animal (215,216). These *in situ* interactions are important since pure *in vitro* studies (where the alveolar macrophages are collected from normal animals, infected in culture and then examined for defects in phagocytosis) do not necessarily reflect the phagocytic derangements observed in macrophages retrieved from virus-infected lungs (217-229) and described herein. This is an important distinction to make since it has led to divergent considerations of the mechanisms by which viruses alter phagocyte function. This dichotomy between *in vivo* and *in vitro* results is not surprising since factors such as interferon, antibody, complement, lymphocytes and most likely other intermediate helper or suppressor components generated by the virus in the animal are not present *in vitro*. Thus, it should be pointed out that mechanisms may differ from one model or set of circumstances to another and apparent conflicts in results may reflect real differences between models rather than accuracy of experimental work.

In addition to what is currently known about the mechanisms by which viral infections suppress host defenses and pave the way to bacterial superinfections, there exists a whole series of imponderables commonly referred to as *host factors,* which undoubtedly also contribute to viral-bacterial interactions in the lung. Inhalation of air pollutants, smoking, alcoholic intoxication, stress, and a myriad of other exogenous factors are known to impair pulmonary antibacterial defenses (21) as are endogenous factors which include genetic endowment, nutritional status, preexisting disease conditions and specific immune status. These host variables, whether inherited or acquired through life experiences may act as concomitant stressors in concert with viral infections to further aggravate the antibacterial defenses of the lungs.

Few data are available on the incidence of secondary bacterial infections. Clinical studies suggest that the frequency might be as high as 40 percent (2,3,180,230,231). This value appears to correlate well with animal models of virus pneumonia. Several experimental studies have demonstrated that members of the normal upper respiratory tract flora appear and multiply in the lung parenchyma in approximately one-third of the animals during viral pneumonitis (94,232-234). It has been our experience that the incidence varies with the severity of the infection; generally, a greater percentage of mice with severe viral pneumonia become superinfected with endogenous respiratory tract flora than of animals with a milder form of the viral infection.

The observation that not all viral pneumonias predispose to secondary bacterial superinfections suggests that conditions must be appropriate for the phenomenon to occur. This undoubtedly involves the interplay of many factors until a threshold is reached when the antibacterial defenses of the lungs are sufficiently overwhelmed for bacterial infections to ensue. Undoubtedly the magnitude of the virus-induced alterations is an important factor.

Qualitatively this means that all the defenses may have to be affected by the virus infection for the inception of bacterial superinfection. For example, lung macrophage dysfunction alone might not be sufficient to cause secondary bacterial complications if the upper respiratory tract were not colonized with potentially pathogenic bacteria. Alternatively, inhalation of a cloud of bacteria at this time would assure the delivery of the microbes into the deep lung to initiate infection. Finally, as mentioned above, host factors and other noninfectious influences which impinge upon the resistance of the host may also have a role in the formula which determines whether the virus-infected host will develop secondary bacterial complications.

References

1.   Mackowiak PA:Microbial synergism in human health. New England J Med 289:21-26 and 83-87, 1978.

2.   Loosli CG:Synergism between respiratory viruses and bacteria. Yale J Biol Med 40:522-540, 1967.

3.   Loosli CG:Influenza and the interaction of viruses and bacteria in respiratory infections. Medicine 52:369-384, 1973.

4. Stuart-Harris CH:The influenza viruses and the human respiratory tract. Rev Infect Dis 1:592-599, 1979.

5. Ansfield MJ, Woods DE, Johanson WG Jr.:Lung bacterial clearance in murine pneumococal pneumonia. Infect Immun 17:195-204, 1977.

6. Berendt RF:Relationship of method of administration to respiratory virulence of *Klebsiella pneumoniae* for mice and squirrel monkeys. Infect Immun 20:581-583, 1978.

7. Jay SJ, Johanson WG Jr., Pierce AK, Reisch JS:Determinants of lung bacterial clearance in normal mice. J Clin Invest 57:811-817, 1976.

8. Jakab GJ:Factors influencing the immune enhancement of intrapulmonary bactericidal mechanisms. Infect Immun 14:389-398, 1976.

9. Onofrio JM, Shulkin AN, Heidbrink PJ, Toews GB, Pierce AK:Pulmonary clearance and phagocytic cell response to normal pharyngeal flora. Am Rev Respir Dis 123:222-225, 1981.

10. Rehm SR, Gross GN, Pierce AK:Early bacterial clearance from murine lungs; species-dependent phagocytic response. J Clin Invest 66:194-199, 1980.

11. Ruppert D,Jakab GJ, Sylwester DL, Green GM:Sources of variance in the measurement of intrapulmonary killing of bacteria. J Lab Clin Med 87:544-558, 1976.

12.   Sato Y, Izumiyama K, Sato H, Cowell JL, Mannclark DR:Aerosol infection of mice with *Bordetella pertussis.* Infect Immun 29:261-266, 1980.

13.   Southern PM Jr., Mayes BB, Pierce AK, Sanford JP:Pulmonary clearance of *Pseudomonas aeruginosa.* J Lab Clin Med 76:548-559, 1970.

14.   Southern PM Jr., Pierce AK, Sanford JP:Comparison of the pulmonary bactericidal capacity of mice and rats against strains of *Pseudomonas aeruginosa.* Appld Microbiol 21:377-378, 1971.

15.   Southern PM Jr., Pierce AK, Sanford JP:Clearance of *Serratia marcescens* from lungs of normal mice.   Infect Immun 3:187-188, 1971.

16.   Brownstein DG, Smith AL, Johnson EA:Sendai virus infection in genetically resistant and susceptible mice. Am J Pathol 105:156-163, 1981.

17.   Brownstein DG:Genetics of natural resistance to Sendai virus infection in mice.   Infect Immun 41:308-312, 1983.

18.   Lindenmann J, Deuel E, Fanconi S, Haller O:Inborn resistance of mice to myxoviruses: macrophages express phenotype *in vitro.* J Exp Med 147:531-540, 1978.

19.   Parker JC, Whiteman MD, Richter CB:Susceptibility of inbred and outbred mouse strains to Sendai virus and

prevalence of infection in laboratory rodents. Infect Immun 19:123-130, 1978.

20. Green GM:Host variables in pulmonary responses to environment, in Lee DHK (ed): Environmental Factors in Respiratory Disease. New York, NY, Academic Press, 1972.

21. Huber GL, LaForce MF, Johanson WG Jr.:Experimental models and pulmonary antimicrobial defenses, in Brain JD, Proctor DF, Reid LM (eds): Respiratory Defense Mechanisms Part II. New York, NY, Marcell Dekker, Inc., 1977.

22. Jakab GJ, Green GM:Variations in pulmonary antibacterial defenses among experimental animals. Infect Immun 11:601-602, 1975.

23. Sherman M, Goldstein E, Lippert W, Wennberg R:Neonatal lung defense mechanisms: a study of the alveolar macrophage system in neonatal rabbits. Am Rev Respir Dis 116:433-440, 1977.

24. Verhoef J, Verbrugh HA:Host determinants in staphylococcal disease. Ann Rev Med 32:107-122, 1981.

25. Couch RB:The effects of influenza on host defenses. J Infect Dis 144:284-291, 1981.

26. Jastrand C, Tunevall G:The significance of bacterial superinfection in influenza. Scand J Infect Dis 6:137-144, 1974.

27.   Jakab GJ:Pulmonary defense mechanisms and the interaction between viruses and bacteria in acute respiratory infections.   Bull Europ Physiopath Resp 13:119-135, 1977.

28.   Jakab GJ:Interactions between Sendai virus and bacterial pathogens in the murine lung: a review. Lab Anim Sci 31:170-177, 1981.

29.   Green GM, Jakab GJ, Low RB, Davis GS:Defense mechanisms of the respiratory membrane.   Am Rev Respir Dis 115:479-514, 1977.

30.   Kazmierowski JA, Aduan RP, Reynolds HY:Pulmonary host defense: coordinated interaction of mechanical, cellular and humoral immune systems of the lung.   Bull Europ Physiopath Resp 13:103-116, 1977.

31.   Reynolds HY:Lung host defenses: a status report. Chest 75 (suppl):239-242, 1979.

32.   Wilkie BN:Respiratory tract immune response to microbial pathogens.   J Am Vet Med Assoc 181:1074-1079, 1982.

33.   Heath RB:The pathogenesis of respiratory viral infection.   Postgrad Med J 55:122-127, 1979.

34.   Green GM, Kass EH:The role of the alveolar macrophage in the clearance of bacteria from the lung.   J Exp Med 119:167-176, 1964.

35.   Goldstein E, Lippert W, Warshauer D:Pulmonary alveolar macrophage. Defender against bacterial infection of the lung. J Clin Invest 54:519-528, 1974.

36.   Goldstein E, Bartlema HC:Role of the alveolar macrophage in pulmonary bacterial defense. Bull Europ Physiopath Resp 13:57-67, 1977.

37.   Kim M, Goldstein E, Lewis JP, Lippert W, Warshauer D:Murine pulmonary alveolar macrophage; rates of bacterial ingestion, inactivation, and destruction. J Infect Dis 133:310-320, 1976.

38.   Coonrod DJ, Yoneda K:Comparative role of complement in pneumococcal and staphylococcal pneumonia. Infect Immun 37:1270-1277, 1982.

39.   Cybulski MI, Movat H:Experimental bacterial pneumonia in rabbits: polymorphanuclear leukocyte margination and sequestration in rabbit lungs and quantitation and kinetics of 52 Cr-labeled polymorphonuclear leukocytes in *E-coli*-induced lung lesions. Exp Lung Res 4:47-66, 1982.

40.   Heidbrink PJ, Toews GB, Gross GN, Pierce AK:Mechanism of complement-mediated clearance of bacteria from the murine lung. Am Rev Respir Dis 125:517-520, 1982.

41.   Larsen GL, Mitchell BC, Harper TB, Henson PM:The pulmonary response of C5 sufficient and deficient mice to *Pseudomonas aeruginosa.* Am Rev Respir Dis 126:306-311, 1982.

42.   Lipscomb MF, Onofrio JM, Nash EJ, Pierce AK, Toews GB:A morphological study of the role of phagocytes in the clearance of *Staphylococcus aureus* from the lung.   J Reticuloendothel Soc 33:420-442, 1983.

43.   Onofrio JM, Toews GB, Lipscomb MF, Pierce AK:Granulocyte-alveolar-macrophage interaction in pulmonary clearance of *Staphylococcus aureus.* Am Rev Respir Dis 127:335-341, 1983.

44.   Pierce AK, Reynolds RC, Harris GD:Leukocytic response to inhaled bacteria.   Am Rev Respir Dis 116:679-684, 1977.

45.   Rehm SR, Gross GN, Hart DA, Pierce AK:Animal model of neutropenia suitable for the study of dual-phagocyte systems.   Infect Immun 25:299-303, 1979.

46.   Rehm SR, Coonrod JD:Early clearance of pneumococci from the lungs of decomplemented rats.   Infect Immun 36:24-29, 1982.

47.   Rylander R, Sneall MC, Garcia I:Pulmonary cell response patterns after exposure to airborne bacteria. Scand J Respir Dis 56:195-200, 1975.

48.   Astry CL, Warr GA, Jakab GJ:Impairment of polymorphonuclear leukocyte immigration as a mechanism of alcohol-induced suppression of pulmonary antibacterial defenses.   Am Rev Respir Dis 128:113-117, 1983.

49.   Densen P, Mandell GL:Phagocyte strategy vs. microbial tactics. Rev Infect Dis 2:817-838, 1980.

50.   Orskov F:Virulence factors of the bacterial cell surface. J Infect Dis 137:630-633, 1978.

51.   Peterson PK, Quie PG:Bacterial surface components and the pathogenesis of infectious diseases. Ann Rev Med 32:29-43, 1981.

52.   Baseler MW,Fogelmark B, Burrell R:Differential toxicity of inhaled Gram-negative bacteria. Infect Immun 40:133-138, 1983.

53.   Blackwood LL, Stone RM, Iglewski BH, Pennington JE:Evaluation of *Pseudomonas aeruginosa* exotoxin A and elastase as virulence factors in acute lung injury. Infect Immun 39:198-201, 1983.

54.   Blackwood LL, Pennington JE:Influence of mucoid coating on clearance of *Pseudomonas aeruginosa* from lungs. Infect Immun 32:443-448, 1981.

55.   Hsieh S, Goldstein E, Lippert W, Margulies L:Effect of protein A on the antistaphylococcal defense mechanisms of the murine lungs. J Infect Dis 138:754-759, 1978.

56.   Lyerly DM,Kreger A:Importance of *Serratia* protease in the pathogenesis of experimental *Serratia marcescens* pneumonia. Infect Immun 40:113-119, 1983.

57. Gross GN, Rehm SR, Toews GB, Hart DA, Pierce AK:Lung clearance of *Staphylococcus aureus* strains with differing protein A content: protein A effect on *in vivo* clearance. Infect Immun 21:7-9, 1978.

58. Johanson WG Jr., Jay SJ, Pierce AK:Bacterial growth *in vivo*. An important determinant of the pulmonary clearance of *Diplococcus pneumoniae* in rats. J Clin Invest 53:1320-1325, 1974.

59. Toews GB, Gross GN, Pierce AK:The relationship of inoculum size to lung bacterial clearance and phagocytic cell response in mice. Am Rev Respir Dis 120:559-566, 1979.

60. Cryz SJ Jr., Furer E, Germanier R:Passive protection against *Pseudomonas aeruginosa* infection in an experimental leukopenic mouse model. Infect Immun 40:659-664, 1983.

61. Jakab GJ, Green GM:Immune enhancement of pulmonary bactericidal activity in murine virus pneumonia. J Clin Invest 52:2878-2884, 1973.

62. Smith RH, Babiuk LA, Stockdale PHG:Intranasal immunization of mice against *Pasteurella multocida*. Infect Immun 31:129-135, 1981.

63. Sordelli DO, Cerquetti MC, Hooke AM, Bellanti JA:Enhancement of *Pseudomonas aeruginosa* lung clearance

after local immunization with temperature-sensitive mutant. Infect Immun 39:1275-1290, 1983.

64. Kazmierowski JA, Gallin JI, Reynolds HY:Mechanism for the inflammatory response in primate lungs. Demonstration and partial characterization of an alveolar macrophage-derived chemotactic factor with preferential activity for polymorphonuclear leukocytes. J Clin Invest 59:273-281, 1977.

65. Larsen GL, Mitchell BC, Henson PM:The pulmonary response of C5 sufficient and deficient mice to immune complexes. Am Rev Respir Dis 123:434-439, 1981.

66. Hudson AR, Kilburn KH, Halprin GM, McKenzie WN:Granulocyte recruitment to airways exposed to endotoxin aerosols. Am Rev Respir Dis 115:89-95, 1977.

67. Larsen GL, Henson PM:Mediators of inflammation. Ann Rev Immunol 1:335-359, 1983.

68. Morrison DC, Kleine LF:Activation of the classical and properdin pathway of complement by bacterial polysaccharides (LPS). J Immunol 118:362-366, 1977.

69. Hoshino A, Takenaka H, Mizukoshi O, Imanishi J, Kishida T, Tovey MG:Effect of anti-interferon serum on influenza virus infection in mice. Antiviral Res 3:59-65, 1983.

70. Wyde PR, Wilson MR, Cate TR:Interferon production by leukocytes infiltrating the lungs of mice during primary influenza virus infection. Infect Immun 38:1249-1255, 1982.

71. Zee YC, Osebold JW, Dotson WM:Antibody responses and interferon titers in the respiratory tracts of mice after aerosolized exposure to influenza virus. Infect Immun 25:202-207, 1979.

72. Hicks JT, Ennis FA, Kim E, Verbonitz M:The importance of an intact complement pathway in recovery from a primary viral infection: influenza in decomplemented and in C5-deficient mice. J Immunol 121:1437-1445, 1978.

73. Onions DE:The immune response to virus infections. Vet Immunol Immunopathol 4:237-277, 1983.

74. Virelizier JL:Host defenses against influenza virus; the role of anti-hemagglutinin antibody. J Immunol 115:434-439, 1975.

75. Virelizier JL, Allison AC, Schild GC:Immune responses to influenza in the mouse, and their control of the infection. Br Med Bull 35:65-68, 1979.

76. Blandford G, Heath RB:Studies on the immune response and pathogenesis of Sendai virus infection of mice. II. The immunoglobulin class of plasma cells in the bronchial sub-mucosa. Immunol 26:667-671, 1974.

77.   Charlton   D,   Blandford   G:Immunoglobulin class-specific antibody response in serum, spleen, lungs, and bronchoalveolar washings after primary and secondary Sendai virus infection of germ-free mice.   Infect Immun 17:521-527, 1977.

78.   Scott GH, Walker JS:Immunoglobulin-bearing cells in lungs of mice infected with influenza virus.   Infect Immun 13:1525-1527, 1976.

79.   Lucas SJ, Barry DW, Kind P:Antibody production and protection against influenza virus in immunodeficient mice. Infect Immun 20:115-119, 1978.

80.   Anderson MJ, Pattison JR, Cureton RJR, Argent S, Heath RB:The role of host responses in the recovery of mice from Sendai virus infection.   J Gen Virol 46:373-379, 1980.

81.   Leung KN, Ada GL:Induction of natural killer cells during influenza virus infection.   Immunobiol 160:352-366, 1981.

82.   Reiss Cs, Schulman JL:Cellular immune responses of mice to   influenza virus infection.   Cell   Immunol 56:502-509, 1980.

83.   Wells MA, Ennis FA, Daniel S:Cytotoxic T-cell and antibody responses to influenza infection of mice. J Gen Virol 43:685-690, 1979.

84. Yap KL, Ada GL:Cytotoxic T cells in the lungs of mice infected with influenza A virus. Scand J Immunol 7:73-80, 1978.

85. Yap KL, Ada GL:The recovery of mice from influenza A virus infection: adoptive transfer of immunity with influenza virus-specific cytotoxic T lymphocytes recognizing a common virion antigen. Scand J Immunol 8:413-420, 1978.

86. McMichael AJ, Gotch FM, Noble GR, Beare PA:Cytotoxic T-cell immunity to influenza. New Engl J Med 309:13-17, 1983.

87. Wells MA, Albrecht P, Ennis FA:Recovery from a viral respiratory infection. I. Influenza pneumonia in normal and T-deficient mice. J Immunol 126:1036-1041, 1981.

88. Wells MA, Ennis FA, Albrecht P:Recovery from a viral respiratory infection. II. Passive transfer of immune spleen cells to mice with influenza pneumonia. J Immunol 126:1042-1046, 1981.

89. Wells MA, Daniel S, Djeu JY, Kiley SC, Ennis FA:Recovery from a viral respiratory tract infection. IV. Specificity of protection by cytotoxic T lymphocytes. J Immunol 130:2908-2914, 1983.

90.   Sissons JGP, Schreiber RD, Cooper NR, Oldstone MBA:The role of antibody and complement in lysis of virus-infected cells.   Med Microbiol Immunol 170:221-227, 1982.

91.   Ennis A:Some newly recognized aspects of resistance against and recovery from influenza. Arch Virol 73:207-217, 1982.

92.   Ada GL, Leung KN, Ertl H:An analysis of effector T cell generation and function in mice exposed to influenza or Sendai viruses.   Immunol Rev 58:5-24, 1981.

93.   Green GM:Patterns of bacterial clearance in murine influenza.   Antimicrob Agents Chemother 1965:26-29, 1966.

94.   Jakab GJ, Dick EC:Synergistic effect in viral-bacterial infection: combined infection of the murine respiratory tract with Sendai virus and *Pasteurella pneumotropica*. Infect Immun 8:762-768, 1973.

95.   Jakab GJ:Effect of sequential inoculation of Sendai virus and *Pasteurella pneumotropica* in mice.   J Am Vet Med Assoc 164:723-728, 1974.

96.   Jakab GJ:Suppression of pulmonary antibacterial activity following Sendai virus infection in mice: dependence on virus dose.   Arch Virol 48:385-390, 1975.

97.   Harford CG, Leidler V, Hara M:Effect of the lesion due to influenza virus on the resistance of mice to inhaled pneumococci.   J Exp Med 89:53-69, 1949.

98.   Harford CG, Hara M:Pulmonary edema in influenzal pneumonia of the mouse and the relation of fluid in the lung to the inception of pneumococcal pneumonia.   J Exp Med 91:245-263, 1950.

99.   Harford CG, Hamlin A:Effect of influenza virus on cilia and epithelial cells in the bronchi of mice. J Exp Med 95:173-187, 1952.

100.   Camner   P,   Jarstrand   C,   Philipson K:Tracheobronchial clearance in patients with influenza. Am Rev Respir Dis 108:131-135, 1973.

101.   Creasia DA, Nettesheim P, Hammons AS:Impairment of deep lung clearance by influenza virus infection. Arch Env Health 25:197-201, 1973.

102.   Jakab GJ, Green GM:Effect of hypersensitivity pneumonitis on the pulmonary defense mechanisms of guinea pig lungs.   Infect Immun 7:39-45, 1973.

103.   Jakab GJ, Green GM:Pulmonary defense mechanisms in consolidated and nonconsolidated regions of lungs infected with Sendai virus.   J Infect Dis 129:263-270, 1974.

104.   Jakab GJ, Green GM:The effect of Sendai virus infection on bactericidal and transport mechanisms of the murine lung.   J Clin Invest 51:1989-1998, 1972.

105.   Warshauer D, Goldstein E, Akers T, Lippert W, Kim M:Effect of influenza viral infection of the ingestion and

killing of bacteria by alveolar macrophages. Am Rev Respir Dis 115:269-277, 1977.

106.   Jakab GJ, Green GM:Defect in intracellular killings of *Staphylococcus aureus* within alveolar macrophages in Sendai virus-infected murine lungs. J Clin Invest 57:1533-1539, 1976.

107.   Warr GA, Jakab GJ, Hearst JE:Alterations in lung macrophage immune receptor(s) activity associated with viral pneumonia. J Reticuloendothel Soc 26:357-366, 1979.

108.   Warr GA, Jakab GJ:Alterations in lung macrophage antimicrobial activity associated with viral pneumonia. Infect Immun 26:492-497, 1979.

109.   Jakab GJ, Warr GA, Sannes PL:Alveolar macrophage ingestion and phagosome-lysosome fusion defect associated with virus pneumonia. Infect Immun 27:960-968, 1980.

110.   Taylor RN, Dietz TM, Maxwell KW, Marcus S:Effect of influenza virus infection on phagocytic and cytopeptic capacities of guinea pig macrophages. Immunol Commun 3:439-455, 1974.

111.   Silverberg BA, Jakab GJ, Thomson RG, Warr GA, Boo KS:Ultrastructural alterations in phagocytic functions of alveolar macrophages after parainfluenza virus infection. J Reticuloendothel Soc 25:405-416, 1979.

112.   Jakab GJ:Mechanisms of virus-induced bacterial superinfections of the lung. Clin Chest Med 2:59-66, 1981.

113.   Warr GA, Jakab GJ, Chan TW, Tsan MF:Effects of viral pneumonia on lung macrophage lysosomal enzymes. Infect Immun 24:577-579, 1979.

114.   Kleinerman ES, Snyderman R, Daniels CA:Depression of human monocyte chemotaxis by herpes simplex and influenza viruses. J Immunol 113:1562-1567, 1974.

115.   Kleinerman ES, Snyderman R, Daniels CA:Depressed monocyte chemotaxis during acute influenza infection. Lancet 2:1063-1066, 1975.

116.   Kleinerman ES, Daniels CA, Polisson RP, Snyderman R:Effects of virus infection on the inflammatory response. Depression of macrophage accumulation in influenza-infected mice. Am J Pathol 65:373-382, 1976.

117.   Pike MC, Daniels DA, Snyderman R:Influenza-induced depression of monocyte chemotaxis: reversal by levamisole. Cell Immunol 32:234-238, 1977.

118.   Ruutu P, Vaheri A, Kosunen TU:Depression of human neutrophil motility by influenza virus *in vitro.* Scand J Immunol 6:897-906, 1977.

119.   Warr GA, Jakab GJ:Pulmonary inflammatory responses during viral pneumonia and secondary bacterial infection. Inflammation 7:93-104, 1983.

120. Wyde PR, Cate TR:Cellular changes in lungs of mice infected with influenza virus: characterization of the cytotoxic responses. Infect Immun 22:423-429, 1978.

121. Wyde PR, Peavy DL, Cate TR:Morphological and cytochemical characterization of cells infiltrating mouse lungs after influenza infection. Infect Immun 21:140-146, 1978.

122. Abramson JS, Giebink GS, Mills EL, Quie PG:Polymorphonuclear leukocyte dysfunction during influenza virus infection in chinchillas. J Infect Dis 143:836-845, 1981.

123. Abramson JS, Giebink GS, Quie PG:Influenza A virus-induced polymorphonuclear leukocyte dysfunction in the pathogenesis of experimental pneumococcal otisi media. Infect Immun 36:289-296, 1982.

124. Ruutu T, Kosunen T:Phagocytic activity of neutorphilic leukocytes of A2 influenza patients. Acta Path Microbiol Scand (Sec B) 79:67-72, 1971.

125. Martin RR, Couch RB, Greenberg SB, Cate TR, Warr GA:Effects of infection with influenza virus on the function of polymorphonuclear leukocytes. J Infect Dis 144:279, 1981.

126. Sawyer WD:Interaction of influenza virus with leukocytes and its effect on phagocytosis. J Infect Dis 119:541-556, 1969.

127.   Nugent KM, Pesanti EL:Effect of influenza infection on the phagocytic and bactericidal activities of pulmonary macrophages. Infect Immun 26:651-657, 1979.

128.   Mills J:Effects of Sendai virus infection on function of cultured mouse alveolar macrophages. Am Rev Respir Dis 120:1239-1244, 1979.

129.   Carthew P, Sparrow S:Sendai virus in nude and germ-free rats. Res Vet Sci 29:289-292, 1980.

130.   Sullivan JL, Mayner RE, Barry DW, Ennis FA:Influenza virus infection in nude mice. J Infect Dis 133:91-94, 1976.

131.   Wyde PR, Couch RB, Mackler BF, Cate TR, Levy MB:Effects of low- and high-passage influenza virus infection in normal and nude mice. Infect Immun 15:221-229, 1977.

132.   Berlin BS, Cochran KW:Delay of fatal pneumonia in X-irradiated mice inoculated with mouse-adapted influenza virus, PR8 strain. Rad Res 31:343-351, 1967.

133.   Blandford G:Studies on the immune response and pathogenesis of Sendai virus infection of mice. III. The effects of cyclophosphamide. Immunol 28:871-883, 1975.

134.   Finnie JC, Aston WP, O'Shaughnessy MV, Stewart RB:The effect of decomplementation on the infectious course of Sendai virus in mice. Can J Microbiol 28:474-477, 1982.

135.   Hurd J, Heath RB:Effect of cyclophosphamide on infection in mice caused by virulent and avirulent strains of influenza virus. Infect Immun 11:886-889, 1975.

136.   Cate TR, Mold NG:Increased influenza pneumonia mortality of mice adoptively immunized with node and spleen cells sensitized by inactivated but not live virus. Infect Immun 11:908-914, 1975.

137.   Jakab GJ, Warr GA:Lung defenses against viral and bacterial challenges during immunosuppression with cyclophosphamide in mice.   Am Rev Respir Dis 123:524-528. 1981.

138.   Shimomura E, Suzuki F, Ishida N:Characterization of cells infiltrating the lungs of X-irradiated and nude mice after influenza virus infection.   Microbiol Immunol 26:129-138, 1982.

139.   Singer SH, Noguchi P, Kirschstein RL:Respiratory diseases in cyclophosphamide-treated mice.   II.   Decreased virulence of PR8 influenza virus.   Infect Immun 5:957-960, 1972.

140.   Suzuki F, Ohya J, Ishida N:Effect of antilymphocyte serum on influenza virus infection in mice. Proc Soc Exp Biol Med 146:78-84, 1974.

141.   Robinson TWE, Cureton RJR, Heath RB:The effect of cyclophosphamide on Sendai virus infection of mice. J Med Microbiol 2:137-145, 1969.

142.   Jakab GJ:Immune impairment of alveolar macrophage phagocytosis during influenza virus pneumonia.   Am Rev Respir Dis 126:778-782, 1982.

143.   Jakab GJ, Warr GA:The participation of antiviral immune mechanisms in alveolar macrophage dysfunctions during viral pneumonia.   Bull Europ Physiopath Resp 19:173-178, 1983.

144.   Jakab GJ, Warr GA:Immune-enhanced phagocytic dysfunction in pulmonary macrophages infected with parainfluenza 1 (Sendai) virus.   Am Rev Respir Dis 124:575-581, 1981.

145.   Bowen HA, Lyles DS:Structure of Sendai viral proteins in plasma membranes of virus-infected cells. J Virol 37:1079-1082, 1981.

146.   Buechi M, Bachi TH:Microscopy of internal structures of Sendai virus associated with the cytoplasmic surface of host membranes.   Virol 120:349-358, 1982.

147.   Burns WH, Allison AC:Surface antigens of virus-infected cells, in Poste G, Nicolson GL (eds): Virus Infection and the Cell Surface. Elsevier/North-Holland Biomedical Press, 1977.

148.   Hackett CJ, Askonas BA:H-2 and viral haemagglutinin expression by influenza-virus-infected cells; the proteins are close but do not cocap.   Immunol 45:431-438, 1982.

149.   Kohama MT, Cardenas JM, Seto JT:Immunoelectron microscopic study of the detection of the glycoproteins of influenza and Sendai viruses in infected cells by the immunoperoxidase method.   J Virol Meth 3:293-301, 1981.

150.   Lindenmann J:Host antigens in enveloped RNA viruses, in Post G, Nicolson GL (eds):   Virus Infections and the Cell Surface.   Elsevier/North-Holland Biomedical Press, 1977.

151.   Shaw MW, Lamon EW, Compans RW:Surface expression of a nonstructural antigen on influenza A virus-infected cells.   Infect Immun 34:1065-1067, 1981.

152.   Brier AM, Wohlenberg C, Rosenthal J, Mage M, Notkins AL:Inhibition or enhancement of immunological injury of virus-infected cells.   Proc Nat Acad Sci 68:3073-3077, 1971.

153.   Forman J:The specificity of thymus-derived T-cells in cell-mediated reactions.   Transplan Rev 29:145-163, 1976.

154.   Sissons JGP, Oldstone MBA:Antibody-mediated destruction of virus-infected cells.   Adv Immunol 29:209-255, 1980.

155.   Hosaka Y, Fukami Y, Yasuda Y, Bonilla JA:Complement-dependent antiviral monospecific antibody-mediated lysis of murine cells coated with Sendai

virus or its envelope component.   Infect Immun 27:355-363, 1980.

156.   Yilma T, Zee YC, Osebold JW:Immunofluorescence determination of the pathogenesis of infection with influenza virus in mice following exposure to aerosolized virus.   J Infect Dis 139:458-464, 1979.

157.   Griffin FM:Effects of soluble immune complexes on Fc receptor- and C3b receptor-mediated phagocytosis by macrophages.   J Exp Med 152:905-919, 1980.

158.   Kavai M, Sandor M, Szegedi GY, Fust G, Gergely J:Effect of soluble immune complexes of Fc and C3 receptor-dependent phagocytosis by human monocytes. Immunol 44:599-606, 1981.

159.   Michl J, Unkeless JC, Pieczonka M, Silverstein SC:Modulation of Fc receptors of mononuclear phagocytes by immobilized antigen-antibody complexes.   J Exp Med 157:1746-1757, 1983.

160.   Rabinovitch M, Manejias RE, Nussenzweig V:Selective phagocytic paralysis induced by immobilized immune complexes.   J Exp Med 142:827-838, 1975.

161.   Blandford G:Arthus reaction and pneumonia.   Br Med J 1:758-759, 1970.

162.   Pernice W, Schmitz H, Schindera F, Behrens F, Sedlacek HH:Antigen-specific detection of immune complexes

in patients with hepatitis B, influenza A and rubella. Behring Inst Mitt 64:102-108, 1979.

163.   Astry CL, Jakab GJ:Influenza virus-induced immune complexes suppress alveolar macrophage phagocytosis.   J of Virology.   In press..

164.   Blandford G, Charlton D:Studies of pulmonary and renal immunopathology after nonlethal primary Sendai viral infection in normal and cyclophosphamide-treated hamsters. Am Rev Respir Dis 115:305-314, 1977.

165.   Scherzer H, Ward PA:Lung injury produced by immune complexes of varying composition.   J Immunol 121:947-952, 1978.

166.   Ward PA:Immune complex injury of the lung. Am J Pathol 97:85-91, 1979.

167.   Daniele RP, Henson PM, Fantone CJ III, Ward PA, Dreisin RB:Immune complex injury of the lung.   Am Rev Respir Dis 124:738-755, 1981.

168.   Johnson KJ, Ward PA:Biology of disease. Newer concepts in the pathogenesis of immune complex-induced tissue injury.   Lab Invest 47:218-226, 1982.

169.   Sanford BA, Shelokov A, Ramsay MA:Bacterial adherence to virus-infected cells: a cell culture model of bacterial superinfection.   J Infect Dis 137:176-181, 1978.

170.   Fainstein V, Musher DM:Bacterial adherence to pharyngeal cells in smokers, nonsmokers, and chronic bronchitics. Infect Immun 26:178-182, 1979.

171.   Johanson WG Jr., Woods DE, Chaudhuri T:Association of respiratory tract colonization with adherence of Gram-negative bacilli to epithelial cells.   J Infect Dis 139:667-673, 1979.

172.   Davidson VE, Sanford BA:Adherence of *Staphylococcus aureus* to influenza A virus-infected Madin-Darby canine kidney cells cultures. Infect Immun 32:118-126, 1981.

173.   Davidson VE, Sanford BA:Factors influencing adherence of *Staphylococcus aureus* to influenza A virus-infected cell cultures.   Infect Immun 37:946-955, 1982.

174.   Huang AS, Okorie TG:Surface analysis by bacterial adherence to virus-infected cells.   J Infect Dis 140:147-151, 1979.

175.   Selinger DS, Reed WP, McLaren LC:Model for studying bacterial adherence to epithelial cells infected with viruses. Infect Immun 32:941-944, 1981.

176.   Sanford BA, Davidson VE, Ramsay MA:Fibrinogen-mediated adherence of group A *Streptococcus* to influenza A virus-infected cell cultures.   Infect Immun 38:513-520, 1982.

177.   Jones WT, Menna JH:Influenza type A virus-mediated adherence of type 1a group B streptococci to mouse tracheal tissue *in vivo.* Infect Immun 38:791-794, 1982.

178.   Ramphal R, Small PM, Shands JW Jr., Fischlschweiger W, Small PA Jr.:Adherence of *Pseudomonas aeruginosa* to tracheal cells injured by influenza infection or by endotracheal intubation.   Infect Immun 27:614-619, 1980.

179.   Fainstein V, Musher DM, Cate TR:Bacterial adherence to pharyngeal cells during viral infection.   J Infect Dis 141:172-176, 1980.

180.   Smith CB, Golden C, Klauber MR, Kanner R, Renzetti A:Interactions between viruses and bacteria in patients with chronic bronchitis.   J Infect Dis 134:552-561, 1976.

181.   Loosli CG, Stinson SF, Ryan DP, Hertweck MS, Hardy JD, Serebrin R:The destruction of type 2 pneumocytes by airborne influenza PR8-A virus; its effect of surfactant and lecithin content of the pneumonic lesions of mice. Chest 67 (Suppl):7S-14S, 1975.

182.   Stinson SF, Ryan DP, Hertweck MS, Hardy JD, Hwang-Kow SY, Loosli CG:Epithelial and surfactant changes in influenzal pulmonary lesions.   Arch Path Labs Med 100:147-153, 1976.

183. LaForce FM, Kelly WJ, Huber GL:Inactivation of staphylococci by alveolar macrophages with preliminary observations on the importance of alveolar lining material. Am Rev Respir Dis 108:784-790, 1973.

184. LaForce FM:Effect of alveolar lining material on phagocytic and bactericidal activity of lung macrophages against *Staphylococcus aureus.* J Lab Clin Med 88:691-699, 1976.

185. Juers JA, Rogers RM, McCurdy JB, Cook WW:Enhancement of bactericidal capacity of alveolar macrophages by human alveolar lining material. J Clin Invest 58:271-275, 1976.

186. Coonrod DJ, Yoneda K:Detection and partial characterization of antibacterial factor(s) in alveolar lining material of rats. J Clin Invest 71:129-141, 1983.

187. LaForce FM, Boose DS:Sublethal damage of *Escherichia coli* by lung lavage. Am Rev Respir Dis 124:733-737, 1981.

188. Harris GD, Woods DE, Fine R, Johanson WG Jr.:The effect of intraalveolar fluid on lung bacterial clearance. Lung 158:91-100, 1980.

189. Nugent KM, Pesanti EL:Nonphagocytic clearance of *Staphylococcus aureus* from murine lungs. Infect Immun 36:1185-1191, 1982.

190.   Green GM, Kass EH:The influence of bacterial species on pulmonary resistance to infection in mice subjected to hypoxia, cold stress, and ethanolic intoxication. Br J Exp Pathol 46:360-366, 1965.

191.   Green GM, Kass EH:Factors influencing the clearance of bacteria by the lung.   J Clin Invest 43:769-776, 1964.

192.   Hall WJ, Douglas RG:Pulmonary function during and after common respiratory infections.   Ann Rev Med 31:233-238, 1980.

193.   Smith CB, Kanner RE, Golden CA, Klauber MR, Renzetti AD:Effect of viral infections on pulmonary function in patients with chronic obstructive pulmonary diseases. J Infect Dis 141:271-280, 1980.

194.   Rodgers B, Mims CA:Interaction of influenza virus with mouse macrophages.   Infect Immun 31:751-757, 1981.

195.   Kavet RI, Brain JD:Methods to quantify endocytosis: a review.   J Reticuloendothel Soc 27:201-221, 1980.

196.   Markham RJF, Wilkie BN:Interaction between *Pasteurella haemolytica* and bovine alveolarmacrophages. Cytotoxic effect on macrophages and impaired phagocytosis. Am J Vet Res 41:18-22, 1980.

197. Maheswaran SK, Berggren KA, Simonson RR, Ward GE, Muscoplar CC:Kinetics of interaction and fate of *Pasteurella hemolytica* in bovine alveolar macrophages.   Infect Immun 30:254-262, 1980.

198.   Markham   RJF,   Ramnaraine   MLR,   Muscoplat CC:Cytotoxic effect of *Pasteurella haemolytica* on bovine polymorphonuclear leukocytes and impaired production of chemotactic factors by *Pasteurella haemolytica*-infected alveolar macrophages. Am J Vet Res 43:285-288, 1982.

199.   Shewen PE, Wilkie BN:Cytotoxin of *Pasteurella haemolytica* acting on bovine leukocytes.   Infect Immun 35:91-94, 1982.

200.   Yates WDG:A review of infectious bovine rhinotracheitis,   shipping   fever   pneumonia   and viral-bacterial synergism in respiratory disease of cattle. Can J Comp Med 46:225-263, 1982.

201.   Bendixen PH, Shewen PE, Rosendal S, Wilkie BN:Toxicity of *Haemophilus pleuropneumoniae* for porcine lung macrophages, peripheral blood monocytes, and testicular cells. Infect Immun 33:673-676, 1981.

202. McGee MP, Kreger A, Leake ES, Harshman S:Toxicity of staphylococcal alpha toxin for rabbit alveolar macrophages. Infect Immun 39:439-444, 1983.

203.   Green HL, Green GM:Differential suppression of pulmonary antibacterial activity as the mechanism of selection of a pathogen in mixed bacterial infection of the lung. Am Rev Respir Dis 98:819-824, 1968.

204.   Nayak DP, Kelley GW, Underdahl NR:The effect of varied inoculums on the distribution and progression of influenza virus (S-15) in lungs of mice. Am J Vet Res 26:984-990, 1965.

205.   Goldstein E, Akers T, Prato C:Role of immunity in viral-induced bacterial superinfections of the lung. Infect Immun 8:757-761, 1973.

206.   Jakab GJ:Recurrent impairment of pulmonary antibacterial defenses induced by sequential infection with parainfluenza 1 (Sendai) virus and influenza A virus. Submitted for publication.

207.   Carthew P, Gannon J:Secondary infection of rat lungs with *Pasteurella pneumotropica* after Kilham rat virus infection. Lab Anim 15:219-221, 1981.

208.   Gardner ID:Effect of influenza virus infection on susceptibility to bacteria in mice. J Infect Dis 142:704-707, 1980.

209.   Goldstein E, Buhles WC, Akers TG, Vedros N:Murine resistance to inhaled *Neisseria meningitidis* after infection with an encephalomyocarditis virus. Infect Immun 6:398-402, 1972.

210.   Hamilton JR, Overall JC, Glasgow LA:Synergistic effect on mortality in mice with murine cytomegalovirus and *Pseudomonas aeruginosa, Staphylococcus aureus,* or *Candida albicans* infections. Infect Immun 14:982-989, 1976.

211.   Klein JO, Green GM, Tilles JG, Kass EH, Finland M:Effect of intranasal reovirus infection on antibacterial activity of mouse lung. J Infect Dis 119:43-50, 1969.

212.   Myerowitz RL, Michaels RH:Mechanism of potentiation of experimental *Haemophilus influenzae* type B disease in infant rats by influenza A virus. Lab Invest 44:434-441, 1981.

213.   Howard CJ, Stott EJ, Taylor G:The effect of pneumonia induced in mice with *Mycoplasma pulmonis* on resistance to subsequent bacterial infection and the effect of a respiratory infection with Sendai virus on the resistance to *Mycoplasma pulmonis.* J Genl Microbiol 109:79-87, 1978.

214.   Hugh R, Huangs KY, Elliott TB:Enhancement of bacterial infection in mice by Newcastle disease virus. Infect Immun 3:488-493, 1971.

215.   Mogensen SC:Viral interaction with phagocyte functions, in O'Grady F, Smith H (eds):   Microbial Perturbation of Host Defenses.   New York, NY, Academic Press, 1981.

216.   Sweet C:Viral interference with nonspecific nonphagocytic defenses, in O'Grady F, Smith H (eds): Microbial Perturbation of Host Defenses.   New York, NY, Academic Press, 181. 981.

217.   Abramson JS, Lyles DS, Heller KA, Bass DA:Influenza A virus-induced polymorphonuclear leukocyte dysfunction.   Infect Immun 37:794-799, 1982.

218.   Abramson JS, Mills EL, Giebink GS, Quie PG:Depression of monocyte and polymorphonuclear leukocyte oxidative metabolism and bactericidal capacity by influenza A virus.   Infect Immun 35:350-355, 1982.

219.   Abramson JS, Lewis JC, Lyles DS, Heller KA, Mills EL, Bass DA:Inhibition of neutrophil lysosome-phagosome fusion associated with influenza virus infection *in vitro.* J Clin Invest 69:1393-1397, 1982.

220.   Busse WW, Sosman JM:Altered luminol-dependent granulocyte chemiluminescence during an *in vitro* incubation with an influenza vaccine.   Am Rev Respir Dis 123:654-658, 1981.

221.   Debets-Ossenkopp Y, Mills EL, van Dijk WC, Verbrugh HA, Verhoef J:Effect of influenza virus on phagocytic cells.   Eur J Clin Microbiol 1:171-177, 1982.

222.   Fisher TN, Ginsberg HS:The reaction of influenza viruses with guinea pig polymorphonuclear leukocytes. II.

The reduction of white blood cell glycolysis by influenza viruses and receptor-destroying enzyme (RDE). Virol 2:637-655, 1956.

223.   Fisher TN, Ginsberg HS:The reaction of influenza viruses with guinea pig polymorphonuclear leukocytes. III. Studies on the mechanisms by which influenza viruses inhibit phagocytosis. Virol 2:656-664, 1956.

224.   Gardner ID, Lawton JWM:Depressed human monocyte function after influenza virus infection *in vitro.* J Reticuloendothel Soc 32:443-448, 1982.

225.   Ginsberg HS, Blackmon JR:Reactions of influenza viruses with guinea pig polumorphonuclear leukocytes. I. Virus-cell interactions. Virol 2:618-636, 1956.

226.   Larson HE, Blades R:Impairment of human polymorphonuclear leukocyte function by influenza virus. Lancet 1:283, 1976.

227.   Larson HE, Parry RP, Gilchrist C, Luquetti A, Tyrrell DAJ:Influenza viruses and staphylococci *in vitro:* some interactions with polymorphonuclear leukocytes and epithelial cells. Br J Exp Pat 58:281-288, 1977.

228.   Merchant DJ, Morgan HR:Inhibition of the phagocytic action of leukocytes by mumps and influenza viruses. Proc Soc Exp Biol Med 74:651-653, 1950.

229.   Rodgers BC, Mims CA:Influenza virus replication in human alveolar macrophages. J Med Virol 9:177-184, 1982.

230.   Eikoff   TC:Sero-epidemiologic   studies   on meningococcal   infection   with   indirect   hemagglutination test. J Infect Dis 123:519-526, 1971.

231.   Fekety FR Jr., Caldwell J, Gump D, Johnson JE, Maxson W, Mulholland J, Thoburn R:Bacteria, viruses, and mycoplasmas in acute pneumonia in adults. Am Rev Respir Dis 104:499-507, 1971.

232.   Phillips PA, Stanley NF, Waltern MNI:Murine disease induced by avian reovirus. Aust J Exp Biol Med Sci 48:277-284, 1970.

233.   Sellers RF, Schulman J, Bouvier C, McCune R, Kilbourne ED:The influence of influenza virus infection on exogenous staphylococcal and endogenous murine bacterial infecton of the bronchopulmonary tissues of mice. J Exp Med 114:237-255, 1961.

234.   Yealland SJ, Heath RB:The significance of secondary Gram-negative coliform infection of the lungs of mice with influenzal pneumonitis. Br J Exp Pathol 59:48-51, 1978.

Models for Bovine Respiratory Disease

L. A. Babiuk, Ph.D.

Department of Veterinary Microbiology
Western College of Veterinary Medicine
University of Saskatchewan
Saskatoon, Saskatchewan, Canada S7N 0W0

S. D. Acres, D.V.M., Ph.D.

Veterinary Infectious Disease Organization
University of Saskatchewan
Saskatoon, Saskatchewan, Canada S7N 0W0

Introduction

Bacterial colonization of the lower respiratory tract of healthy animals including cattle and man is a relatively rare event. However, in individuals suffering from a variety of diseases, including virus infections, colonization occurs rapidly. Thus it has been estimated that 90 percent of bacterial pneumonias develop after a viral infection or some other form of debilitation. Furthermore, individuals suffering from a viral pneumonia have a 40 percent chance of subsequently developing bacterial pneumonia (1,2). It has been suggested that the reasons for the increase in bacterial colonization of the lung are related to changes in the surface properties of epithelial cells lining the respiratory tract and resulting modifications to the local physiological environment.

These two changes allow greater numbers of bacteria to adhere to the surface of epithelial cells in the upper respiratory tract (URT) as well as to replicate at a faster rate. This increased rate of adherence and replication may result in the production of microcolonies which can then enter the lower respiratory tract (3).   If these microcolonies are enclosed by mucus and bacterial glycocalyx, they will be more difficult to phagocytize than individual bacteria and will be resistant to attack by antibodies or antibiotics (4).   In addition to the form and rate of bacteria entering the lung, the rate of bacterial clearance from the lung will determine whether or not colonization and disease occur.   Bacterial clearance can also be reduced or impaired by viral infections as well as other factors.

Some of the factors which can make animals more susceptible to bacterial colonization are management induced.   For example, present day management systems often stress animals and this presumably makes them more susceptible to bacterial colonization and also promotes transfer of pathogens between animals.   These pathogens further alter the respiratory tract environment and compromise the host's immune system allowing the development of bovine respiratory disease.   It must be emphasized that this is a disease complex involving a large number of interactions between the different stressors and pathogens with the host. For example, the cumulative effects of several stress factors acting synergistically or additively may be important, whereas one acting in isolation may not be sufficient to increase susceptibility (5). Thus, if one tries experimentally to induce susceptibility to shipping fever by transportation or environmental changes alone, it may not work. However, if several of these stress factors are combined, it might.

Considering these factors, we would like to propose that for infection of the lung and subsequent development of bacterial pneumonia to occur, a number of events are important. It is likely that not all of these events occur in every animal, or to the same degree in each animal or even in the same sequence. However, they do represent some of the known pathogenic mechanisms which result in pneumonia. Since *Pasteurella haemolytica,* particularly type 1A, is the most common bacterium isolated from cases of respiratory disease in North America, we will focus our attention on this organism. However, the following hypothetical sequence of events may also apply to other bacteria which occasionally cause pneumonia.

Observations

Colonization of the Upper Respiratory Tract

It appears that the first step involved in initiation of bovine respiratory disease is colonization of the URT by *Pasteurella haemolytica,* particularly the nasal-pharyngeal area including the tonsillar crypts.   The bacteria can remain localized in the URT for a long time but for some reason the level or degree of growth is limited and the animal does not exhibit any ill effects.   In fact, in many instances they may be so sequestered that regular swabbing does not reveal any *Pasteurella haemolytica*. The reasons why the bacteria remain localized are not well known; however, a variety of host immunological and physiological factors as well as bacterial characteristics are probably involved. However, under certain conditions they do migrate from the URT to the lung.   Whether this is due to factors which increase the rate of proliferation in the URT, decrease the rate of clearance or both remains to be determined. Preliminary observations suggest that stress and changes in environment caused by weaning, transportation and mixing may be sufficient to increase the rate of detection of *Pasteurella haemolytica* in the URT (unpublished results, also G. Frank, this Symposium) and this is often followed by movement down the trachea into the lung where rapid proliferation and production of disease occurs.

In man, increased colonization of the oropharynx with Gram-negative organisms followed by pneumonia has been correlated with reduced levels of fibronectin on the surface of epithelial cells (6). The quantities of cell-surface fibronectin vary with the physiological state of the cell as well as the environment. Viral infection tends to cause death of mature cells which have high levels of fibronectin on their surfaces. Replacement with immature dividing cells might result in lower levels of fibronectin leading to colonization by Gram-negative organisms (6,7). Furthermore, cell surface proteases could degrade fibronectin on adjacent cells and possibly favor adherence of Gram-negative bacteria. Additionally, cell death occurring as a result of virus infection could release intracellular proteases. Once sufficient numbers of bacteria are present, they could also produce proteases and further decrease fibronectin levels and favor additional colonization (6,8). None of these possibilities have been investigated in calves infected with *Pasteurella haemolytica*.

Bacterial Colonization of the Lower Respiratory Tract

Movement of bacteria from the URT to the lung can occur by a number of mechanisms. The most obvious method is by aerosolization of the organisms present in the URT and inhalation into the lungs. Since infected animals do contain bacteria in their airways, this appears to be a feasible method of entry (9) particularly if it continues for many hours or days. Entry of bacteria into the lungs of animals whose upper respiratory tracts are not colonized could also occur by breathing aerosolized bacteria from infected cohabitants. Entry into the lung could also occur by progressive colonization down the trachea with bacterial secretions, such as cytotoxin, impairing the action of cilia until the organism eventually reaches the lung. Thirdly, bacteria present in the upper respiratory tract could also be aspirated into the lung. Aspiration of bacterial microcolonies enclosed in mucus (10) or bacterial glycocalyx, which is present in large amounts on some strains of *Pasteurella haemolytica* (11), could render them more resistant to normal lung defense mechanisms such as phagocytosis, antibodies and surfactants (3).

Requirements for Disease

Two factors are essential for colonization of the lung and for disease to occur: (1) a susceptible host and (2) an environment conducive to the uncontrolled growth of *Pasteurella haemolytica* (Figure 1). As pointed out above, infection will not necessarily lead to disease because many cattle have large quantities of *Pasteurella haemolytica* present in their upper respiratory tracts for long periods of time without developing pneumonia. Presumably these bacteria enter the lung in low numbers and are efficiently and rapidly removed by lung immune mechanisms. Therefore, in addition to the mere presence of the organism, the local physiological environment must be such that the bacteria can grow in an uncontrolled manner. In many instances the events that lead to uncontrolled growth are varied and multifactorial, and specific factors may interact in a very complex fashion to make the animal susceptible (Table 1).

Figure 1. Requirements for respiratory disease

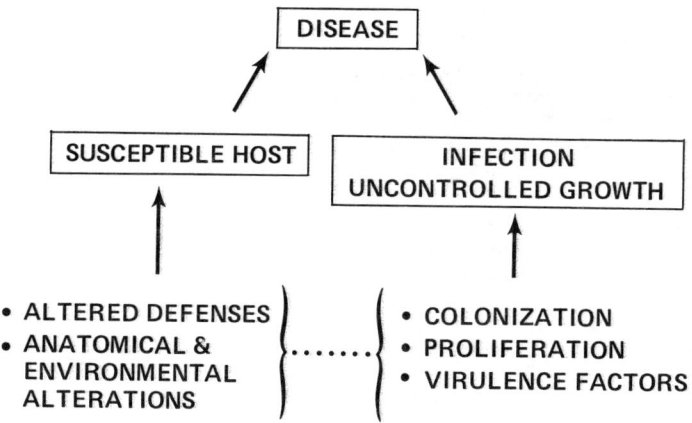

Table 1. Factors influencing colonization of the lung

1. Virus infections — alter:
    - mucociliary clearance
    - bronchotracheal secretions
    - bacterial adherence — fibronectin
    - local iron levels
    - macrophage functions
    - neutrophil functions
    - lymphocyte functions

2. Respiratory tract environment
    - levels of Fe^{++} and Zn^{++}
    - mucosal surfaces — mucus
        - — quantity
        - — quality
    - lysozyme
    - antibody

3. Bacterial characteristics
    - cytotoxin(s)
    - capsules
    - fimbriae
    - enzymes
    - cation sequestering mechanisms
    - endotoxin
    - plasmids

Some of the factors that can influence the susceptibility of cattle to increased colonization are altered defense mechanisms. These defenses can be impaired by a variety of factors including stress and viral infections. In addition to altering defense mechanisms, many factors which make the host more susceptible to infection may alter the environment of the respiratory tract in such a way that they also promote growth of the bacteria. In each case, there is a relationship between whether the host is susceptible and whether colonization and proliferation occur. For example, it is becoming increasingly evident that adherence to mucosal surfaces is often required for colonization by bacteria, and that colonization appears to be a prerequisite for production of disease (4,12-14). This is especially true in the gastrointestinal tract where bacteria are removed rapidly from mucosal surfaces unless they adhere. Whether bacteria adhere or not can be influenced both by the organism as well as its environment (15). Even though the bacterium may have the genetic potential to produce an adhesin, such as a fimbrial antigen, which mediates attachment, the environment may influence the amount of adhesin produced or its binding capacity. In bacteria that produce a capsule, the extent of adhesion may also be influenced by the quantity and quality of the capsule which in turn may be influenced by environmental factors. For example, a hyaluronic acid capsule will reduce adherence because of its high-charge density and net repulsion between the bacteria and the animal cell (16). However, in the presence of divalent cations such as zinc, these charges may be reduced such that adhesion is enhanced (17,18) and this may explain how zinc increases bacterial virulence. It is known that zinc levels are altered during virus infection but whether specific virus infections increase available zinc at the mucosal surface remains to be determined (16,19).

Virus infections appear to enhance adherence and colonization by both Gram-positive and Gram-negative bacteria (20-22). The exact mechanism whereby virus infection leads to increased adherence is probably multifactorial ranging from direct or anatomical surface alteration of the host cell membrane, to induction of bacterial receptors on exposed surfaces, to alteration of the extracellular environment which indirectly allows bacterial attachment. In addition, the mechanisms whereby viruses alter adherence of bacteria may depend on whether the bacterium is a Gram-positive or Gram-negative organism. It has been suggested that virus infections also alter the secretion of bactericidal or bacteriostatic factors by epithelial cells of the respiratory tract (23), thereby encouraging rapid growth of the adherent bacteria.

Once large quantities of bacteria are present in the upper respiratory tract they can form microcolonies which can enter the lung by aspiration (24) or as a result of reduced mucociliary clearance (25). In the lung these microcolonies are difficult to phagocytize and are resistant to attack by antibodies and antibiotics (4). In fact, when phagocytes encounter such microcolonies, they may become "frustrated" in their attempts to phagocytize them and discharge their toxic enzymes into the surrounding tissue (26). In addition, the bacteria may release cytotoxins which impair or destroy phagocytic cells thus further preventing clearance and inducing lung injury which in turn creates a better environment for the bacteria to replicate.

Another factor involved in the respiratory tract environment which may influence whether bacteria colonize and produce microcolonies or not is the actual mucosal surface to which the bacteria will have to attach. For instance, if the mucosal surface is intact and the epithelial cells are unaccessible to the adhesins produced by the bacterium, the mucocillary motion could rapidly remove the bacterium from the respiratory tract. Other factors such as enzymes and antibodies which coat the bacteria and prevent their attachment to epithelial cells will definitively have an effect on colonization of the lungs or respiratory tract. However, not just any antibody against the organism will be protective but the antibody must be directed against the specific bacterial adhesin.

The final factors which contribute to colonization of the lung are the characteristics of *Pasteurella haemolytica* itself. Most pathogenic bacterial species possess specific attributes of virulence which are essential in disease pathogenesis. Some of the characteristics of *Pasteurella haemolytica* are listed in Table 1; however, it must be stressed that little is known about the importance of these factors in the pathogenesis of pneumonia and their contribution to virulence.

In recent years evidence has been accumulating which suggests that the cytotoxin (or cytotoxins) produced by *Pasteurella haemolytica* is one of the important virulence factors. The cytotoxin reduces the immune competence of the lung by damaging or destroying several types of immune cells including alveolar macrophages, lymphocytes and neutrophils (27-30). Cytotoxin production is high in log-phase bacterial cultures but low in stationary-phase cultures and this may be one of the reasons why pneumonia can be reproduced in calves by intratracheal inoculation of log-phase but not stationary-phase cultures of *Pasteurella haemolytica.* Presumably when log-phase cultures are used they contain enough preformed cytotoxin and/or the bacteria produce enough very rapidly after inoculation to impair the immune response long enough for bacteria to establish a foothold in the lung.

Most strains of *Pasteurella haemolytica* are encapsulated to some degree and some appear to produce abundant quantities of glycocalyx (11). The anti-phagocytic role of bacterial capsules is well-known and it is likely that they play a similar role in protecting *Pasteurella haemolytica* in the respiratory tract. Fimbriae (pili) are present on some strains of *Pasteurella multocida* isolated from rabbits and appear to play a role in colonization of the respiratory tract in that species (31). Some strains of *Pasteurella haemolytica* are also fimbriated (Biberstein, personal communication); however, it is not yet known if they are virulence factors. In other bacterial species, fimbriae act as important attachment and anti-phagocytic mechanisms. Hence, it is possible that the fimbriae seen on *Pasteurella haemolytica* perform one or both of these functions in the lung.

Recently, various enzymes have been shown to be associated with virulence (32,33). Some of these, such as neuraminidase, have also been shown to be present in different serotypes of *Pasteurella haemolytica* (34). However, there have been no published reports attempting to correlate virulence with ability to produce neuraminidase. In addition, the role of endotoxin in the pathogenesis of pneumonia is poorly understood. Finally, it is possible that certain organisms or isolates of organisms have better cation-sequestering mechanisms which can trap iron or zinc even if it happens to be present in the environment in very low concentrations. Therefore, extensive hemorrhaging, or iron release as a result of cell death, would not be essential for the organisms to be able to colonize and rapidly build up within the lungs.

Models of Bacterial Pneumonia

Direct Deposition of Pasteurella haemolytica into the Lung

It is possible to induce pneumonia in cattle by depositing bacteria directly into the lung by intratracheal or transthoracic injection (35-38). These methods, and modifications of them, bypass the defense and clearance mechanisms of the URT and therefore they overcome the requirement for proliferation and colonization of the URT. Furthermore, they are most consistent when large quantities of log-phase bacteria are inoculated. Since log-phase cultures produce large quantities of cytotoxin and perhaps capsular material, this could mean that a certain amount of cytotoxin or capsular material is necessary to impair host defense mechanisms sufficiently to allow the bacteria to become established. Once established, the release of enzymes and other metabolites from phagocytic cells can produce an environment favorable for bacterial growth and reduced clearance, production of more cytotoxin and more cell death which eventually tip the balance in favor of the bacterium. Although these models are useful for the evaluation of vaccines (4,38) and antibiotics, as well as being helpful in understanding some of the bacterial-host interactions, they may not simulate the natural situation since it is unlikely that such large numbers of bacteria hardly ever enter the lung at one time under natural situations. However, it must be emphasized that it is not known how many bacteria enter the lung under natural conditions. Only rarely is it possible to induce pasteurellosis by intranasal instillation or aerosolization of *Pasteurella haemolytica* alone without some other insult. Under these circumstances, the bacteria that enter the lung are quickly cleared--within four hours--with only a transient fever and neutrophil infiltration into the lung

(39). These results suggest that the small numbers of bacteria that are aerosolized into the lung under these circumstances can be readily cleared.

Models which Impair Host Defenses

It is possible to favor bacterial growth by interferring with the host defense mechanisms by a variety of methods. For example, this can be achieved by creating lung edema and by chemical or viral immunosuppression (40). Thus, induction of pulmonary edema by endotoxin can dramatically reduce the clearance of *Pasteurella haemolytica* from the lung (40). These models predominantly affect the clearance of bacterium from the lower respiratory tract but have limited effects on URT colonization and clearance. Steroids and stress also reduce clearance in the respiratory tract but may also affect mucus secretions, mucociliary clearance and subsequent deposition of bacteria into the lung (10), thereby approaching what may occur under natural conditions. Exposing the respiratory tract to acetic acid is another method that has been used to alter mucociliary clearance mechanisms (Robinson, this Symposium).

The observation that virus infections can enhance bacterial pneumonia has prompted a number of groups to use combinations of viruses and bacteria as a means of producing the disease.   In many instances it has been shown that the virulence of the virus, the initial virus dose, as well as the route of infection may influence the extent of viral-bacterial synergistic interactions (41).   In most of these models, the best results are obtained if the virulent viruses are aerosolized to ensure rapid infection of the entire respiratory tract.

Viral damage has been shown to lower the activity of a variety of bactericidal mechanisms of the lung (2,31,42) especially those involving macrophages and neutrophils (Table 2).

Table 2. Effect of viral infection on macrophage and neutrophil activity

1. Macrophage dysfunction
   - chemotaxis
   - Fc receptors
   - phagocytosis
   - phagosome-lysome fusion
   - intracellular killing
   - decreased lysosome levels
   - decreased monokine production

2. Neutrophil dysfunction
   - chemotaxis
   - altered maturity
   - H_2O_2 release
   - chemiluminescence

Alveolar macrophages present in lavage fluids from virus-infected lungs often have decreased Fc receptor activity. However, a more important defect is the inability of macrophages to kill ingested bacteria (2,43-47). The reason for the decreased killing is due, at least in part, to inhibition of phagosome-lysosome fusion (25). Reduced killing may also be explained by the presence of local edema which creates anaerobic conditions detrimental to the phagocytic and bactericidal capacity of the alveolar macrophage (48). In addition to the bactericidal activity, the alveolar macrophage is very important in aiding recruitment of neutrophils by production of chemotactic factors (49-51). It has been shown recently that virus infection can reduce the production of these chemotactic factors by alveolar macrophages, and therefore could dramatically reduce neutrophil recruitment into the lung (39,52,53).

Virus infection also alters neutrophil and lymphocyte function (54,55) as well as neutrophil population (52) or mobility (56,57). In some cases, the neutrophil could be infected by the virus (58) or the mere interaction of the virus with the neutrophil would be sufficient to induce neutrophil dysfunction (36,59,60). If sufficient numbers of neutrophils are infected, this could easily explain neutropenia and altered mobility *in vivo.* The importance of neutrophils in clearing Gram-negative bacteria has been shown in animals and humans which are rendered neutropenic and which exhibit decreased PMN migration rates into lungs and increased susceptibility to pneumonia (61,62). Since many viruses can spread systemically, causing viremia, it is possible that the presence of virus or viral glycoproteins may trigger oxidative metabolism of the neutrophil and then cause subsequent neutrophil dysfunction, as has been suggested to occur in influenza virus infections (53,59,63).

Lymphocytes can be important in both recovery as well as in immunopathological processes in the host (64). If alveolar macrophages express viral antigens on their surface, either due to replication or phagocytosis of the antigen, cytotoxic T cells could be directed against the macrophages and further impair their functions (65-68). Finally, it is possible that certain subpopulations of T lymphocytes, such as suppressor cells, may influence susceptibility and reactivity against a virus infection. Whether it is coincidental or not, T suppressor cell activity appears to peak at approximately the time that maximum susceptibility to bacteria superinfection occurs following exposure to bovine herpesvirus 1 (BHV-1) (55).

Furthermore, treatment of animals with low levels of cyclophosphamide circumvents viral-bacterial synergistic interactions (69). The doses of cyclophosphamide used mainly affect the induction of thymus-derived T suppressor cells (70). Moreover, these suppressor cells have been implicated in the depression of cell-mediated immune responses following infection with influenza and respiratory syncytial virus (71) and susceptibility more closely resembles the induced suppression of cell-mediated immunity rather than of virus shedding and lesion development.

In BHV-1-*Pasteurella haemolytica* infections, an aerosol dose of at least 10^6 PFU of virus per animal is required to induce sufficient immunosuppression and environmental alterations of the lung by four days post-infection to allow the bacteria to produce pneumonia (41). Similarly, when influenza and Sendai virus are used in mice, the severity of the disease is directly correlated to the input virus (2). In most of these models, the maximum susceptibility is at least partially correlated to anatomical or pathological changes occurring throughout the airways including the upper and lower respiratory tracts. Thus maximum damage, as well as maximum susceptibility to bacteria, occurs between four to seven days after infection. In the case of the BHV-1/*Pasteurella haemolytica* model, this time also correlates well with the maximum temperature response of calves. Thus the peak temperature response occurs between three to five days and starts decreasing rapidly thereafter if animals are infected with virus only. If, however, animals are challenged with bacteria at this time, the temperature response does not decrease but increases approximately 1° C and remains elevated until the animals die. In animals that die early, there is still evidence of viral tracheobronchiolitis but animals that die later (longer than twelve days after virus infection) have very little evidence of viral infection and virus may not be isolated from infected lungs. Thus in many cases of pneumonia, the role of the specific virus involved may go unrecognized in natural field situations. These models combine both the physical and anatomical alterations of the URT which produce environmental conditions conducive to bacterial growth and presumably reduces mucociliary action and alters clearance of bacteria from the lungs. Thus virus infections can increase the rate of replication of the bacteria in the URT (72, Babiuk unpublished results), thereby increasing the numbers of bacteria that can enter the lung, as well as reduce clearance from the lung.

In addition to viral-bacterial interactions, there is also evidence for bacterial-bacterial interactions (73). Infection with mycoplasma appears to enhance the colonization of cattle with *Pasteurella haemolytica*. Whether this occurs as a result of the mycoplasma altering the host-cell epithelial surfaces or lowering defense mechanisms is not presently known but it is possible that under natural conditions various factors such as stress can increase mycoplasma replication which in turn create the environment conducive for *Pasteurella haemolytica* colonization and growth.

Recently, Gilmour *et al.* (74) successfully reproduced pneumonic pasteurellosis in calves and sheep by intravenous injection of agar into animals followed by an aerosol challenge of *Pasteurella haemolytica*. In these cases, the agar produced emboli and thrombi in arterial vessels of the lung in addition to classical lesions of pneumonic pasteurellosis. This model presumably does not affect the upper respiratory tract but creates foci in the lung in which the bacteria may localize and grow and also may prevent the proper infiltration of phagocytic cells into the lung. To date no information is available as to the effect of these agar thrombi on leukocyte infiltration and phagocytosis of bacteria in the lung but it is presumed that they interfere with proper clearance of the bacteria and, therefore, promote colonization and proliferation of the lung with the aerosolized bacterium. Once the bacteria overwhelms the animal, the lesions are similar to those observed in the field.

Models which Alter Bacterial Characteristics

It may be possible to decrease bacterial phagocytosis in the lung by creating microcolonies of bacteria embedded in agar beads.   Although this has not been reported for *Pasteurella haemolytica,* it has been shown to induce pneumonia in rats with *Pseudomonas aeruginosa* (75).   Incorporation of the bacteria in agar beads, followed by intratracheal injection, deposits the organism in the lung. The size of these beads is such that they cannot be phagocytized but they are still small enough to allow diffusion of nutrients into the bead to allow rapid bacterial growth and toxin production. Once the organisms proliferate to a specific extent, then they reach such high numbers that the normal clearance mechanisms of the lung cannot clear the bacterium and pneumonia subsequently results.

Iron is known to play a significant role in bacterial growth and pathogenesis (76,77), and some organisms produce iron chelators to help trap the iron required for their growth. Although the production of iron chelators is not correlated directly with virulence, the presence of these chelators or abundance of iron offers a definitive replicate advantage for the organism. In the case of *Pasteurella multocida,* we have been able to decrease the number of organisms required to kill 50 percent of mice from 10^4 organisms/mouse to 10 organisms/mouse (unpublished results). However, similar attempts with *Pasteurella haemolytica* were not as successful, indicating considerable differences between these two organisms. Nevertheless, iron supplementation combined with alteration of defense mechanisms such as occurs following virus infection might aid in reproducing the disease in laboratory animals. However, this may not be sufficient if cytotoxin is important for disease production since *Pasteurella haemolytica* cytotoxin has no effect on rodent leukocytes. In cattle, where *Pasteurella haemolytica* is capable of colonizing and inducing disease, it is possible that increased levels of iron alone may be sufficient to increase pathogenicity and virulence under field conditions.

Injury to Lungs via Inflammatory Processes

Viruses may act as initiators of disease by allowing the bacteria to colonize the respiratory tract and by killing various cells. Bacterial toxins are directly toxic to selected cell populations (27,30,78). In addition, however, a vast amount of tissue damage occurring in pneumonia is due to the host's response to the agents. Leukocytes are one of the major mediators of tissue injury due to their accumulation and release of biological mediators at the sites of injury (26). Some of the same mediators that are required for bacteriocidal activity in the cell are detrimental to the host when released extracellularly. The release of lysosomal enzymes can occur most frequently when leukocytes are overwhelmed with a bacterial load such as occurs in pneumonia (79) or by extracellular bacterial cytotoxins released into the environment (28-30,78,80). However, release is also induced by membrane perturbation and membrane potential changes (81-83). These changes result in a "respiratory burst" and release of toxic oxygen metabolites and arachidonic acid (84,85). It is not the intent of this paper to review in detail all the various mediators of inflammation, enzymes, mediators of increased permeability, vasoactive substances, et cetera, that are released into the lung during an inflammatory process since this has been done recently (26), except to say that these can help to clear the organism. However, if allowed to continue in an uncontrolled fashion, these may lead to further lung pathology and possibly death of the individual.

Summary

In summary, a number of models have been used to study bovine respiratory disease with each model significantly aiding in the understanding of the pathogenesis of this disease complex. It must be emphasized that this is a complex wherein many factors interact to either produce no disease or severe pneumonia. If the organisms possess the factors essential for colonization and growth in the respiratory tract and the host is susceptible, then disease will occur (Table 3).

Table 3. Relationship of host immunity and bacterial virulence to induction of pneumonia

Presence of Virulence Factors	Hosts Lung Immunity	
	Intact	Impaired
—	—	±
+	+	+++

However, even if the host is susceptible, if the organism does not possess the ability to colonize, it is highly unlikely that the animal will suffer any serious ill effects. At present it appears that considerable knowledge concerning the immune responses of the host is available but almost nothing is known about the physiology and genetics of *Pasteurella haemolytica,* the organism most often isolated from the lungs of cattle suffering from respiratory disease. The observation that the majority of cases of pneumonia are produced by one serotype (A1) of *Pasteurella haemolytica* suggests that this strain, or isolates of this strain, have some unique properties worth investigating. Once more is known about the regulation of cytotoxin production, fimbriae, capsule formation and other factors including identification of the antigens involved in producing protective antibodies (86), then it may be possible to more judiciously design better vaccines to aid in the control of this economically important disease.

References

1.   Finland M, Peterson OL, Strauss E:Staphylococcic pneumonia occurring during an epidemic of influenza. Arch Int Med 70:183-205, 1942.

2.   Jakab GJ:Immune impairment of alveolar macrophage phagocytosis during influenza virus pneumonia. Am Rev Resp Dis 126:776-782, 1982a.

3.   Lam J, Chan R, Lam K, Costerton JW:Production of mucoid microcolonies by *Pseudomonas aeruginosa* within infected lungs in cystic fibrosis.   Infect Immun 28:546-556, 1980.

4.   Corstvet RE, Ranciera RJ, Newman P:Vaccination of calves with *Pasteurella multocida* and *Pasteurella haemolytica.* Am Assoc Vet Lab Diagnos 7, 1978.

5.   Nugent KN, Pesanti EL:Chronic glucocorticosteroid therapy impairs staphylococcal clearance from murine lungs. Am Rev Res 125(S):173-185, 1982.

6.   Woods DE, Strauss DS,Johanson WG, Bass JA:Role of fibronectin in prevention of adherence of *Pseudomonas aeruginosa* to buccal cells.   Infect Dis 143:784-790, 1981.

7.   Hynes RO, Bye JM:Density and cell cycle dependence of cell surface proteins in hamster fibroblasts. Cell 3:113-120, 1974.

8.   Yamada KM, Weston JA:Isolation of a major cell surface glycoprotein from fibroblasts.   Proc Natl Acad Sci USA 71:3492-3496, 1974.

9.   Grey CL, Thomson RG:*Pasteurella haemolytica* in the tracheal air of calves.   Can J Comp Med 35:121-128, 1971.

10.   Nugester WJ, Klepser RG:Experimental studies on possible mechanisms of certain predisposing factors in lobar pneumonia.   AmJ Path 13:642-643, 1937.

11.   Gentry MJ, Corstvet RE, Panciera RJ:Extraction of capsular material from *Pasteurella hemolytica*. Am J Vet Res 43:2070-2073, 1982.

12.   Aly R, Shinefield HI, Strauss WG, Maibach HI:Bacterial adherence to nasal mucosal cells. Infect Immun 17:546-549, 1977.

13.   Beachey EH:Bacterial adherence: adhesin-receptor interactions mediate the attachment of bacteria to mucosal surfaces. J Infect Dis 143:325-345, 1981.

14.   Costerton JW, Irvin RT, Cheng KJ:The role of bacterial surface structures in pathogenesis.   CRS Critical Rev Microbiol, 8:303-338, 1981.

15.   Williams RC, Gibbons RJ:Inhibition of streptococcal attachment to receptors on human buccal epithelial cells by antigenically similar salivary glycoproteins.   Infect Immun 11:711-718, 1975.

16.   Beisel WR:Trace elements in infectious processes. Med Clin North Am 60:831-849, 1976.

17.   Sugarman B:Effect of heavy metals on bacterial adherence.   J Med Microbiol 13:351-354, 1980.

18.   Sugarman B, Epps LR, Stenback WA:Zinc and bacterial adherence.   Infect Immun 37:1191-1199, 1982.

19.   Falchuk KH:Effect of acute disease and ACTH on serum zinc proteins.   N Engl J Med 296:1129-1134, 1977.

20.   Davison VE, Sanford BA:Adherence of *Staphylococcus aureus* to influenza A virus-infected MDBK cells.   Infect Immun 32:1118-1126, 1981.

21.   Ramphal R, Small PM, Sands JW:Adherence of *Pseudomonas aeruginosa* to tracheal cells injured by influenza infection or by endotracheal intubation.   Infect Immun 27:614-619, 1980.

22.   Sanford BA, Shelokov A, Ramsay MA:Bacterial adherence to virus-infected cells: a cell model of bacterial superinfection.   J Infect Dis 137:176-181, 1978.

23.   Pijoan C, Campos M, Ochoa G:Effect of a hog cholera vaccine strain on the bactericidal activity of porcine alveolar macrophages.   Rev Latin Microbiol 22:69-72, 1980.

24.   Johanson WG, Pierce AK, Sanford JG:Changing pharyngeal bacterial flora of hospitalized patients. N Engl J Med 281:1137-1140, 1969.

25.   Jakab GJ:Viral-bacterial interactions in pulmonary infection.   Adv Vet Sci Comp Med 26:155-171, 1982.

26.   Slauson DO:The mediation of pulmonary inflammatory jury.   Adv Vet Sci Comp Med 26:99-154, 1982.

27.   Koehler KL, Markham RJF, Muscoplat CC, Johnson DW:Evidence of cytocidal effects of *Pasteurella haemolytica* on bovine peripheral blood mononuclear leukocytes. Am J Vet Res 41:1690-1693, 1980.

28. Maheswaran SK, Berggren JCC, Simonson RR, Ward GE, Muscoplat CC:Kinetics of interaction and fate of *Pasteurella haemolytica* in bovine alveolar macrophages. Infect Immun 30:254-262, 1980.

29. Markham RJF, Ramnaraine ML, Muscoplat CC:Cytotoxic effect of *Pasteurella haemolytica* on bovine polymorphonuclear leukocytes and impaired production of chemotractic factors by *Pasteurella haemolytica*-infected alveolar macrophages. Am J Vet Res 43:285-288, 1982.

30. Markham RJF, Wilkie BN:Interaction between *Pasteurella haemolytica* and bovine alveolar macrophages: cytotoxic effects on macrophages and impaired phagocytosis. Am J Vet Res 41:18-22, 1980a.

31. Glorioso JC, Jones GW, Rush HG, Pentler LJ, Darif A, Coward JE:Adhesion of type A *Pasteurella multocida* to rabbit pharyngeal cells and its possible role in rabbit respiratory tract infections. Infect Immun 35:1103-1109, 1982.

32. Milligan TW, Baker CJ, Strauss DC, Mattingly SJ:Association of elevated levels of extracellular neuraminidase with clinical isolates of type III group B streptococci. Infect Immun 21:738-746, 1978.

33. Ray PK:Bacterial neuraminidase and altered immunological behavior of treated mammalian cells. Adv Appl Microbiol 21:227-267, 1977.

34.   Frank GH, Tabatabai LB:Neuraminidase activity of *Pasteurella haemolytica* isolates.   Infect Immun 32:1119-1122, 1981.

35.   Friend SCE, Wilkie BN, Thomson RG, Branum DA:Bovine pneumonic pasteurellosis: experimental induction in vaccinated and nonvaccinated calves.   Can J Comp Med 41:77-83, 1977.

36.   Friend SCE, Thomson RG, Wilkie BN:Pulmonary lesions induced by *Pasteurella hemolytica* in cattle.   Can J Comp Med 41:219-223, 1977.

37.   Newman PR, Corstvet RE, Panciera RJ:Distribution of *Pasteurella haemolytica* in the bovine lung following vaccination and challenge exposure as an indicator of lung resistance. Am J Vet Res 43:417-422, 1982.

38.   Wilkie BN, Markham RJF, Shewan PE:Response of calves to challenge with *Pasteurella haemolytica* after parental or pulmonary vaccination.   Am J Vet Res 41:1773-1778, 1980.

39.   McGuire R, Babiuk LA:Evidence for defective neutrophil function in lungs of calves exposed to infectious bovine rhinotracheitis virus.   Vet Immunol Immunopath, in press.

40.   Gilka F, Thomson RG, Savan M:The effect of edema, hydrocortisone acetate, concurrent viral infection and

immunization on the clearance of *Pasteurella hemolytica* from the bovine lung. Can J Comp Med 38:251-259, 1974.

41. Yates WDG:Viral-bacterial pneumonia. Ph.D. Thesis, University of Saskatchewan, Saskatoon, 1982.

42. Jakab GJ, Dick EC:Synergistic effect in viral-bacterial infection: combined infection of the murine respiratory tract with Sendai virus and *Pasteurella pneumotropica.* Infect Immun 8:762-768, 1973.

43. Goldstein E, Buhles WC, Akers TC, Vedros N:Murine resistance to inhaled *Neisseria meningitidis* after infection with an encephalomyocarditis virus. Infect Immun 6:398-402, 1972.

44. Jakab GJ, Warr GA, Sannes PL:Alveolar macrophage ingestion and phagosome-lysosome fusion defect associated with virus pneumonia. Infect Immun 27:960-968, 1980.

45. Silverberg BA, Jakab GJ, Thomson RG, Warr GA, Boo KS:Ultrastructural alterations in phagocytic functions of alveolar macrophages after parainfluenza virus infections. J Reticuloendothel Soc 25:405-416, 1979.

46. Taylor RN, Dietz TM, Maxwell KW, Marcus S:Effect of influenza virus infection on phagocytic and cytopeptic capacities of guinea pig macrophages. Immunol Comm 3:439-455, 1974.

47.   Warr GA, Jakab GJ:Alteration in lung macrophage antimicrobial activity associated with viral pneumonia. Infect Immun 26:492-497, 1979.

48.   Green GM, Kass EH:The role of the alveolar macrophage in the clearance of bacteria from the lung. J Expt Med 119:167-175, 1964.

49.   Gadek JE, Hunninghake GW, Zimmerman RL, Crystal RG:Regulation of the release of alveolar macrophage-derived neutrophil chemotactic factor. Am Rev Resp Dis 121:723-733, 1980.

50.   Hunninghake GW, Gallin JI, Fauci AS:Immunologic reactivity of the lung. Am Rev Res Dis 117:15-23, 1978.

51.   Merril WW, Naegeel GP, Matthay RA, Reynolds HY:Alveolar macrophage-derived chemotactic factor. J Clin Invest 65:268-276, 1980.

52.   Bale JF, Kern ER, Overall JC, Glasgow LA:Enhanced susceptibility of mice infected with murine cytomegalovirus to pathogenesis and altered inflammatory response.   J Infect Dis 145:525-531, 1982.

53.   Yourtee EL, Bia FL, Griffith BP, Root RK:Neutrophil response and function during cytomegalovirus infection in guinea pigs. Infect Immun 36:11-16, 1982.

54.   Abramson JS, Giebink GS, Mills EL, Quie PG:Polymorphonuclear leukocyte dysfunction during influenza

virus infection in chinchillas.   J Infect Dis 143:836-845, 1981.

55.   Filion L, McGuire R, Babiuk LA:The suppressive effects of BHV-1 on bovine leukocyte functions. Infect Immun, in press, 1983.

56.   Nelson RD, McCormack RT, Fiegel VD, Simmons RL:Chemotactic deactivation of human neutrophils: evidence for monospecific and specific components.   Infect Immun 22:441-444, 1978.

57.   Ruutu P, Vaheri A, Kosunen TU:Depression of human neutrophil viability by influenza viurus *in vitro.* Scand J Immunol 6:897-907, 1977.

58.   Rinaldo CR, Stussel TP, Black PH, Hursch MS:Polymorphonuclear leukocyte function during cytomegalovirus mononucleosis.   Clin Immunol Immunopath 12:331-334, 1979.

59.   Abramson JS, Lewis JC, Lyles DS:Inhibition of neutrophil lysosome-phagosome fusion associated with influenza virus infection *in vitro.* J Clin Invest 69:1393-1397, 1982a.

60.   Faden H, Sutyla P, Ogra DL:Effect of viruses on luminol-dependent chemiluminescence of human neutrophils. Infect Immun 24:673-678, 1979.

61.   Kurrle E, Bhaduri S, Keieger D, Gaus W, Heimple H, Pflieger H, Arnold R, Vanek E:Risk factors for infection of the oropharynx and respiratory tract in patients with acute leukemia. J Infect Dis 144:128-136, 1981.

62.   Rehm SR, Gross GN, Pierce AK:Early bacterial clearance from murine lungs.   J Clin Invest 66:194-199, 1980.

63.   Abramson JS, Mills EL, Gienbink GS, Quie PS:Depression of monocyte and polymorphonuclear leukocytes oxidative metabolism and bacteriocidal capacity by influenza A virus. Infect Immun 35:350-355, 1982.

64.   Rouse BT, Babiuk LA:Mechanisms of viral immunopathology. Adv Vet Sci Comp Med 23:103-136, 1979.

65.   Forman AJ, Babiuk LA:Effect of infectious bovine rhinotracheitis virus infection on bovine alveolar macrophage function. Infect Immun 35:1041-1047, 1982.

66.   Nugent KM, Pesanti EL:Effect of influenza infection on the phagocytic and bactericidal activities of pulmonary macrophages. Infect Immun 26:651-657, 1979.

67.   Shanley JD, Pesanti EL:Replication of murine cytomegalovirus in lung macrophages: effect on phagocytosis of bacteria. Infect Immun 29:1152-1159, 1980.

68.   Yilma T, Zee YC, Osebold JW:Immunofluorescence determination of the pathogenesis of infection with

influenza virus in mice following exposure to aerosolized virus. J Infect Dis 139:458-464, 1979.

69. Jakab GJ, Warr GA:Lung defenses against viral and bacterial challenges during immunosuppression with cyclophosphamide in mice. Am Rev Resp Dis 123:524-528, 1981a.

70. Chiorazzi N, Fox D, Katz DH:Hapten-specific IgE antibody responses in mice VI selective enhancement of IgE antibody production by low doses of x-irradiation and by cyclophosphamide. J Immunol 117:1629-1635, 1976.

71. Roberts NJ:Different effects of influenza virus, respiratory syncytial virus and Sendai virus on human lymphocytes. Infect Immun 35:1142-1146, 1982.

72. Jericho KWF, Langford EV:Pneumonia in calves produced with aerosols of bovine herpesvirus-1 and *Pasteurella haemolytica.* Can J Comp Med 42:269-277, 1978.

73. Houghton SB, Gourlay RN:Synergism between *Mycoplasma bovis* and *Pasteurella haemolytica* in calf pneumonia. Vet Record 113:41-42, 1983.

74. Gilmour NJL, Angus KW, Donachie W, Fraser J:Experimental pneumonia pasteurellosis in sheep and cattle. Vet Record 110:406-407, 1982.

75. Cash HA, Woods DE, McCullough B, Johanson WG, Bass JA:A rat model of chronic respiratory infection with *Pseudomonas aeruginosa.* Am Rev Resp Dis 119:453-459, 1979.

76. Hatch GE, Slade E, Boykin E:Correlation of effects of inhaled versus intratracheally injected metals and susceptibility to respiratory infections in mice. Am Rev Resp Dis 124:167-173, 1981.

77. Miles AA, Khimji L:Enterobacterial chelators of iron: their   occurrence,   detection   and   relation   to pathogenicity. J Med Microbiol 8:477-490, 1975.

78. Markham RJF, Wilkie BN:Influence of broncho alveolar washing supernatant and stimulated lymphocyte supernatants on uptake of *Pasteurella haemolytica* by cultural bovine alveolar macrophages.   Am J Vet Res 41:443-446, 1980b.

79. Hawkins   HK:In   Trump   BF,   Arstila   AU (eds):Pathobiology of Cell Membranes, vol. 2. New York, NY, Academic Press, 1980, pp. 251-285.

80. Berggren KA, Baluyat CS, Simonson RR, Bemrick WJ, Maheswaran, SK:Cytotoxic effects of *Pasteurella haemolytica* on bovine neutrophils. Am J Vet Res 42:1383-1388, 1981.

81. Henson PM, McCarthy K, Larsen GL, Webster RO, Giclas PC, Dreisin RB, King TE, Shaw JO:Complement fragments, alveolar macrophages and alveolitis.   Am J Pathol 97:93-110, 1979.

82. Korchak HM, Weissman G:Changes in membrane potential of human granulocytes antecedes the metabolic

responses to surface stimulation. Proc Natl Acad Sci USA 75:3818-3822, 1978.

83.   Weissman G, Korchak HM, Perez HD, Smolem JE, Goldstein IM, Hoffstein ST:Leukocytes as secretory organs of inflammation. Adv Inflam Res 1:95-112, 1979.

84.   DeChatelet LR, Mullikins D, McCall CE:The generation of superoxide anion by various types of phagocytes. J Infect Dis 131:443-446, 1975.

85.   Samuelsson B, Hammarstrom S, Burgeat P:Pathways of arachidonic acid metabolism.   Adv Inflam Res 1:405-412, 1979.

86.   Wood WB:Studies on the mechanism of recovery in pneumonococcal pneumonia: I.   The action of type specific antibody upon the pulmonary lesion of experimental pneumonia. J Exp Med 73:201-222, 1941.

Pathogenesis of Pneumonia in Feedlot Cattle

R. G. Thomson, Dip. A.C.V.P., M.V.Sc., D.V.M., Ph.D.

Department of Veterinary Pathology
Western College of Veterinary Medicine
University of Saskatchewan
Saskatoon, Saskatchewan, Canada S7N 0W0

The program outline of this meeting clearly emphasizes the significance of respiratory tract infections as one of the, if not the most important diseases in the feedlot industry. However, it is not easy to obtain a clear overview of the problem. Perhaps we who are involved in isolated areas of research on the problem confuse ourselves along with those who are not directly involved. Should we not define the problem and rank the significant components in importance? What is the respiratory problem in the real world of the feedlot?

The intent of this presentation is to describe the respiratory tract lesions of the most important diseases, point out their differential features and describe their pathogenesis.

The feedlot operator and veterinarian face two major practical problems aside from trying to prevent respiratory diseases in the first place. One is to find the very acute cases of pneumonia before they die. The fact that these cases are so difficult to find before it is too late indicates the very rapid course of the disease. The second problem is to provide adequate therapy, in time, to those cases which can be found by observing clinical signs and which should be treatable and able to gain weight efficiently following therapy.

It is essential that an accurate assessment be made by postmortem examination of pulmonary lesions in any animals which die, either with or without therapy. Are the problems and the lesions really those of the disease that was anticipated? Are the cases being found in time? Is the treatment adequate?

It is necessary to recognize and identify the significant pulmonary lesions caused by specific agents. A veterinarian in feedlot practice must be able to make these determinations. However, many have difficulty in assessing the lesions in dead animals and deciding which of the major etiological agents are significant and what their influence is at a particular point in the course of what may seem to be a spectrum of clinical signs and lesions. It is possible to accurately age and identify the lesions in acute cases which die. Aging the lesions will determine if the major problem is failure to find the cases in time for therapy. To just culture microorganisms from the lung lesions is to avoid determining what is really happening in the lungs. Let us review the lesions most often found in acute respiratory disease in feedlot cattle; but first we must establish the criteria and terminology.

Jubb and Kennedy present a very practical description of the three main morphological types of lung lesions in cattle (1). Figure 1 conveys the essence of each in general terms. *Bronchopneumonia* is an anteroventral dark, firm, lobular lesion which involves inflammation of and within bronchi, bronchioles and alveoli. *Fibrinous pneumonia* is an anteroventral dark, hard, swollen, lobar lesion involving inflammation primarily in terminal airways, alveoli and interlobular tissue. The presence of fibrin indicates severe vascular damage with much edema, hemorrhage and exudation. There has literally been an explosion deep in the lung parenchyma. *Interstitial pneumonia* is generalized in the lung, tan to pink to red, rubbery and wet, often with noticeable separation of lobules by edema, with the main lesion being in the alveolar walls which are thickened. The acute lesions of each type are very characteristic (2,3), (Table 1).

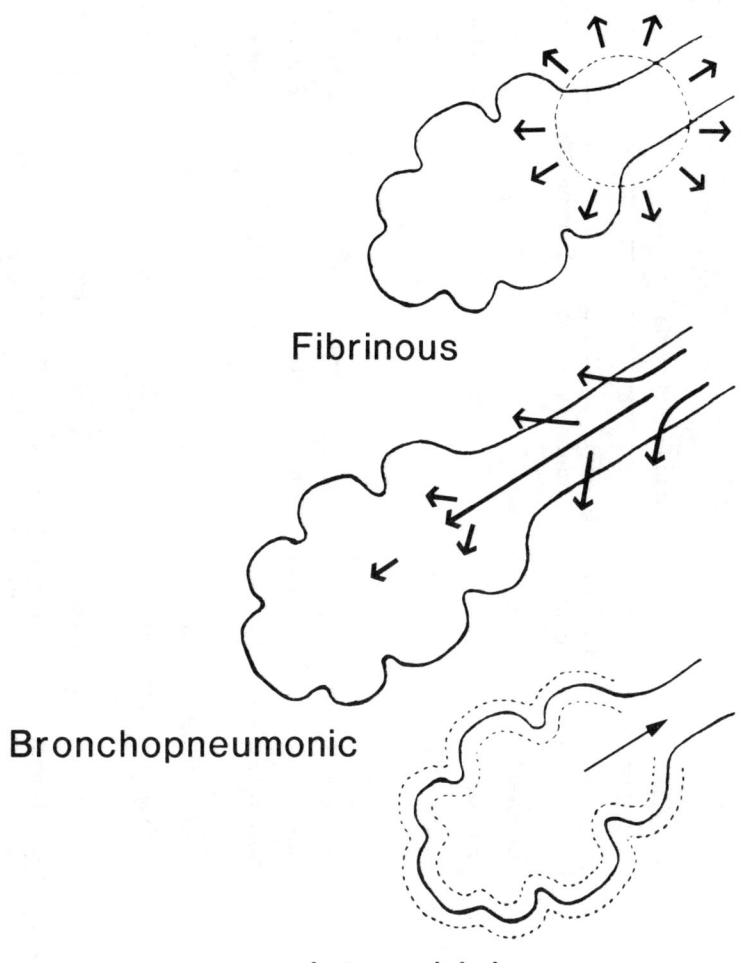

Fibrinous

Bronchopneumonic

Interstitial

Figure 1. The three main morphological types of lung lesions in cattle.

Table 1. Acute gross pneumonic lesions in feedlot cattle

Features		Type of Pneumonia			
	Fibrinous	Fibrinous-broncho	Bronchopneumonia	Necrotizing Bronchiolitis	Interstitial
Location	Anteroventral	Anteroventral	Anteroventral	Anteroventral	Entire lung
Color	Dark red	Dark red	Dark	Dark	Reddish-tan
Fibrin — surface — interlobular	Present Present Present	Present — variable	Absent	Absent	Absent
Size	Swollen	Swollen or normal	Normal	Normal or swollen	Swollen
Texture	Hard	Firm	Rubbery to firm	Rubbery to firm	Rubbery
Cut surface	Dry, marbled	Marbled, wet, red	Wet, red	Dark with pale bronchiolar pattern	Wet, lobules separated
Trachea	Normal or froth	Normal or froth	Normal or froth	Froth and necrotic debris	Froth
Bronchioles	Froth	Froth and exudate	Exudate	Necrotic debris	No lesions
Coagulation necrosis	Present	Variable	Absent	Usually absent	Absent
Cause	Past. hemolytica	Past. hemolytica + multocida + virus	Past. multocida + virus	IBR Virus Past. multocida Past. hemolytica	Toxicity

The most important pneumonia caused by microbiological agents is the fulminating acute fibrinous pneumonia caused by *Pasteurella hemolytica* and which is highly fatal.   The distinctive feature of these lesions is the pattern of coagulation necrosis of the lung parenchyma.   Such acute lesions are probably of three or four days' duration. Affected animals are difficult to identify clinically in time for therapy to be effective.

Acute bronchopneumonias have less or no fibrin, less or no coagulation necrosis, more fluid in the exudate and are likely to have mixtures of *P. hemolytica* and *P. multocida,* with the latter predominating, possibly with evidence of viral infection.

Toxic agents arriving in the lung via the blood damage alveolar walls which result in interstitial pneumonias, such as "acute atypical interstitial pneumonia of cattle." The acute lesions of the latter disease are very characteristic.

The lesions of acute fibrinous or fibrinous bronchopneumonia of a week or more duration usually appear as bronchopneumonia, often with areas of coagulation necrosis (sequestration) present as raised, hard, irregular areas.   These are often confused with abscesses.   In those lesions which have had a significant *viral* component there may be chronic bronchiolitis including obliterative and/or peribronchial fibrosis with nonspecific alveolar exudation.

It is rare to see specific evidence of virus infection, such as inclusion bodies, in acute lesions of fatal cases of fibrinous pneumonia. Rarely parainfluenza-3 viral inclusions can be observed. If *necrotizing bronchiolitis* is present, infectious bovine rhinotracheitis viral inclusions may be seen. Usually they are no longer visible in naturally-occurring cases at the time of death. The significance of recognizing the lesions of IBR viral-induced necrotizing bronchiolitis is often not appreciated. When this lesion is dominant in the lungs, that specific IBR viral problem must be recognized and dealt with. Failure to recognize the gross bronchiolar lesions leads to great frustration, particularly in so-called treatment failures. Specific morphological evidence of lesions of mycoplasma, bovine virus diarrhea (BVD) virus, adenovirus, chlamydia or respiratory syncytial virus are very rarely recognized or confirmed (4).

The review by Yates of the evidence for involvement of various agents in feedlot pneumonia is the most comprehensive and complete to date (5). It is truly a major landmark in bovine respiratory literature.

The emphasis of this paper will now be on a discussion of the pathogenesis of the *P. hemolytic*-induced induced lesions. *P. hemolytica* is the cause of acute fatal cases of severe fibrinous pneumonia (1,6,7,8). Viruses may assist by weakening the antibacterial defenses but are not necessary for these lesions. The emphasis on *P. hemolytica* started with the works of Carter (9) and Biberstein (10). It has taken nearly 25 years for the significance of this organism to be generally accepted. Several laboratories are now concentrating on the toxin produced by *P. hemolytica* as the factor which injures the lung and causes the fibrinous pneumonia (11,12).

P. hemolytica is part of the normal nasal flora in cattle. Magwood *et al.,* (13) defined the components of the normal bacterial nasal flora of cattle and also developed a method to quantitate the flora on the surfaces of the nasal mucosa. This method became a major tool in assessing the nasal flora in shipped animals under field conditions (7,14). Frank has examined the bovine nasal bacterial flora in more detail since then and will discuss this subject at this conference (15).

Our laboratory investigated the differences between animals shipped from western to central Canada, and which developed clinical respiratory diseases and compared them

to those which did not develop clinical respiratory disease
(16). We tried to determine what was happening to and in
the animals in the real world under natural conditions.
Animals were purchased on arrival and sampled over various
time intervals for body temperature, plasma fibrinogen,
nasal flora, serum antibody and leukocyte profiles. Many
animals were killed after one week of sampling and the
lungs recovered to assess the amount and type of pneumonia
present. Lung scores, i.e., the amount of pneumonia
present, were established by using a scale of the physical
area of lungs affected with pneumonia. Each lobe was
scored from 0 to 5. Thus the maximum score was 35, i.e.,
4x5=20 for the right lung, and 3x5=15 for the left lung,
with a range for an animal of 0 to 35.

Cattle were classified as sick (S) or well (W) based on
the level of body temperature and plasma fibrinogen.
Levels of serum antibody, lung scores, nasal flora
(quantitative and qualitative) were compared between S and
W groups. None were treated. In general, sick animals had
lower serum antibody to *P. hemolytica* and high levels of *P.
hemolytica* in nasal flora on arrival, whereas there was
little difference between S and W in serum antibody levels
to PI-3 virus. We concluded that S animals were more
susceptible to the effects of *P. hemolytica* and had much

higher levels of *P. hemolytica* in their nasal flora. Recent
comparisons of methods of identifying specific serum
antibody to *P. hemolytica* indicates that our methods were
probably not accurate (L. Filion, personal communication).
Serological evidence of protection by immunity is
undergoing reevaluation.

It was necessary to determine if there was a
relationship between the high levels of *P. hemolytica* on the
nasal mucosa and the numbers being breathed into the lung
from the nasal mucosa. Using an Anderson air sampler in an
isolated environment, animals with high numbers on their
nasal mucosa did breathe them into the lung, generally in
relationship to the numbers present in the nasal mucosa.
Numbers of organism and particle sizes were determined in
tracheal air.   The organisms were constant in the oral
cavity but were not breathed out in expired air (14).

This set the stage for investigation of the normal
clearance of bacteria from the lungs of cattle and also
whether viruses could influence normal bacterial clearance.
Lillie (17) transposed the methods of studying the
clearance of *Staph. aureus* in mice to the determination of
normal clearance of *P. hemolytica* in calves. It was
remarkably similar. Experiments using mice indicated that
certain viruses could reduce bacterial clearance in

viral-infected mice about one week after the virus infection. Lopez converted this technology to the determination of viral influences or *P. hemolytica* clearance in calves. Parainfluenza-3 (PI-3) virus did impair the bacterial pulmonary clearance of *P. hemolytica* in calves seven days after the viral infection and the defect corrected after eleven days (18). However, further work by Lopez *et al.* (19) indicated that BVD virus and *Mycoplasma bovis* do not interfere with bacterial clearance.

Elegant work by Jakab (20) and others unfolded the specific mechanisms by which Sendai virus interferes with the clearance of *Pasteurella pneumontropica* in mice, a model which has similarities to the PI-3-*P. hemolytica* model in cattle. Jericho, Stockdale and Yates have experimentally demonstrated bacterial clearance defects in cattle using IBR virus and PI-3 virus (5). Other papers cover this general topic in detail at this conference (Babiuk and Jakab).

The real problem is carrying out effective immunization of the respiratory tract with either the viral agents, which might influence the clearance of *P. hemolytica,* or to immunize directly with *P. hemolytica* (21). The paper by Wilkie at this conference will address that topic.

The focus keeps coming back to *P. hemolytica* as the most significant organism in causing the acute fatal fibrinous pneumonia in feedlot cattle. *P. multocida* is not likely primary but will be present secondarily, either in viral-induced lesions or in some *P. hemolytica*-induced lesions. Schiefer *et al.* (22) have pointed out that in field cases of acute fibrinous pneumonia, *P. hemolytica* is present in pure culture. However, in cases where evidence of viral infections are present, particularly in bronchioles, *P. multocida* dominates.

But let us return to the beginning. The real problem is the sudden build-up of *P. hemolytica* in the nasal flora and its descent into the lungs in large numbers in a susceptible animal. The impression might be gained that the "infection" is highly contagious. But is it? Grey (14) found that the animals with high numbers of organisms in the nasal flora did not breathe them out, but did have them in their oral cavities. A pertinent observation in feedlots is that fibrinous pneumonia does not sweep through the feedlot like an epizootic but rather it centers on certain pens. Is it really contagious? Could it be that certain stresses in cattle alter the nasal pharyngeal ecosystem to allow *P. hemolytica* to dominate and be breathed into the lung? That in fact is what seems to happen in certain other species. In addition, aspiration of pharyngeal flora is apparently a common occurrence in humans (23) and the pneumonia starts in the areas where aspirates would land--anteroventral in animals and distal in humans. Dalton (24) indicates that a throat swab is as accurate as a lung swab in determining the cause of bacterial pneumonia. Weinstein indicates that pharyngeal bacterial flora builds rapidly prior to entry into the lung (25).

Kainer (26) points out several factors by which the bovine respiratory tract is particularly prone to infection, including probable aspiration and the high speed of particles impacting on respiratory surfaces.

Bacteria on mucosal surfaces exist in a very complex ecosystem. Different species associate with each other in a fluid mosaic of glycocalyx and the relationships of organisms change with their various growth phases. Microcolonies exist in the glycocalyx (26). The glycocalyx can exclude phages, sera, antibody macrophages and clearance mechanisms (27). Pure cultures on mucosal surfaces are an artifact. Virus infection, stress and antibiotics alter the relationships of organisms to each other and to the cells near them. Most bacteria must attach to a cell to cause it harm. Bacteria attach to the cells by specific host receptor sites called adhesins. Such attachments are genetically determined and this accounts for the apparent specificity of certain infections of certain tissues in certain species. Many of the disease-causing bacteria are part of normal flora, i.e., *E. coli* in the intestine and urinary tract and *P. hemolytica* and *P. multocida* in the respiratory tract. Thus the tissue specificity of infection resides in attachments which are called adhesins on the fimbria of Gram-negative bacteria and fibrillae of Gram-positive bacteria.

Three questions arise regarding pathogenesis. Do bacteria adhere to cells by specific receptors? Is adhesion a requirement for causing disease? Can infection be blocked by preventing adhesins from functioning? The answer is yes to all three. Pigs with K88 *E. coli* intestinal receptors are genetically immune to disease caused by that organism. Pathogens must (a) compete, (b) colonize, (c) have appropriate receptors, (d) build a population, (e) compete, and (f) persist. Persistence is the key to success (28,29).

Pseudomonas aeruginosa builds in the pharynx of stressed human patients because of depletion of membrane fibronectin by host cell proteases which allows the bacteria to adhere to the cells (30). Perhaps this applies to *P. hemolytica* and cattle.   This area of investigation is essential to determine the pathogenesis of the fatal fibrinous pneumonias in cattle caused by *P. hemolytica*. We may have been looking in the wrong place for the key event.

The search for the magic immunogen continues, but which one is it--the toxin, an adhesin or an unknown?

Another major factor in pathogenesis is to determine the influence of management practices on the pneumonias.   The Bruce County Beef Project has assisted in evaluation of certain influences (31).   Mixing groups of animals, vaccinating on arrival and feeding corn silage increased the risk of disease, and when all three occurred in the same groups of animals, the incidence and risk of respiratory disease was increased considerably.

A major question for the industry and for reseachers is to determine the best long-term strategy for reducing losses.   The two best prospects are to alter management practices which contribute to respiratory diseases, or to put a major effort into potential vaccination programs. Vaccines have not been effective when tested under field conditions (32).   (This must come as a great surprise to producers.)   Which should it be? The long-term detailed research program on epidemiology by the Alberta Department of Agriculture will be very influential in determining future directions.   That project involves very detailed observation and analysis of the management practices and diseases in several large feedlots.

In summary, the agents which cause the respiratory disease in feedlots are known, the general circumstances and management practices which allow the agents to cause respiratory disease are known, and good management practices which can largely prevent major respiratory disease problems are known.   The problems are in the execution of good management practices (including accurate records), in establishing early accurate clinical and pathological diagnoses of what is happening in sick and dead cattle and in developing effective prevention procedures.   That is the defensive task.   The offenders, *Pasteurella* organisms and viruses, will take what they are given for as long as we let them.

References

1.   Jubb KVF, Kennedy PC:Pathology of Domestic Animals, Vol. 1, ed. 2.   New York, Academic Press, Inc., 1970, pp. 164-166.

2.   Thomson RG:The pathogenesis and lesions of pneumonia in cattle.   Continuing Education Article No. 7, Comp on Cont Educ 3:11, S403-S412, 1981.

3. Jensen R, Pierson RE, Braddy PM, Sarri DS, Lauerman H, Collier JR, Keyvanfar H, Collier JR, Horton DP, McChesney AE, Benitez A, Christie RM:Shipping fever pneumonia in yearling feedlot cattle. J Am Vet Med Assoc 169:500-506, 1976.

4. Rehmtulla AJ:A study of naturally occurring lung lesions in shipping fever of cattle. Thesis, University of Guelph, 1978.

5. Yates WDG:A review of infectious bovine rhinotracheitis, shipping fever pneumonia and viral-bacterial synergism in respiratory disease of cattle. Can J Comp Med 46:225-263, 1982.

6. Rehmtulla AJ, Thomson RG:A review of the lesions in shipping fever of cattle. Can Vet J 22:1-8, 1981.

7. Thomson RG:The pathogenesis of shipping fever in cattle. Respiratory session. Proceedings. 13th Annual Convention, American Association of Bovine Practitioners, Toronto, 103-112, 1980.

8. Lillie LE:The bovine respiratory disease complex. Can Vet J 15:233-242, 1974.

9. Carter GR:Some remarks on shipping fever in Canada. Can J Comp Med 20:289-293, 1956.

10. Biberstein EL, Gills M, Knight H:Serological types of *Pasteurella haemolytica.* Cornell Vet 50:283-300, 1960.

11.   Benson ML, Thomson RG, Valli VEO:The bovine alveolar macrophage II. *In vitro* studies with *Pasteurella haemolytica.* Can J Comp Med 42:368-369, 1978.

12.   Markham RJF, Wilkie BN:Interaction between *Pasteurella haemolytica* and bovine alveolar macrophages: Cytotoxic effect on macrophages and impaired phagocytosis. Am J Vet Res 41:18-22, 1980.

13.   Magwood SE, Barnum DA, Thomson RG:Nasal bacterial flora of calves in healthy and in pneumonia-prone herds. Can J Comp Med 33:237-243, 1969.

14.   Grey CL, Thomson RG: *Pasteurella haemolytica* in the tracheal air of calves. Can J Comp Med 35:212-128, 1971.

15.   Frank GH: *Pasteurella haemolytica* and respiratory disease in cattle. Proceedings. 83rd Annual Meeting, U.S. Animal Health Assoc, 153-160, 1979.

16.   Thomson, RG, Chander S, Savan M, Fox ML:Investigation of factors of probable significance in the pathogenesis of pneumonic pasteurellosis in cattle. Can J Comp Med 39:194-207, 1975.

17.   Lillie LE, Thomson RG:The pulmonary clearance of bacteria by calves and mice. Can J Comp Med 36:129-136, 1972.

18.   Lopez A, Thomson RG, Savan M:The pulmonary clearance of *Pasteurella hemolytica* in calves infected with

bovine parainfluenza-3 virus. Can J Comp Med 40:385-391, 1976.

19. Lopez A, Maxie MG, Savan M, Ruhnke HL, Thomson RG, Barnum DA:The pulmonary clearance of *Pasteurella haemolytica* in calves infected with bovine virus diarrhea or *Mycoplasma bovis.* Can J Com Med 46:302-306, 1982.

20. Jakab GJ:Mechanisms of virus-induced bacterial superinfection of the lung. Clinics in Chest Medicine 2:59-65, 1981.

21. Wilkie BN:Respiratory tract immune response to microbial pathogens. J Am Vet Med Assoc 181:No. 10, 1074-1079, 1982.

22. Schiefer B, Ward GE, Moffat RE:Correlation of microbiological and histological findings in bovine fibrinous pneumonia. Vet Path 15:313-321, 1978.

23. Lindsey JO, Pierce AK:An examination of the microbiologic flora of normal lung of the dog. Amer Review of Respiratory Disease, 117:501-505, 1978.

24. Dalton, HP, Muhovich M, Escobar MR, Allison MJ:Pulmonary infection due to disruption of the pharyngeal bacterial flora by antibiotics in hamsters. Amer J Path 76:469-479, 1974.

25. Weinstein L, Goldfield M, Chang T:Infections occurring during chemotherapy: a study of their frequency,

types and predisposing factors. N Engl J Med 251:247-254, 1954.

26. Costerton JW, Irvin RT, Cheng K-J:The role of surface structures in pathogenesis. CRC Critical Reviews in Microbiology, 303-338, 1981.

27. Beachey EH:Bacterial adherence: adhesion-receptor interactions mediating the attachment of bacteria to mucosal surfaces. J Infect Dis 143:325-345, 1981.

28. Waldemar G, Johanson JR, Higuchi JH, Caudhuri TR, Woods DE:Bacterial adherence to epithelial cells in bacillary colonization of the respiratory tract. American Review of Respiratory Disease, 121:55-63, 1980.

29. Glorioso JC, Jones GW, Rush HG, Pentler LJ, Carif CA, Coward JE:Adhesion of type A *Pasteurella multocida* to rabbit pharyngeal cells and its possible role in rabbit respiratory tract infections. Infection and Immunity 35:1103-1109, 1982.

30. Beachey EH (ed):Bacterial adherence, in Receptors and Recognition, series B, volume 6. London, Chapman and Hall, 1980, pp. 441-458.

31. Martin SW, Meek AH, Davis DG, Johnson JA, Curtis RA:Factors associated with morbidity and mortality in feedlot calves. The Bruce County beef project, year two. Can J Comp Med 45:103-112, 1981.

32. Martin SW:Vaccination: is it effective in preventing respiratory disease or influencing weight gains in feedlot calves? Can Vet J 24:10-19, 1983.

Bacteria as Etiologic Agents in Bovine Respiratory Disease

Glynn H. Frank, D.V.M., Ph.D.

National Animal Disease Center
Agricultural Research Service, U.S. Department of Agriculture
P.O. Box 70
Ames, Iowa 50010

Introduction

It is common for outbreaks of acute bovine respiratory disease (BRD) to occur within two weeks after calves arrive at a feedyard. Most affected calves recover from the disease, but some die. The disease can become chronic. The cost in treatment and in lost productivity is the greatest disease loss the beef cattle industry suffers. Upon necropsy, the lungs usually have lesions of a fibrinous bacterial pneumonia. At first, the bacteria isolated from the pneumonic lungs were suspected of being the cause of BRD, but their role was questioned after investigations began.

Reasons for doubt included: inability to cause the disease with *Pasteurella* alone; isolation of *Pasteurella* from healthy cattle; the tendency of the disease to occur following stresses related to marketing and transportation; and confusing results on efficacy of *Pasteurella* bacterins and immune serum (1).

Over the last 25 years, investigators have found many other agents associated with BRD. However, none of them filled the role of the sole etiologic agent. We now realize the complexity of the situation and can take a more realistic look at the role of bacteria as etiologic agents in BRD.

Several review articles address the subject (1-7). It is difficult to determine the role of a suspected agent in BRD. A broad spectrum of agents have been isolated and many of these cause only asymptomatic infections in the healthy, unstressed host. Even experimental infections result in mild, transient signs of BRD at best. Therefore, many agents are implicated only by a long history of frequent isolation from clinical cases. However, the problem is in distinguishing between saprophytes or commensals and those that are important primary or secondary etiologic agents. In the case of BRD, most etiologic agents do not express their full virulence in the healthy calf unless other disease agents are actively involved.

Observations on the Role of Bacteria in BRD

The usual bacterial flora of pneumonic bovine lungs has been determined by an accumulation of observations over years of study. Several species of bacteria have been isolated, but the most commonly isolated species were *Pasteurella haemolytica* and *P. multocida* and *Mycoplasma.*

Reports on the bacterial flora of healthy lung tissue vary as to whether known pathogens are found. Collier *et al.* (8) found no known pathogens in the lungs, tracheas and bronchial lymph nodes of healthy cattle at slaughter. Soil and fecal bacteria were isolated in small numbers, but it was concluded that the bacteria were recently inhaled transients. Others isolated *P. haemolytica* and *P. multocida* from both pneumonic and nonpneumonic lungs, but isolated smaller numbers of the pathogens from nonpneumonic lungs (9).

The bacterial nasal flora of healthy, unstressed cattle consists of a large population of a wide variety of mixed species. Over prolonged sampling intervals of individual cattle, shifts in the predominant species in the nasal flora occur (10). We have observed that the general background flora varies even within a single group of cattle.

The nasal flora of cattle undergoing acute BRD will often contain *P. haemolytica* serotype 1 as the predominant species (5,11). *P. multocida* is widely distributed and is often found in the nasal passages of both healthy calves and those undergoing BRD. The predominant serotype is Carter's Type A (2), or Heddleston's type 3 (12).

Several other species of bacteria are sometimes isolated from pneumonic lungs as well as from the tissues of the upper respiratory tract of normal cattle. Their involvement in BRD has not been studied to the extent that the *Pasteurella* species have. Therefore, little is known about the role these less-frequently isolated bacteria have in BRD.

Haemophilus somnus causes thromboembolic meningo encephalomyelitis (TEME) of cattle. The subject of TEME and other disease syndromes associated with *H. somnus* have been reviewed (13,14). *Haemophilus somnus* itself is a virulent pathogen that causes a septicemia in cattle. The resulting varied manifestations of disease have been referred to as the "*Haemophilus somnus* complex" (13). One form of the complex is respiratory disease (13,15). As a result, *H. somnus* is isolated from cattle with bronchopneumonia and fibrinous pneumonia, but its involvement in typical BRD is unclear (14).

Corynebacterium pyogenes is frequently isolated from pneumonic lungs as well as from healthy tissues from the upper respiratory tract. It is a known pathogen often found in abscesses of cattle, swine, sheep and goats, but its involvement in BRD is unknown.

Mycoplasmas are isolated with great frequency from cattle with BRD. At least twelve mycoplasma species have been isolated from the respiratory tracts of cattle (16). Those most frequently isolated are *M. bovirhinis*, *M. bovis*, *M. dispar* and *Ureaplasma species* (16,17). They are isolated both from pneumonic lungs and from the respiratory tracts of healthy calves (17,18). Several species have caused lesions of pneumonia in gnotobiotic calves, but the role of mycoplasmas in BRD has not been determined (17,18).

From all observations and experimental evidence, *P. haemolytica* and *P. multocida* are the most important bacteria involved in BRD. It has been generally stated that *P. multocida* is frequently carried in the nasal passages of healthy calves, but that the carrier rate in calves undergoing BRD is not significantly higher than that of normal calves. *Pasteurella haemolytica* in contrast, is found much more frequently in calves undergoing BRD than in healthy calves. In a long-term study of bacterial colonization of the nasal passages of several herds of cattle, *P. haemolytica* seemed to have active cycles of nasal colonization, while *P. multocida* was isolated at a more constant rate (10). Thomson *et al.* (19,20), found higher mean colony counts of *P. haemolytica* in the nasal passages of sick calves than in well calves, but there were not significant differences in mean colony counts of *P. multocida* between the two groups. Therefore, summarizing from the limited information available, *P. multocida* is an important pathogen involved in BRD. However, the carrier rate of *P. multocida* and its numbers in the nasal passages do not seem to fluctuate with the incidence of stress or with BRD as in the case of *P. haemolytica.*

In a study correlating histological findings in lungs from natural BRD cases with the species of *Pasteurella* isolated, *P. haemolytica* was associated with fibrinous pleuropneumonia, while *P. multocida* was associated with fibrinous bronchopneumonia (21). However, since the disease occurred naturally, all agents contributing to the lesions were not known. While it is recognized that both *P. haemolytica* and *P. multocida* have important roles in the BRD complex, most in-depth experimental and field information concerns *P. haemolytica.* Relatively little deals specifically with *P. multocida.* The remainder of the paper will deal with the involvement of *P. haemolytica* in BRD.

Experimental Observations

Pasteurella haemolytica usually causes no problem in the healthy, unstressed calf. Our attempts to colonize the nasal passages of healthy calves have not resulted in their carrying detectable numbers of *P. haemolytica* for long periods of time. Aerosol exposures of calves with *P. haemolytica* freshly isolated from frozen pneumonic lung caused either no clinical reaction or a one-day fever response. Usually *P. haemolytica* were isolated from the nasal passages for one-two days or less (22). The immediate, brief febrile response has been described by others (23,24). On rare occasions, aerosol exposure with *P. haemolytica* alone caused clinical illness with prolonged shedding (23,25) and death (23).

In studies at Guelph on lung clearance of *P. haemolytica* by healthy calves, 90 percent of the bacteria put into the lungs were cleared within four hours (26). The healthy, unstressed calf is so efficient at clearing *P. haemolytica* that there is not much margin left for improvement.

To establish *P. haemolytica* infections in the lung, investigators have subjected calves to stressful situations or to concomitant infections with viral agents or have damaged or bypassed the protective mechanisms in the upper respiratory tract. Common methods to stress calves have included exposure to rapidly fluctuating hot and cold temperatures, forced exercise or transport. The most commonly used viruses for experimental combination infections have been parainfluenza-3 (PI-3) virus or infectious bovine rhinotracheitis (IBR) virus (5).

Others have injected *P. haemolytica* directly into the lung (27). These methods have led to some degree of success in allowing *P. haemolytica* to become established in the lung and lesions to develop. Similar models are used to test the efficacy of immunizing products.

Pasteurella haemolytica can reside at undetectable levels in the nasopharynx for long periods of time. In several instances, our calves exposed to PI-3 virus or to IBR virus one month after an exposure to and clearing of *P. haemolytica* began shedding detectable numbers of *P. haemolytica* several days after they became clinically ill. In our experience, this was not repeatable enough to design experiments based on the phenomenon (22).

To establish nasal colonization with *P. haemolytica,* we determined that exposing calves to broth cultures of the bacteria intranasally five days after a PI-3 virus or an IBR virus infection was a reproducible method. The procedure usually resulted in prolonged shedding of high numbers of *P. haemolytica* in the nasal mucus. The usual termination of the nasal infection was an abrupt cessation of shedding of *P. haemolytica* rather than a gradual decrease in the number shed, and an immediate return of the normal preexposure nasal flora (22).

Field Observations

In a two-year study of the development of BRD in calves going through the marketing process, we made several key observations (11). Few calves at the farm-of-origin carried detectable numbers of *P. haemolytica* in the nasal passages. On the farm-of-origin, almost all *P. haemolytica* isolates were serotype 2. The nasal carrier rate increased at the auction barn and was markedly high at the feedyard, after the calves had been transported 1600 kilometers. Shortly after arrival at the feedyard, during the episodes of acute BRD, 80-100 percent of the *P. haemolytica* isolates from the nasal passages were serotype 1. Similar numbers of both sick and well cattle were carrying *P. haemolytica* serotype 1 in the nasal passages. In most of the nasal carriers, *P. haemolytica* serotype 1 was the predominant species in the nasal flora. We isolated only serotype 1 from the lungs of the calves that died from acute BRD. Serum titers to serotype 1 followed the course of transit, disease and convalescence. Serum titers to serotype 2 fluctuated independently of such factors.

The sudden rapid proliferation of *P. haemolytica* in the nasopharynx of stressed or sick calves is a phenonemon that was observed only recently (5). During the earliest studies, most nasal swab samples were collected from calves during disease outbreaks. Both healthy and diseased calves in the groups would have been shedding large numbers of *P. haemolytica* at that time. Such findings probably gave the impression that *P. haemolytica* was readily found in the nasal passages of healthy calves. Before serotyping studies were done routinely, the concept was that the same *P. haemolytica* as that involved in BRD could be readily isolated from the nasal passages of healthy calves.

Pasteurella haemolytica serotype 1 is isolated almost exclusively from the nasal passages of calves suffering from BRD at the feedyard and from pneumonic lungs (5,14). Other serotypes are rarely isolated from cattle with BRD (5). There are nine established serotypes plus isolates which cannot be typed of the biotype A of *P. haemolytica* and they are readily found in the nasal passages of healthy sheep in the United States (28). Serotype 2 is probably not an important pathogen in BRD. It is, however, a frequent cause of pneumonia in sheep. The reason for the difference of serotype occurrence in cattle and sheep is not apparent.

Proposed Mechanism of Pasteurella Pneumonia

From our observations on nasal colonization with *P. haemolytica*, we know that under certain conditions *P. haemolytica* can proliferate rapidly in the nasal passages, increasing from undetectable numbers to become the major portion of the nasal flora. After the increase of *P. haemolytica* in the nasal passages, it is likely that greater numbers will travel through the trachea in droplet form and enter the lungs (29). Healthy, unstressed calves are not usually affected by *P. haemolytica* but when the calf's condition allows rapid replication of its endogenous *P. haemolytica* in the nasal passages, the calf is likely to be susceptible to small numbers of exogenous *P. haemolytica* as well. The rapid proliferation in the nasal passages can occur after the stress of transportation or as a result of virus-induced clinical illness (11,22). Since the conditions under which the rapid proliferation occurred had systemic rather than local effects on the host, the same conditions might allow *P. haemolytica* to proliferate rapidly in the lungs and cause pneumonia.

Epizootiologic studies that have employed serotyping have added to our knowledge on the involvement of *P. haemolytica* in BRD. They allow us to focus our efforts on a narrower group within the *P. haemolytica.* However, serotyping as a tool in epizootiologic studies now is of limited value, since serotype 1 is almost exclusively involved in BRD. A further breakdown within the serotype 1 group would make more detailed epizootiologic studies possible.

Conclusion

The following are some specific, critical questions remaining that if answered would enhance the possibility of reducing the involvement of *P. haemolytica* in BRD.

1. Where and how does *P. haemolytica* serotype 1 live in the upper respiratory tract of the healthy calf?

2. What mechanism allows the rapid selected proliferation of *P. haemolytica* serotype 1 in the nasal passages?

3. What are the interactions of *P. haemolytica* serotype 1 with the host within the lung?

4. What are the best methods for determining the efficacy of immunizing products?

Finally, if *P. haemolytica* serotype 1 were completely eliminated, would BRD be the same problem as exists at present? Would the void left by *P. haemolytica* serotype 1 be filled by another serotype of *P. haemolytica* or by another bacterium?

References

1. Hamdy AH, Morrill CC, Hoyt HH:Shipping fever of cattle. North Central Regional Research Bulletin 165, Ohio Agricultural Research and Development Center, Research Bulletin 975, Wooster, Ohio, 1965.

2.   Carter GR:*Pasteurella* infections as sequelae to respiratory viral infections. J Am Vet Med Assoc 163, part 2:863-864, 1973.

3.   Lillie LE:The bovine respiratory disease complex. Can Vet J 15:233-242, 1974.

4.   Gilmour NJL:The role of pasteurellae in respiratory diseases of cattle, in Martin WB (ed): Current Topics in Veterinary Medicine, Respiratory Diseases in Cattle, vol. 3, The Hague, Martinus Nijhoff, 1978, pp. 356-362.

5.   Frank GH:*Pasteurella haemolytica* and respiratory disease in cattle. Proc US Anim Health Assoc 83:153-160, 1979.

6.   Rhemtulla AJ, Thomson RG:A review of the lesions in shipping fever of cattle. Can Vet J 22:1-8, 1981.

7.   Yates WDG:A review of infectious bovine rhinotracheitis, shipping fever pneumonia and viral-bacterial synergism in respiratory diseases of cattle. Can J Comp Med 46:225-263, 1982.

8.   Collier, JR, Rossow CF:Microflora of apparently healthy lung tissue of cattle. Am J Vet Res 25:391-393, 1964.

9.   Allan EM:Pulmonary bacterial flora of pneumonic and nonpneumonic calves, in Martin WB (ed): Current Topics in Veterinary Medicine, Respiratory Diseases in Cattle, vol. 3. The Hague, Martinus Nijhoff, 1978, pp. 345-355.

10.   Magwood SE, Barnum DA, Thomson RG:Nasal bacterial flora of calves in healthy and in pneumonia-prone herds. Can J Comp Med 33:237-243, 1969.

11.   Frank GH, Smith PC:Prevalence of *Pasteurella haemolytica* in transported calves. Am J Vet Res 44:981-985, 1983.

12.   Blackburn BO, Heddleston KL, Pfow CJ:*Pasteurella multocida* serotyping results (1971-1973).   Avian Dis 19:353-356, 1975.

13.   Brown LN, Dillman RC, Dierks RE:The *Haemophilus somnus* complex. Proc US Anim Health Assoc 74:94-108, 1970.

14.   Stephens LR, Little PB, Wilkie BN,*et al.:*Infectious thromboembolic meningoencephalitis in cattle: a review. J Am Vet Med Assoc 178:378-384, 1981.

15.   Panciera RJ, Dahlgren RR, Rinker HB:Observations on septicemia of cattle caused by a *Haemophilus*-like organism. Path Vet 5:212-226, 1968.

16.   Ernø H:Mycoplasmas involved in bovine pneumonia, in Martin WB (ed): Current Topics in Veterinary Medicine, Respiratory Diseases in Cattle, vol 3. The Hague, Martinus Hijhoff, 1978, pp. 279-283.

17.   Gourlay RN, Howard CJ:Isolation and pathogenicity of mycoplasmas from the respiratory tract of calves, in Martin WB (ed): Current Topics in Veterinary Medicine,

Respiratory Diseases in Cattle, vol 3. The Hague, Martinus Nijhoff, 1978, pp. 295-304.

18.   Stalheim OHV:Mycoplasmal respiratory disease of ruminants: a review and update. J Am Vet Med Assoc 182:403-406, 1983.

19.   Thomson RG, Benson ML, Savan M:Pneumonic pasteurellosis of cattle: microbiology and immunology. Can J Comp Med 33:194-206, 1969.

20.   Thomson RG, Chander S, Savan M, et al.:Investigation of factors of probable significance in the pathogenesis of pneumonic pasteurellosis in cattle. Can J Comp Med 39:194-207, 1975.

21.   Schiefer B, Ward GE, Moffatt RE:Correlation of microbiological and histological findings in bovine fibrinous penumonia. Vet Pathol 15:313-321, 1978.

22.   Frank GH:Unpublished data, 1983.

23.   Baldwin DE, Marshall RG, Wessman GE:Experimental infection of calves with myxovirus parainfluenza-3 and Pasteurella hemolytica. Am J Vet Res 28:1773-1782, 1967.

24.   Friend SCE, Wilkie BN, Thomson RG, et al.:Bovine pneumonic pasteurellosis: experimental induction in vaccinated and nonvaccinated calves. Can J Comp Med 41:77-83, 1977.

25.   Collier JR, Chow TL, Benjamin MM, *et al.*:The combined effect of infectious bovine rhinotracheitis virus and *Pasteurella hemolytica* on cattle.   Am J Vet Res 21:195-198, 1960.

26.   Lillie LE, Thomson RG:The pulmonary clearance of bacteria by calves and mice.   Can J Comp Med 36:129-137, 1972.

27.   Newman PR, Corstvet RE, Panciera RJ:Distribution of *Pasteurella haemolytica* and *Pasteurella multocida* in the bovine lung following vaccination and challenge exposure as an indicator of lung resistance.   Am J Vet Res 43:417-422, 1982.

28.   Frank GH:Serotypes of *Pasteurella haemolytica* in sheep in the midwestern United States.   Am J Vet Res 43:2035-2037, 1982.

29.   Grey CL, Thomson RG:*Pasteurella haemolytica* in the tracheal air of calves.   Can J Comp Med 35:121-128, 1971.

Viruses as Etiologic Agents of Bovine Respiratory Disease

Bruce D. Rosenquist, D.V.M., Ph.D.

Department of Veterinary Microbiology
College of Veterinary Medicine
University of Missouri
Columbia, Missouri 65211

Introduction

Since the title of this paper is "Viruses as Etiologic Agents of Bovine Respiratory Disease," this provides an opportunity to briefly discuss at the outset two subjects which seldom, it seems to me, get discussed. These two subjects are (1) requirements for a virus to be established as a "pathogen," and (2) why a unified, multidisciplinary, nationwide (multiregional) approach must be undertaken to eventually clarify the etiology of acute bovine respiratory disease (BRD) in North America.

First, most acute respiratory disease in humans is caused by viruses and, similarly in cattle, viruses are blamed for the majority of cases of acute respiratory disease. Cattle are susceptible to infection with many pathogenic viruses and often these viruses infect in various combinations. An extensive list of viruses has now been isolated from cattle with acute BRD. I think that we in veterinary medicine are often too reluctant to accept some viruses as pathogens, sometimes insisting on fulfilling Koch's postulates as originally written. It has been stated that "insistence on their fulfillment before causality is accepted with a new agent in relation to a disease should be abandoned."

Some hindrances to establishing causal involvement of a given virus in a given respiratory syndrome include: causal involvement may be apparent only in certain years, or during certain times of the year, or in certain age groups of animals, or in certain types of populations of animals (considering here host susceptibility differences, immunological status), or in certain geographical locations, or under certain environmental conditions. In some cases, two or more agents or factors are needed to produce disease. Thus, in addition to the agent involved (the primary emphasis of Koch's postulates), the circumstances under which infection occurs and the influence of the host response in determining whether disease develops needs to be considered.

Under experimental conditions, it may be difficult or impossible to include all the factors involved in production of clinical signs of BRD after exposure to a suspected pathogen--yet this should not exclude a virus from being considered a pathogen under the right conditions. I am not suggesting that all of the viruses considered here are equally pathogenic, but I think a case can be made for all of them causing clinical signs of respiratory disease in appropriate cattle under the right circumstances.

The second subject is the desirability of a nationwide (more accurately multiregional) effort to clarify the etiology of BRD. A true picture of the role all these agents play in the various clinical syndromes of bovine respiratory disease in the United States will eventually require nationwide, well-coordinated studies. At this time, however, I do not visualize the requisite funding for a project of the required magnitude. Well-supported regional undertakings sustained over a period of several years, such as the "Virus Watch Programs" in humans done to detect viral infections and determine associated clinical illnesses and epidemiologic data, would yield invaluable data were it conducted properly with experienced personnel in all appropriate disciplines. These should include veterinarians in private practice, academic clinicians, animal scientists, epidemiologists, virologists, bacteriologists, immunologists, pathologists and biostaticians. A science writer would be an added plus (Table 1). I should add politicians.

Table 1. Personnel for bovine "virus watch" program

Cattle owners
Practicing veterinarians
Academic clinicians
Animal scientists (various disciplines)
Epidemiologists
Virologists
Bacteriologists
Immunologists
Pathologists
Biostaticians
Science writers (?)

Nor should the value of participation by interested "lay" personnel such as feedlot operators, cow-calf cattlemen, dairymen, et cetera, be overlooked. Indeed, without their cooperation, any such study would yield less than it was capable of.

Some members of the NC-107 Technical Committee (Bovine Respiratory Diseases), as well as others, did make a limited attempt in this direction in 1976 and 1977. This was the so-called (barnyard name) Tennessee/Texas shipping fever project. It attempted to define the serologic and microbiologic status of calves before, and at various times after, shipment from the farm-of-origin to final destination in a feedlot. It involved scientists with differing expertise in a half-dozen states. The cooperation was voluntary and not separately funded for all cooperators. Although valuable information was obtained (which would not have been possible without the cooperation of various individual scientists), due to limitations in funding, personnel and the like, much that could have been achieved was not.

This paper is restricted to those viruses and diseases described which cause BRD in the United States. As such, we can identify about ten viruses belonging to six virus families (Table 2).

Table 2. Viruses implicated in bovine respiratory disease in the United States

Name	Family
Infectious bovine rhinotracheitis	Herpesviridae
Malignant catarrhal fever	Herpesviridae
Bovine herpesvirus "Type 4"	Herpesviridae
Adenovirus	Adenoviridae
Parainfluenza 3	Paramyxoviridae
Respiratory syncytial virus	Paramyxoviridae
Bovine virus diarrhea	Togaviridae
Reovirus	Reoviridae
Rhinovirus	Picornaviridae
Enterovirus	Picornaviridae

The importance of each of these viruses as pathogens in the etiology of BRD is subject to debate in many cases and requires further definition.

Observations

Since time is limited and since the literature is abundant concerning infectious bovine rhinotracheitis (IBR), parainfluenza 3 (PI-3), and bovine viral diarrhea (BVD) viruses, while not denying their importance, I would like to spend the majority of time on some of the "less well-recognized or appreciated" members of the BRD complex of viruses.

Infectious Bovine Rhinotracheitis, Bovine Viral Diarrhea, Parainfluenza 3

All recognize the "big three"--IBR, BVD and PI-3--as being ubiquitous bovine viruses. Opinions vary as to their individual roles as respiratory pathogens, and as to whether BVD virus should be included as a respiratory pathogen. The IBR virus is universally accepted as a pathogen in its own right; I agree. Parainfluenza-3 virus causes disease, without a doubt, but perhaps it often requires a bacterium to cause serious (economically important) disease. Bovine virus diarrhea virus, considered by some to cause basically only enteric or systemic disease, is now considered by many to also play a role in causation of respiratory disease and therefore can legitimately be called a "respiratory virus."   Only one serotype of each is recognized and each can produce respiratory disease by itself, as well as predispose cattle to superinfection with bacteria, primarily *Pasteurella* spp.

"Type 4" Bovine Herpesviruses

Serotypes. I am referring here to that group of viruses tentatively classified as such of which the Movar 33/63 isolate from a calf with keratoconjunctivitis is the reference strain.   In the United States, viruses antigenically related to this one have been isolated from cattle with malignant catarrhal fever (not the cause), undifferentiated respiratory disease, tracheitis and pharyngitis, and nonrespiratory conditions.

Importance. This is not known, but they have been shown to be capable of causing disease.

Incidence. Nationwide this is not clear.   A survey in Oklahoma indicated that the virus was not very widespread, since only 7/351 (2 percent) of cattle tested were seropositive by the indirect fluorescent antibody test.

Pathogenicity. Experimental infection of calves has given mixed results and reports range from no apparent infection, to mild upper respiratory tract disease, to frank respiratory disease.

Signs. Reported signs include fever, nasal discharge, conjunctivitis, and mild clinical signs of tracheitis and coughing.

Adenoviruses

Serotypes. Eight serotypes of bovine adenoviruses (BAV) are recognized (ninth candidate) in the world. Not all have been isolated in the United States, nor are all associated with disease.

Importance. It appears that Type 3 is the most important BAV pathogen in the BRD complex in the United States.

Incidence. Where studied, adenoviruses appear to be widespread in the cattle population. In some studies, the majority of adult cattle have been seropositive to Types 1, 2, 3, or 4, and in some instances up to 100 percent were seropositive.

Pathogenicity. In the field, pneumonia or pneumoenteritis has been associated with BAV-3 infection in young calves and in feedlot cattle with acute BRD. The BAV-4 has been isolated from a week-old calf with pneumoenteritis, and an eight-month-old bull with fever and respiratory disease. The BAV-7 has similarly been isolated from calves with pneumonia or pneumoenteritis.

Signs. These may include fever, lacrimal and nasal discharge, diarrhea, conjunctivitis and coughing.

Experimental infections with some serotypes produce similar signs.

Respiratory Syncytial Virus

Serotypes. One serotype is recognized.

Importance. This virus is an important cause of respiratory disease in cattle. Infection with bovine respiratory syncytial virus can explain a number of previously undiagnosed outbreaks of BRD in the United States. This requires investigators looking for it and laboratories capable of performing the required serologic or virologic examinations.

Incidence. Serologic surveys indicate widespread infection among United States cattle. Where such testing has been done, the number of seropositive cattle has ranged from 38 percent to 100 percent. Approximately 88 percent of Missouri beef and dairy calves less than one year of age are seropositive. Virus isolations have been few, due in part to the extreme lability of the virus and the fact that cattle do not appear to excrete the virus for long after the onset of clinical disease.

Pathogenicity. Experimentally, mild signs of BRD can be produced--fever and rhinitis, with or without cough. Some reports indicate more severe experimental disease. This may depend on the route of inoculation--i.e., intranasal versus intranasal and intratracheal combined; in one study only coughing was noted after intranasal inoculation, while severe respiratory signs were produced after intratracheal inoculation. Under field conditions, I think there is no doubt this is an important respiratory pathogen, and clinical signs can be severe.

Signs. Reported signs include fever, rapid respiratory rate, cough and nasal discharge.

Reoviruses

Serotypes. Three serotypes of bovine reoviruses are recognized.

Importance. I really do not know how important reoviruses are. The "orphan" in their name is well-taken. There is serologic evidence that at least some of the serotypes are associated with mild respiratory illness in cattle. No doubt most infections are not apparent. Their importance in causing BRD in the United States is not well established.

Incidence. Reovirus-neutralizing antibodies are very prevalent in bovine sera in the U.S.

Pathogenicity. Experimental infection of calves, especially with Type 1, has produced mild respiratory illness and lung lesions or no signs of disease.

Signs. Reported signs are common to many other respiratory infections--fever, depression, nasal discharge, coughing or no signs at all.

Rhinoviruses

Serotypes. Two serotypes (1 and 2) are officially recognized. All reported isolates to date except one have been Type 1 bovine rhinoviruses.

Importance. Opinions as to their importance in causation of BRD vary. I suppose the majority of veterinary opinion downgrades their importance and pathogenicity. I disagree. In some cases they are the only viruses demonstrable in calves with BRD. Human rhinoviruses are the most common viruses isolated from people with common colds, and also occasionally cause more serious illnesses such as bronchitis.

Incidence. These "nose viruses" are ubiquitous among the United States cattle population wherever incidence has been studied. Seropositive rates to Type 1 bovine rhinovirus (neutralizing antibody) recorded include 95 percent in Maryland cattle and 71 percent in Iowa calves. Approximately 95 percent of Missouri beef and dairy calves less than one year of age are seropositive; the figure approaches 100 percent by twelve months of age.

Reports of their isolation are not many, probably because the cell culture systems used in some diagnostic laboratories do not permit their replication, and because in some cases initial cytopathic effects produced by inoculation of cultures with clinical specimens may be minimal and not recognized by inexperienced personnel (indeed it may not be present until a "blind" passage, which is not practical nor productive in most diagnostic laboratory situations), and also because of their lability to heat and the fact that, even after experimental infection, many calves do not excrete large amounts of virus.

Pathogenicity. After experimental infection, signs have usually been minimal or nonexistent, but not always.

Signs. Fever, lachrimation, nasal discharge, cough and increased respiratory rate may occur.

Enteroviruses

Serotypes. There are seven serotypes of bovine enteroviruses.

Importance. Their etiologic significance as pathogens in BRD has not been determined.

Incidence. These viruses are widespread in the United States cattle population.

Pathogenicity. Experimentally, most attempts to reproduce disease have been fruitless. In the field, perhaps they may act with bacteria to cause pneumonia. Certainly, isolations of enteroviruses from cattle with respiratory disease is not rare, but their etiologic role is unclear.

References

1.   Evans AS:Causation and disease: the Henle-Koch postulates revisited. Yale J Biol Med 49:175-195, 1976.

2.   Kahrs RF:Viral Diseases of Cattle. Ames, Iowa, Iowa State University Press, 1981, 299 pp.

3.   Kurstak E, Kurstak C (eds):Comparative Diagnosis of Viral Diseases, Vol. III, Vertebrate Animal and Related Viruses, Part A - DNA Viruses. New York, Academic Press, 1981, 429 pp.

4.   Kurstak E, Kurstak C (eds):Comparative Diagnosis of Viral Diseases, Vol. IV, Vertebrate Animal and Related Viruses, Part B - RNA Viruses. New York, Academic Press, 1981, 694 pp.

5.   Martin WB (ed):Respiratory Diseases in Cattle. The Hague, Martinus Nijhoff, 1978, 562 pp.

6.   Mohanty SB:Bovine Respiratory Viruses. Adv Vet Sci Comp Med 22:83-109, 1978.

7.   Potgieter LND:Current concepts on the role of viruses in respiratory tract disease of cattle. Bov Pract 12:75-81, 1977.

8.   Proceedings of a Colloquium on Immunity to Selected Infectious Diseases of Cattle.   J Am Vet Med Assoc 163:777-924, 1973.

9.   Proceedings of a Symposium on Immunity to the Bovine Respiratory Disease Complex.   J Am Vet Med Assoc 152:705-940, 1968.

10.   Smith PC, Frank GH, Gillette KG:Viral infections in bovine respiratory diseases in the United States.   Bull Off Int Epiz 88:179-190, 1977.

11.   12th World Congress on Diseases of Cattle, Amsterdam, The Netherlands, Proceedings, Volume 1, 1982.

Chemical Synthesis of Subunit Vaccines

James L. Bittle, D.V.M.

Department of Molecular Biology
Scripps Clinic and Research Foundation
10666 North Torrey Pines Road
La Jolla, California 92037

The North Anerican Symposium on Bovine Respiratory
Disease reviewed the major causes of bovine respiratory
disease and discussed the need for immunological mechanisms
to control these diseases. In this regard, vaccines have
been successfully used to control the major infectious
diseases of the bovine respiratory tract that are shown
below:

1. infectious bovine rhinotracheitis

2. parainfluenza

3. contagious pleuropneumonia

4. *Pasteurella*

Other agents causing bovine respiratory disease are listed
below, but these have not been shown to be significant
enough to warrant vaccine development:

1. respiratory syncytial virus infection

2. adenovirus infection

3. rhinovirus infection

4. herpesvirus infection

5. chlamydial infection

Problems associated with the use of vaccines are that animals occasionally react adversely to the antigens in the vaccines or the antigens do not induce an adequate immune response. Therefore, there is a continual need to produce vaccines that are safer and more effective. To accomplish this task, we must explore improved means of making antigens and of presenting these antigens to the immune system of the host animal.

The present bovine vaccines are of three types and include:

1. *Modified Live Organisms.* Antigens that are made by modifying the virulence of the organism so they multiply in the host and induce antibodies but not disease.

2. *Inactivated Whole Organisms.* Chemically-inactivated antigens that do not replicate in the animal but induce antibody formation.

3. *Subunits.* Subunit vaccines which use the antigenic fraction of an organism but not the infectious nucleic acid or other unnecessary antigens.

The modified vaccines have the advantage of inducing longer-lasting immunity, but may cause disease. The inactivated vaccines are safer, but in general are not as antigenic and must be administered more frequently. Subunit vaccines have not been widely used in cattle until recently when pili vaccines were introduced.

Recent developments in recombinant DNA technology have made possible the identification of surface proteins and their amino acid sequences. From this information, antigenic sites may be identified and made by either chemical or biological synthesis. Our laboratory at the Research Institute of Scripps Clinic has concentrated on chemical synthesis (1,2). This is accomplished by isolating the gene that codes for the desired surface protein. This gene contains the genetic information (nucleotide sequence) which may be translated directly into an amino acid sequence of the surface protein. Peptides from this amino acid sequence may be synthesized chemically, and these may be tested for their ability to induce neutralizing antibodies. Once the proper amino acid sequence of the antigenic site is found, it will often mimic the antigenic site found on the native antigen. These chemically-synthesized antigenic sites are then incorporated into a vaccine. The immunogen may contain a small fraction, approximately 5 percent or less, of the antigen made by using the whole organism, but it is the active site for antibody induction. The degree of antibody stimulation may be determined by the manner in which the peptide is presented to the immune system. Thus, the exact amino acid sequence and its incorporation in an adjuvant system is very important.

In a cooperative effort with Dr. Fred Brown of the Animal Virus Research Institute at Pirbright, England (3), we have found that of the nine peptides made from the 213 amino acid sequence of the VP1 type 0-1 of foot-and-mouth disease virus (Figure 1), two were quite active (Table 1).

AMINO ACID SEQUENCE OF FOOT AND MOUTH DISEASE
VIRUS POLYPEPTIDE VP1 TYPE O (KAUFBEUREN STRAIN)

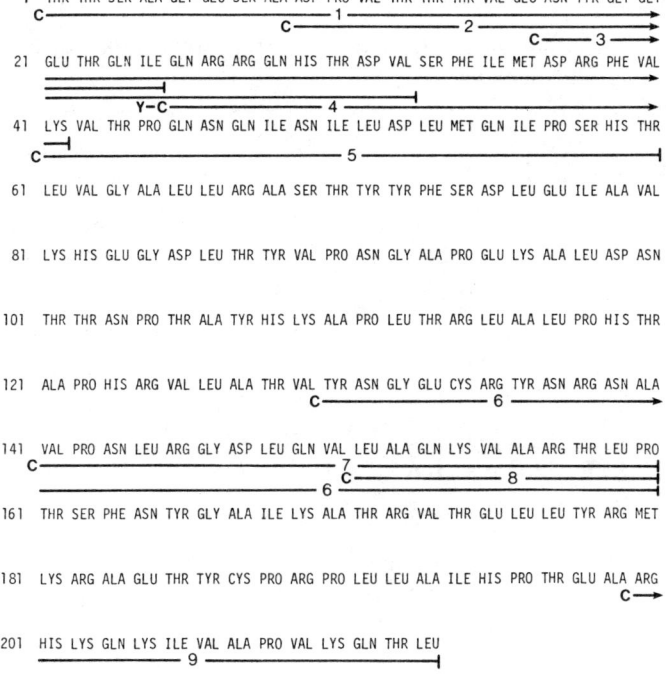

Figure 1.

Table 1. Antibody response in rabbits to foot-and-mouth disease virus VP1 peptides

Peptide No.	Peptide Region	Anti-Peptide Antibody	Neutralization Index, Log 10
1	1–41	480, 480	≲0.9,≲0.7
2	9–24	120, 60	≲0.3,≲0.3
3	17–32	120, 30	≲0.5,≲0.9
4	24–41	60, 960	≲0.5,≲0.9
5	41–60	ND	<1.0,<1.0
6	131–160	320, 320	>4.0,>4.0
7	141–160	480, 480	≲6.3, 4.3
8	151–160	120, 240	1.1, 2.9
9	200–213	1280, 240	3.5, 3.1

One of these sequences, number seven of the nine peptides made from amino acid region 141–160 induced good antibody levels in guinea pigs, and these animals were protected when challenged with a homologous strain of virus (Table 2).

Table 2. Protection of guinea pigs against challenge with FMDV by inoculation with inactivated virus particles or synthetic peptides 141–160 and 200–213

Antigen	Dose (µG)	Adjuvant	Neutralization Index (Log 10)	No. Protected/ No. Challenged
Virus	1	Freund's	2.5 (1.3–2.9)	2/2
	10	Freund's	⩾5.3 (⩾4.5)	4/4
141–160	20	A1 (OH)$_3$	2.1 (0.9–2.7)	3/4
	200	A1 (OH)$_3$	2.7 (1.7–⩾3.7)	3/3
	20	Freund's	2.1 (0.1–2.5)	1/4
	200	Freund's	⩾3.3 (1.5–⩾3.3)	4/4
200–213	20	Freund's	1.1 (NS)	0/4
	200	Freund's	0.5 (ND)	0/4

384 James L. Bittle

We have been able to produce similar antibody responses in cattle that are compatible with protection (Figure 2).

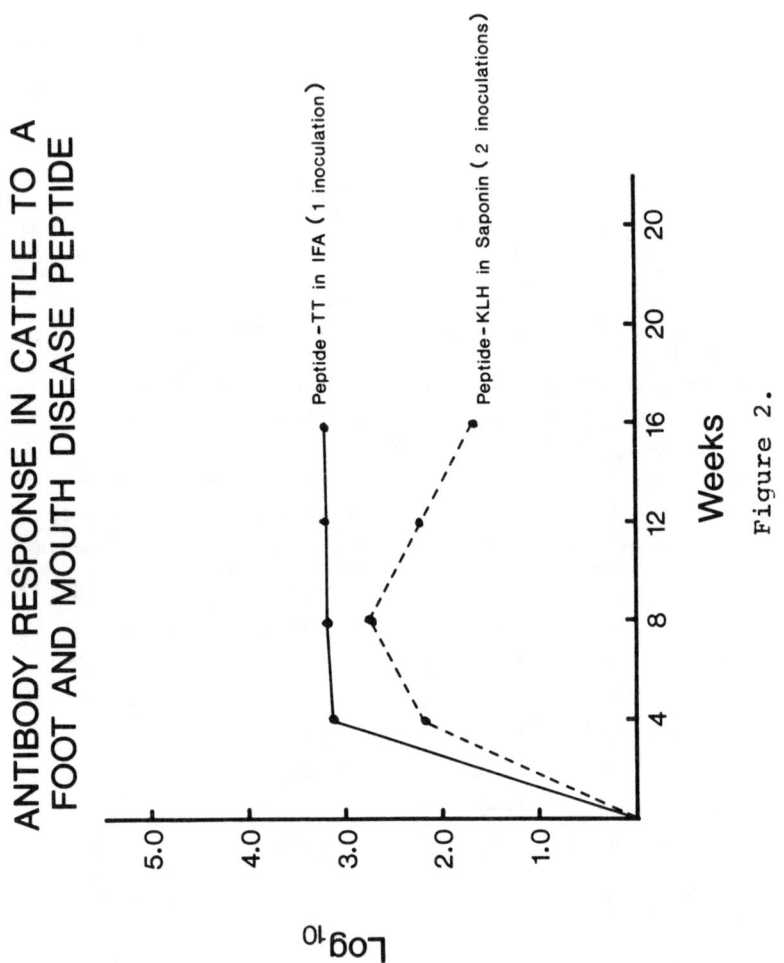

Figure 2.

Studies are in progress to determine the activity of peptides made from sequences of other serotypes and also to show the effectiveness of various dose levels of peptides in cattle.

Enough research has been done, however, to show that an effective synthetic vaccine for foot-and-mouth disease is possible, and it would have several distinct advantages over the present vaccine. These are mainly:

1. the non-infective nature of the synthetic antigen;
2. the improved stability at high temperatures will improve storage and distribution of the vaccine; and
3. the ease of chemical synthesis in vaccine production.

The synthesis may *now* be done in a completely automated form, and from this process, large quantities of peptides made from pure amino acids can be produced. This type of product and production process has many advantages over the biological processes used to make our present vaccines and biosynthetic products.

Foot-and-mouth disease is only one example of many diseases in which chemical synthesis is being used to develop new vaccines for the future (4). These new vaccines will further improve our ability to control disease in man and animals.

References

1. Sutcliffe JG, Shinnick TM, Green N, Liu F-T, Niman HL, Lerner RA:Chemical synthesis of a polypeptide predicted from the nucleotide sequence allows detection of a new retroviral gene product. Nature Vol. 287, 5785:801-805, 1980.

2. Lerner RA:Synthetic vaccines. Scien American, pp. 66-74, 1983.

3. Bittle JL, Houghten RA, Alexander H, Shinnick TM, Sutcliffe JG, Lerner RA:Protection against foot-and-mouth disease by immunization with a chemically synthesized peptide predicted from the viral nucleotide sequence. Nature, vol 298, 5869:30-33, 1982.

4. Bittle JL:Development of chemically synthesized antigens for vaccines. Proceedings of the 86th Ann Mtg of the US Anim Health Assoc, Nashville, Tennessee, 1982.

Biological Synthesis of Subunit Vaccines

Donald O. Morgan, D.V.M., Ph.D.

U.S. Department of Agriculture, Agricultural Research Service
Plum Island Animal Disease Center
P.O. Box 848
Greenport, New York 11944

Summary

Recent advances in biotechnology hold great promise for veterinary medicine, particularly in the area of vaccine development. Peptide vaccines eliminate the danger of the spread of contagion and assure the quality and quantity of vaccine needed for disease control programs. Recombinant DNA technology and organic synthesis provide alternate means of production with the former having an advantage with large polypeptide immunogens. Monoclonal antibodies offer the necessary precision for defining the immunogenic epitopes and relating them to field-strain infectious agents and vaccine sources. Quality control and estimates of vaccine potency will both benefit from the link between "*in vitro* antigenicity" and immunogenicity provided by hybridoma technology. Anti-idiotype vaccines for which monoclonal antibodies could serve as a source of immunogen offer an alternative source for immunogens which are difficult to produce.

Observations

The treatment of choice for infectious diseases is prophylaxis and as a practical matter the immune system is the optimum instrument for achieving this goal. Animals are quite efficient in their ability to develop immunity to disease. Vaccines composed of disease agents in killed or attenuated forms have been developed against a vast spectrum of diseases. Subunits of parasites (1), bacteria (2,3) and viruses (4) have been demonstrated to be effectively immunogenic. Peptides derived from subunits have been used to protect animals (5). Most recently effective vaccines have been formulated from polypeptides synthesized both organically and biosynthetically (6,7,8). Both systems of synthesis are effective and the one to use will be decided by the requirements of the particular goal. Synthesis of large molecules such as one might anticipate in the preparation of polyvalent immunogens should present no large problem to genetic engineering (9); whereas, the products of organic synthesis are rather restricted in size. The following report concerns vaccines produced by recombinant DNA technology using foot-and-mouth disease virus (FMDV) as a model.

Over the past few decades, estimation of the immunogen content of FMDV vaccines has evolved from being based on the infectivity titer prior to inactivation to the more realistic measurement of intact virion content. Subunits of this virion, ranging from 12S protein subunits to polypeptides, have been demonstrated to be quite adequate immunogens (4). However, commonly used dose volumes of FMDV-infected tissue culture harvest, the source of commercial vaccine immunogen, would have to be concentrated beyond practical limits in order to attain the concentration of subunits needed to elicit detectable neutralizing antibody. This observation of a decrease in immunogenicity upon degradation of the infective agent appears true for most derived subunit preparations. A popular explanation for this decrease in immunogenicity between the intact agent (i.e., virion) and its subunits is the mode of presentation to the immune system. It is evident that an epitope whose antigenicity survives the degradation of a virion is not itself changed but it has lost a degree of immunogenicity. If this "setting" or mode of presentation were understood, it is quite reasonable to expect that it could be enhanced as well as detracted from. Perhaps this is the sort of thing that could be achieved through coupling to carrier molecules and immunopotentiators (2). Thus far, most successful subunit vaccines have been heavily dependent upon the use of "adjuvants."   Freunds' complete and incomplete have both been successfully used with FMDV subunits (5,6). Unfortunately both of these preparations may result in highly undesirable vaccine-site reactions.   Research in immunopotentiation both in cell-mediated and humoral immunity is voluminous and beyond the scope of this report.

The capsid of the picornoviridae should provide one of the least complex examples of the conglomerate of epitopes that make up the surface proteins of infectious agents. These epitopes can be divided into two groups, continuous and discontinuous. Structurally, the continuous epitope is the simplest, depending directly upon amino acid sequence; whereas, the discontinuous epitope involves a tertiary or greater degree of structural complexity and could involve amino acids from two different areas of a protein or more than one protein.   Several epitopes of each category have been demonstrated on the FMDV virion.   Both categories of FMDV epitopes are immunogenic as judged by the passive protection conveyed by their identifying antibodies (10,11).   Further, the monoclonal antibody reacting with FMDV passively protected the pig and the mouse, showing that immunity can be achieved with an epitope (12).   Bio- and organically-synthesized peptides, containing continuous epitopes of FMDV, have been shown capable of eliciting virus-neutralizing antibodies and, in addition, vaccination with the biosynthesized peptides has protected cattle and swine from challenge infection (6,7,8).

In order to select a likely "vaccine peptide," the infectious agent must be reduced to an immunogenic fragment of reasonable size. In the case of FMDV, the virion, 12S protein subunit and structural virus protein 1 (VP1) were shown to be immunogenic (11). Viral RNA was used to prepare cDNA which was inserted into plasmids and replicated. The cDNA thus produced was used to develop a nucleotide map of that area of the FMDV genome coding for the viral structural proteins. Amino acid (AA) sequence data from the N-terminal end of VP1 was used to locate this protein on the genome map, thus enabling the derivation of the remaining AA sequence of VP1 and selection of its encoding region. Biosynthesized immunogenic VP1 was obtained from cultures of *E. coli* which had been used to support a specially contructed expression plasmid containing that region of FMDV RNA coding for VP1 (13).

As the immunogenic epitopes or clusters of epitopes of FMDV are more accurately defined, it will be possible to describe and evaluate those of type, subtype and strain specificities. Polyvalent immunogens can be prepared and perhaps increased in immunogenity (i.e., repeating units, et cetera).   The biosynthesis of such potentially large molecules can readily be accomplished through recombinant DNA technology.

All aspects of vaccine production, distribution and delivery will eventually be reshaped by synthetic peptide technology, some subtly and some drastically.   The major ponderable in this situation is just how rapidly one may expect the changes to come about.

Vaccine programs for disease control are often hampered by problems of quantity and quality, two areas which can readily be influenced by peptide vaccines.   The immunogens provided by this technology are less complex (i.e., peptide *versus* virion) and can be accurately defined.   Defined peptides can be assayed with authority, thus assuring batch-to-batch homogeneity.   Immunogenicity should become more predictable based upon previous animal tests of the same peptide.   The number of costly potency tests can be reduced and quality assured.   Production methodology with genetic engineering is such that, once it is set up for an immunogen, shortage of that peptide should not be a problem.   Stable immunogenic peptides can be produced in high concentrations which allow accumulation of emergency stocks, a highly desirable aspect in many disease control programs.   Dose volumes, rather than being dictated by immunogen concentration, can be chosen to suit the delivery system. There exists the potential for a "projectile"-type delivery system which would have advantages on the "range" and with wild animals.

Optimum conformation of immunogens is of paramount importance even in the case of apparently continuous epitopes. A particular amino acid sequence can be immunogenic in one preparation but nonimmunogenic in another. The particular protein can be detected; however, its immunogenicity must be determined in animals until data are available to properly correlate immunogenicity and antigenicity. Consider the immune system (i.e., animal) and the infectious agent as adversaries and it becomes rapidly apparent that the phrase "optimum conformation of immunogen" can be interpreted more than one way. Following this line of reasoning a bit further, one can speculate that in the evolution of a successful infectious agent the prevailing epitope conformation would unlikely be optimum from the standpoint of the immune system. Thus it is not unreasonable to anticipate that superior vaccines can be produced through artificially-enhanced epitope conformation. The optimal exploitation of the advantages of synthetic immunogens is dependent upon determining precisely what is needed for a particular purpose. For example, there are highly antigenic epitopes on infectious agents which are largely irrelevant to vaccines. The surface of the least complex virions is a conglomeration of epitopes and there appear to be several mechanisms of antibody-mediated neutralization of viral infectivity (11). However, the temptation to relate these facts should be resisted in respect to antibody classes and other factors. The foot-and-mouth disease virion has several different epitopes, the corresponding monoclonal antibodies of which can separately (or in a mixture) neutralize the virus (10). Data indicate that the virus is equally vulnerable to the neutralizing activity of these antibodies. It appears unlikely that serum from convalescent (immune) animals would contain equal amounts of these antibodies. For these reasons the terms major and minor antigenic determinants of a virion become confusing except under defined circumstances. On the other hand, with FMDV, for example, certain epitopes occur more frequently among the strains than do others (11). One would surmise that the most catholic immunogenic epitope of FMDV type A would make the most broad spectrum peptide vaccine for type A.

Monoclonal antibodies provide a means by which one can relate "in vitro" antigenicity to immunogenicity. Demonstration that a monoclonal antibody can convey passive immunity to an infectious disease indicates that the corresponding epitope plays a role in immunity (12). Additionally, elicitation of antibodies of the same specificities as the protective "monoclonal" would predict that the eliciting product could be an effective vaccine. Once collections of monoclonal antibodies are prepared and characterized, they will be of enormous benefit to diagnostic and control programs. For example, a hypothetical type X strain Y FMDV could be considered a unique collection of epitopes, some or all of which are shared with other type X viruses. Characterized monoclonal antibodies (developed to type X virus) could be used to determine which, if any, of the FMDV type X strain Y epitopes are related to an "outbreak virus." The epitope or set of epitopes could then be selected from existing immunogen or plasmid stocks (or organically synthesized) and a vaccine formulated for "the outbreak" could be on location in a short time. This scheme is, of course, limited by one's repertoire of "monoclonals and immunogens" but it is potentially much more versatile than anything now available.

In FMDV, antibodies to continuous and discontinuous epitopes are each capable of protecting animals (12,14). However, the relative advantages and disadvantages of the two types of epitopes in vaccines are not known. The continuous epitopes thus far reported have presented no especially prohibitive production problems. On the other hand, it can be anticipated that production of discontinuous epitopes will be a more formidable problem. Immunogenic epitopes of a discontinuous nature (i.e., virion specific) have been demonstrated on FMDV with both polyclonal and monoclonal antibody preparations (4,11).

It was proposed sometime ago that anti-idiotypes elicited by a protective antisera might have epitopes similar to that of the infectious agent (15). Anti-idiotype vaccines have been shown to be efficacious in trypanosomiasis and to prime the immune system to hepatitis B virus surface antigen (16,17). Foot-and-mouth disease "protective" monoclonal antibodies reactive with FMDV virion-specific epitopes are being used as first-stage immunogens in an investigation to evaluate the potential of this technology for eventually eliciting antibodies to the discontinuous epitopes on FMDV.

Peptide vaccines are theoretically applicable to any infectious agent which can be neutralized by the immune system. They are stable, a particular advantage for storage and use under range conditions. Small peptides will ultimately be manufactured by the most economic

method--organic synthesis or recombinant DNA.   In the case
of polypeptides and proteins, such as one might envision
for a multivalent FMDV vaccine, recombinant DNA procedures
appear to be the most suitable.

References

1.   Urban   JF,   Romanowski   RD:Biochemical   and
immunological characterization of functional antigens from
larval stages of *Ascaris suum.* Fed Proc 41:583, 1982.

2.   Audibert F, Jolivet M, Chedid L, *et al.:*Successful
immunization with a totally synthetic diphtheria vaccine.
Proc Nat Acad Sci USA 79:5042-5046, 1982.

3.   Mikesell P, Ivins BE, Ristroph JD, *et al.:*Plasmids,
Pasteur, and anthrax.   ASM News 49:320-322, 1983.

4.   Morgan DO, Moore, DM, McKercher PD:Vaccination
against foot-and-mouth disease, in New Developments with
Human and Veterinary Vaccines.   New York, Alan R. Liss,
Inc., 1980, pp. 169-178.

5.   Bachrach HL, Morgan DO, McKercher PD, *et
al.:*Foot-and-mouth disease virus: immunogenicity and
structure of fragments derived from capsid protein VP_3 and
of virus containing cleaved VP_3 .   Vet Microbiol 7:85-96,
1982.

6.   Kleid DG, Yansura D, Small B, *et al.:*Cloned viral
protein vaccine for foot-and-mouth disease; responses in
cattle and swine.   Science 214:1125-1129, 1981.

7.   Bittle JL, Houghten RA, Alexander H, *et al.*:Protection against foot-and-mouth disease by immunization with a chemically synthesized peptide predicted from the viral nucleotide sequence. Nature 298:30-33, 1982.

8.   Kupper H, Keller W, Kurz S, *et al.*:Cloning of cDNA of major antigen of foot-and-mouth disease virus and expression in *E. coli*. Nature 289:555-559, 1981.

9.   Bachrach HL:Recombinant DNA technology for the preparation of subunit vaccines.   J Am Vet Med Assoc 181:992-999, 1981.

10.   Robertson BH, Morgan DO, Moore DM:A monoclonal antibody against a fragment of the outer capsid protein, VP_1, of foot-and-mouth disease virus which neutralizes infectivity. The 2nd Ann Mtg Am Soc of Virology, Michigan State University, East Lansing, Michigan, 1983.

11.   Morgan DO, Robertson BH, Moore DM, *et al.*:Aphthoviruses: monoclonal antibodies and genetically engineered vaccines in foot-and-mouth disease control programs.   Proceedings of the IV International Conference on Comparative Virology. New York, Marcel Dekker, Inc., 1982, in press.

12.   Morgan DO, Moore DM, Robertson BH, *et al.*: Immunization of swine with defined segments of foot-and-mouth disease virus VP_1 produced by recombinant

DNA procedures. Conf of Res Workers in Animal Diseases, Chicago, Illinois, 1983.

13. Moore DM:Production of a vaccine for foot-and-mouth disease through cloning. Proc of the Beltsville Symposia in Agricultural Res, 1982.

14. Timpone CA:Monoclonal antibodies reactive with FMDV. MS thesis, Library of Coll of Vet Med, Cornell University, Ithaca, New York, 1983.

15. Nisonoff A, Lamoyi E:Implications of the presence of an internal image of the antigen in anti-idiotypic antibodies: possible application to vaccine production. Clin Immunol and Immunopath 21:397-406, 1981.

16. Sacks DL, Esser KM, Sher A:Immunization of mice against African trypanosomiasis using anti-idiotypic antibodies. J of Exper Med 155:1108-1119, 1982.

17. Kennedy RC, Adler-Storthz K, Henkel RD, et al.:Immune response to hepatitis B surface antigen: enhancement by prior injection of antibodies to the idiotype. Science 221:853-855, 1983.

A Molecular Approach to Bacterins

Harland W. Renshaw, D.V.M., Ph.D.

Department of Veterinary Microbiology and Parasitology
Texas A&M University
College Station, Texas 77843

Summary

Increased interest in providing improved preventative medicine programs for both humans and animals has prompted the development of advances in immunoprophylactic technologies. The renewed interest in the development of successful bacterins has occurred because of a growing awareness by biomedical scientists that antibiotics and antimicrobial chemotherapeutic agents will not provide the means to control and eliminate all bacterial diseases. General features of host anti-infectious defense in relation to immune protection against infectious diseases are considered. The most effective immunoprophylactic preparations usually stimulate development of host protective mechanisms in the vaccinated animal that parallel those developed in the infected animal.

The structure and function of bacterial cell walls are considered and current knowledge about the outer membrane proteins of Gram-negative bacteria is discussed. The outer membrane proteins are considered in detail because they represent likely candidate antigens capable of stimulating development of a protective immune response. Matrix porins form transmembrane channels that determine access of solutes to the periplasmic space and cytoplasmic membrane. The potential value of major outer membrane porin proteins as immunogens is considered.

Justifications for a molecular approach to production of bacterins for the bovine respiratory disease complex (BRDC) are indicated. Current knowledge about *Pasteurella haemolytica* leukotoxin is summarized and the potential importance of this exotoxin as a virulence factor is considered. Evidence from studies in this laboratory of outer membrane proteins and leukotoxin from *P. haemolytica* is summarized. It is suggested that a long-term goal of investigators studying the BRDC should be the development of an efficacious subunit bacterin for *P. haemolytica* and *P. multocida.*

Introduction

The principal factors which allow for the development of successful bacterins can be summarized into two categories. These are the demonstration of a specific immunological response which is related to immunity and the extraction of a bacterial antigen which induces the appropriate immunological response when inoculated into the host. The development of immunoprophylactic technologies has received increased attention by biomedical scientists because of a growing awareness that antibiotics and antimicrobial chemotherapeutic agents cannot be relied upon to control and eventually eliminate all infectious diseases (1). However, preventative vaccination is not always effective (2). The recent resurgence of interest in vaccines is interrelated with a re-emergence of interest in the areas of microbial immunology and preventative medicine (1-3).

A little over a century ago it was definitively shown that infectious diseases were caused by microorganisms. It has been suggested that the beginning of modern immunology can be dated to a specific experiment in which Pasteur, using fowl cholera organisms (Pasteurella multocida), performed his fundamental experiments in the attenuation of bacteria in culture and their use as an inoculum to induce immunity (4). When Pasteur did this classical study on acquired immunity there was no information on mechanisms that could explain the appearance and the specificity of the enhanced resistance of the vaccinated host. It is now known that vaccination confers immunity by stimulating a complex series of events culminating in the active development of specific lymphoid cells and their products which are capable of interacting with the infectious agent (2,3,5).

In relationship to the field of preventative medicine, the essential purpose of vaccination is to stimulate a specific immunologic response to an infectious agent or its protective antigens. The expectation is that the vaccinated host will develop protective antibodies in the blood and/or cell-mediated immunity to the infectious agent. Although the protection provided by vaccination may wane with time, adequate residual immunity usually remains so the vaccinated host is capable of responding to future exposure to the same antigenic stimulus with a rapid and heightened return of the immune response (1,3,5).

Development of the optimal vaccination procedure for providing protection for a given infectious agent is a time-consuming and largely empirical process (2,5). Several injections of antigen are frequently required to establish a long-lasting capacity to develop a secondary response to a natural infection or subsequent "booster" vaccination. Generally, vaccine preparations that utilize an adjuvant with soluble antigens are more effective than preparations without adjuvants. During the last few decades there has been a renewed interest in the development of adjuvants and immunopotentiating materials that could be used in conjunction with antigenic preparations to preferentially stimulate development of those immune mechanisms responsible for host resistance to the pathogen (6-8). The route of vaccine administration is frequently determined by convenience. However, in certain disease states it may be advantageous to preferentially activate (i) a systemic immune response, (ii) a local immune response, (iii) a cell-mediated immune response, or (iv) various combinations of the above. It is anticipated that major thrusts will be made during the next several decades to develop improved means for preferentially stimulating different aspects of the immune response.

Immune Protection Against Infectious Diseases

The role and manner of the immune response has been clearly defined in some infectious diseases. In general, methods for prevention of these infections have been readily devised by developing vaccines which are generally considered efficacious. On the other hand some infectious diseases present special problems which have hampered development of effective vaccines. A major impediment to production of safe and effective vaccines for use in many cases in preventive vaccination programs in domestic animals has been a paucity of basic information about the pathogenesis of these diseases. In some cases the host-parasite relationship is so poorly understood that the factors which determine susceptibility and/or resistance to the infection are undefined. In many cases the antigen-antibody reactions involved in microbial infections are not adequately understood. The immune response to some microbial antigens may be weak or absent. The role of acquired cellular resistance and factors derived from T-lymphocytes and macrophages in controlling or preventing certain infectious diseases is not known. Despite the lack of knowledge in many areas that would enhance the capacity to produce effective vaccines, there have been marked advances made in the use of vaccines in both human and veterinary medicine (9). Antibiotics and antimicrobial chemotherapeutic agents have been used rather successfully to control many acute infections, especially those caused by pyogenic cocci. But the high expectations originally held by many for the use of antibiotics and antimicrobial chemotherapeutic agents have not been realized. Biomedical scientists are once again seriously considering the advantages of preventative immunization for controlling acute and chronic infections of man and animals caused by a wide variety of infectious agents.

Many of the major advances made in developing efficacious vaccines have occurred with viruses and bacterial toxins (5). These advances have occurred in part because of the (i) knowledge of the immunogens, (ii) chemical simplicity of the immunogens, and (iii) induction of a specific immunologic response related to immunity. The physical, chemical and biologic properties of a substance are determined by its primary structure. Key chemical groupings (determinant groups) on the substance determine its immunogenicity or capacity to evoke an immune response. The most potent of these determinants are referred to as immunodominant points. Although the majority of immunogens are protein, other chemical classes are also capable of inducing an immune response. Polysaccharides either as pure substances or in combination with proteins or lipids are important bacterial immunogens. It is generally agreed that certain antigens are more effective than others in eliciting a protective immune response. Immunogenicity depends upon the physiochemical properties of the immunogen used, the route and dose of administration and the immune responsiveness of the host. In turn, host-related factors such as age, genetic makeup, nutritional status and general health can influence responsiveness to vaccination as well as resistance to infection (2). Vaccine efficacy is measured by the degree of protection induced in the immunized host following challenge. The most effective vaccines generally stimulate the development of protective mechanisms in the vaccinate that parallel those developed in the infected host. Vaccines currently available in both human and veterinary medicine can be divided into two broad categories consisting of nonreplicative and, replicative vaccines (2,5). The nonreplicative vaccines contain killed or inactivated agents or their products. Most, but not all, currently used bacterial vaccines (bacterins) are included in this category as are toxoids, capsular polysaccharide vaccines and some viral vaccines. The primary immune mechanism that is stimulated by administration of nonreplicative vaccines is serum antibody of the IgG variety. Serum IgG is the immune mechanism most effective in infections with a blood-borne phase in their pathogenesis. Duration of immunity is relatively short and boosters of additional antigen are frequently required to maintain the immune state. Although killed vaccines do not possess the hazards of the live vaccines, they sometimes induce toxic and hypersensitivity reactions. The replicative vaccines are live or attenuated virus or bacterial vaccines. Live attenuated vaccines usually are more effective in the prevention of disease than their inactivated counterparts. Generally these vaccines induce a sequence of immunologic events which mimic those that follow natural infection. The immunogenic potential of a live vaccine is related to its capacity for self-replication in the host. Thus even small infective doses usually lead to appropriate immunogenic responses and booster immunizations are not required. A hazard of replicative vaccines is that they contain live agents which are subject to mutation to more virulent forms. Additionally, the use of replicative vaccines can lead to devastating effects in the compromised host because of concurrent diseases or immune defects.

Depending upon the particular host-bacterial parasite relationship, there are different anti-infectious host defense mechanisms brought to bear on the bacterial pathogen itself or its disease-causing products (3). Bacterial infections have been classified as belonging to three broad categories: (i) the acute highly productive type, (ii) the chronic type exemplified by intracellular parasites, and (iii) toxigenic disease usually associated with acute infections. The relative roles of innate immunity and acquired immunity vary depending upon the nature of the infection. Antitoxic immunity is usually mediated through neutralization by production of specific antibody (antitoxin) and the detoxification process depends upon the formation of toxin-antitoxin complexes that are frequently cleared by phagocytic cell degradation. In instances where the toxin is present in excessive amounts, the toxin-antitoxin complexes can cause injury to the host and may give rise to immunologically-mediated disease. Antibodies produced against endotoxins are usually less protective than those produced against exotoxins. Antibacterial immunity can be mediated by antibody and/or cell-mediated events with immunity in acute infections frequently mediated by antibody and in chronic infections by cellular immune mechanisms.

Bacterial Cell Walls

The outermost layer of the bacterial cell, whether it is the bacterial cell wall or capsules, is that part of the microorganism which makes first contact with the environment (10). These surfaces may be the only points at which important interactions between the bacteria and environment may occur, such as adherence to surfaces or solids, interaction with DNA from another bacterium, or interaction with anti-infectious defense systems of the host's body. Peptidoglycans, a special class of polymers, provide strength to the wall, which is necessary since some bacteria when surrounded by their optimal growth media develop an internal cell pressure as large as 20 atmospheres. In addition to peptidoglycans, the bacterial walls contain a variety of proteins, polysaccharides, lipopolysaccharides and polyol-phosphate compounds distributed in these structures. A large variety of polysaccharides, polypeptides and proteins may be excreted by some bacterial strains forming semi-organized capsules which extend outward from the bacterial cell wall into the microbe's microenvironment. The available evidence suggests that those different substances are important in determining the nature of bacterial cell-environment interactions.

Some bacterial species possess filament-like appendages that are apparently involved in bacterial cell-environment or bacterial cell-bacterial cell interactions. Flagella enable the organism to swim and may be singularly attached at one end of the bacterial cell, or multiply attached around the bacterial cell (11,12). Bacteria use their flagella to move through their environment, in some cases toward needed nutrients and in others away from noxious materials. Fimbriae are long thin projecting filaments on the surface of Gram-negative bacteria which enable the organism to adhere to solid surfaces (13). Sex pili are wider filaments than fimbriae and fewer are formed per bacterial cell (14). They are important in the transfer of chromosomal DNA and extrachromosomal genetic elements (plasmids) between bacteria. Sex pili absorb filamentous

DNA phages at their tips and male-specific RNA phages along their sides.   Sex pili can retract and this may be an important, if not essential, part of the conjugation process whereby cell-to-cell transmission of DNA occurs. A diagrammatic representation of a bacterial cell is presented in Figure 1.

Figure 1.   Diagrammatic representation of bacterial cell structure.

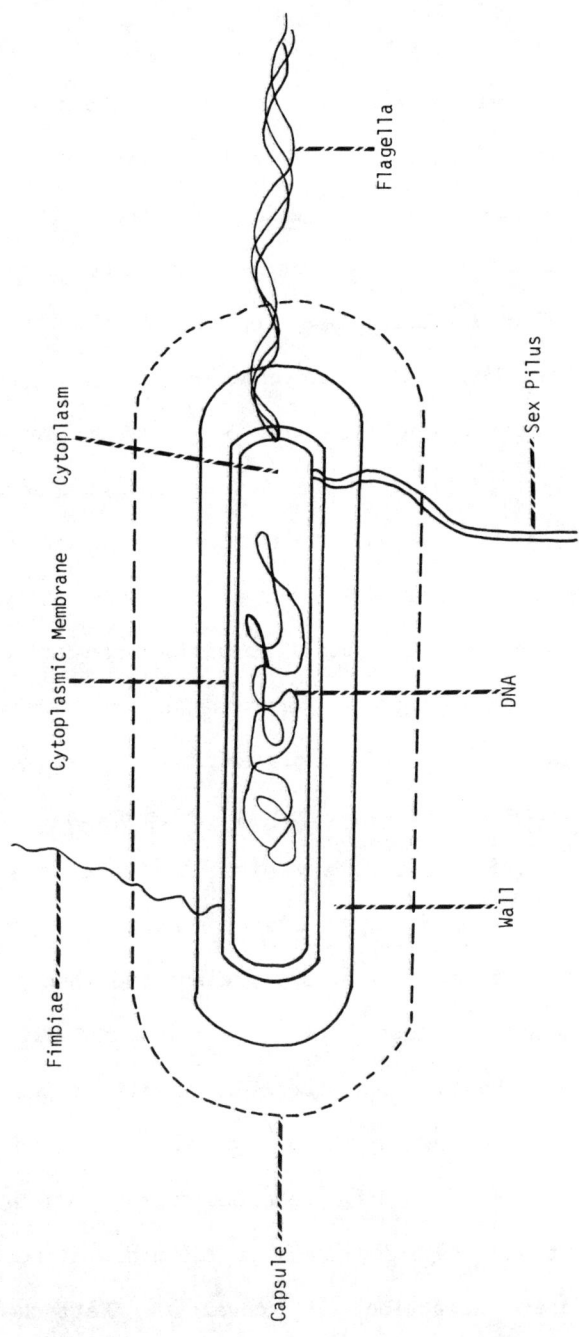

The outer layers of cell walls from Gram-positive and Gram-negative bacteria differ both in their morphology and chemistry (10,15).   The cell walls of Gram-positive bacteria are relatively thick structures morphologically, and chemically they consist of polysaccharides, teichoic and teichuronic acids, and peptidoglycans. The cell walls of Gram-negative bacteria contain an outer membrane with lipopolysaccharides attached to it and an underlying very thin layer of peptidoglycan. Peptidoglycan accounts for 5 to 10 percent of the total dry weight of the wall of Gram-negative organisms, whereas in Gram-positive organisms 50 to 60 percent is usually peptidoglycan and occasionally it may be as high as 90 percent. The peptidoglycans of all bacteria are composed of glycan strands connected by short polypeptide chains consisting of alternating D and L amino acids (10,15,16).   In any given bacterial species only a few kinds of amino acids are present in the peptidoglycan. However, D-alanine is always present and when all bacterial species are considered, a large number of different amino acids are present with some being unique to these polymers. Several different types of peptidoglycans differing in their cross-linking have been described. All Gram-negative bacteria have peptidoglycans of identical structure and the lipoprotein fraction is covalently attached to the peptidoglycan by a unique hydrophobic polypeptide which stretches between the peptidoglycan or murein layer and the outer membrane, apparently acting as an anchor between these two layers. Lipopolysaccharides (LPS) consist of lipid A and complex polysaccharides containing unique sugars (10,15,17). The lipid A fixes the molecule to the outer leaflet of the outer membrane and the molecule often extends long distances from the outer membrane. LPS is also referred to as the endotoxin of Gram-negative bacteria because the firmly bound molecule is only released when the cells are lysed. The toxicity of LPS for animals is associated with the lipid A portion of the molecule and the polysaccharide acts as a major surface antigen (O antigen) of the bacterial cell. A model of the Gram-negative cell envelope is presented in Figure 2.

Figure 2.   Schematic model of Gram-negative cell envelope.

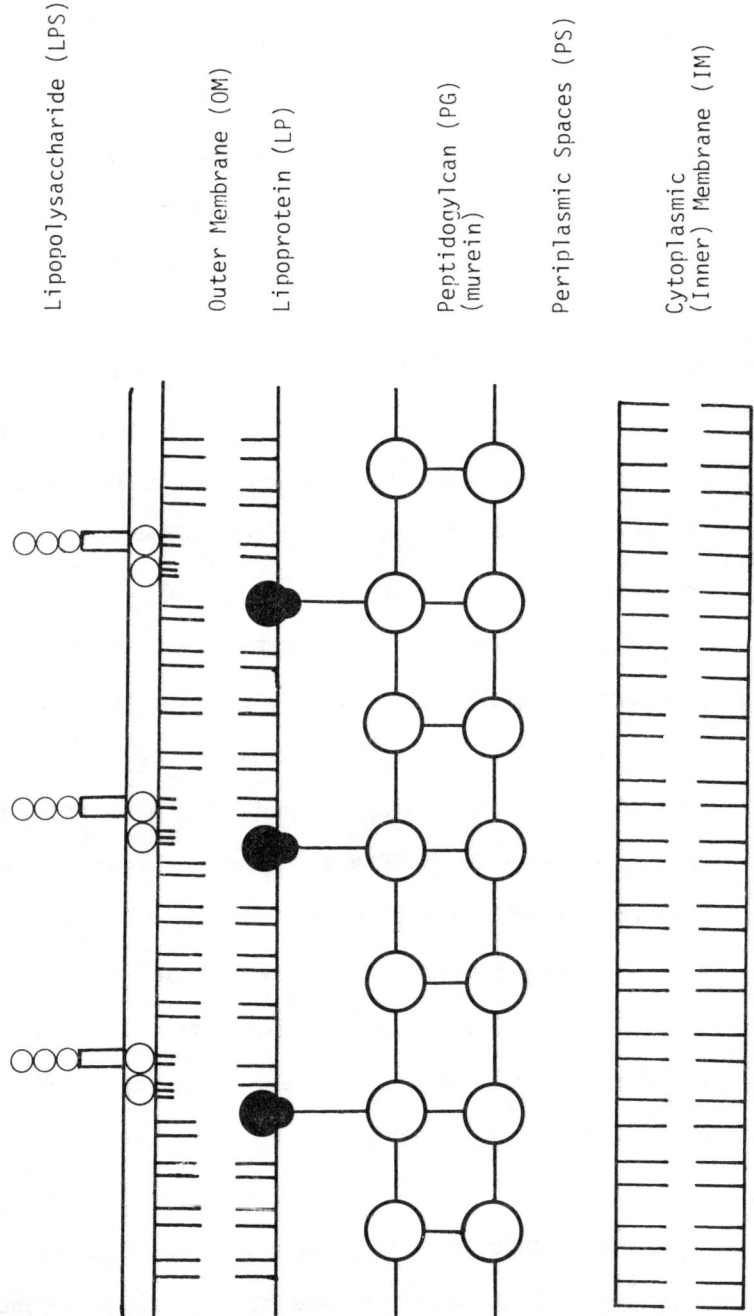

Lipopolysaccharide (LPS)

Outer Membrane (OM)

Lipoprotein (LP)

Peptidoglycan (PG)
(murein)

Periplasmic Spaces (PS)

Cytoplasmic
(Inner) Membrane (IM)

Outer Membrane Proteins of Gram-Negative Bacteria

The outer membrane of Gram-negative bacteria should be of interest to animal disease investigators interested in developing methods to control bacterial infections incriminated in the BRDC. There is a growing volume of work related to the structure, biosynthesis and assembly, and function of the outer membrane of Gram-negative organisms (18). Particular attention has been devoted to outer membrane proteins because they represent likely candidate antigens capable of stimulating development of an adaptive immune response in the infected host (19). Immune responses to outer membrane proteins may play an important role in providing protection against experimental or natural infections. Antibodies made against some of these outer membrane proteins may function as opsonins or bactericidins. Since these proteins are structural constituents of the cell it is unlikely that they function as virulence factors. A few unique proteins termed "matrix" or "major proteins" are present in relatively large amounts in the outer membrane, accounting for as much as 70 percent of the total outer membrane protein (10,18-20).

Numerous functions have been attributed to the outer membrane of Gram-negative bacteria (10,18-22). The outer membrane, in conjunction with the peptidoglycan, may be important in maintaining the structural integrity of the bacterial cell.   The outer membrane acts as a diffusion barrier against various compounds, contains specific uptake systems for nutrients, and nonspecific passive diffusion pores that will accomodate low molecular weight substances. It also provides a protective environment for hydrolytic enzymes and binding proteins located in the area between the cytoplasmic and outer membranes. The outer membrane contains receptors for bacteriophages and colicins and is involved in conjugation and septum formation during cell division.   Whereas a wide range of enzymic activities are associated with the bacterial cytoplasmic membrane, only two enzymic activities, a protease and a phosphatase, have been demonstrated in the outer membrane.

The protein composition of the outer membrane of Gram-negative species differs from that of the cytoplasmic membrane.   When cytoplasmic membranes are dispersed with anionic detergents such as sodium dodecyl sulphate (SDS) and separated by unidirectional polyacrylamide gel electrophoresis (PAGE), some 30 to 40 bands representing different proteins can be resolved when stained with Coomassie Blue (10,18-20). The molecular weights of these proteins range from about 1,500 to several 100,000 daltons.

If the same membranes are dispersed and then separated by two-dimensional electrophoresis, 200 or more proteins and polypeptides can be identified.   The outer membrane of Gram-negative bacteria contains about ten to twenty "minor proteins" and four or five "major proteins."   Although the minor proteins are usually present in limited amounts, under certain growth conditions some of them are synthesized in quantities almost as great as the major proteins.   Most minor proteins have vital roles in bacterial cell growth such as nutrient uptake through the outer membrane.   Many minor proteins, like some major proteins, act as receptors for bacteriophages and colicins. Properties of minor proteins in the outer membrane of Gram-negative organisms are discussed in several excellent reviews (18,23,24).

The major outer membrane proteins of *Escherichia coli* and *Salmonella typhimurium* have been the subject of considerable study during the last several decades (18-24).   The principal classes of structural proteins in the outer membrane of *E. coli* are murein lipoprotein, a heat-modifiable protease-sensitive protein (OmpA or TolG protein), and matrix porins (OmpC or 1a and OmpF or 1b). Parallel studies in a wide variety of Gram-negative bacteria have detected analagous major outer membrane proteins with the exception that in some instances the murein lipoprotein counterpart is absent.

Murein lipoprotein of *E. coli* is an unusual polypeptide consisting of 58 amino acid residues that bears lipid substituents at the N-terminus and is linked by the ϵ-amino group of its C-terminal lysine to the carboxyl group of every tenth to twelfth meso-diaminopimelic acid residue of the peptidoglycan (25). The lipoprotein is apparently highly conserved among the bacterial species studied thus far. A part of the lipoprotein may be exposed to the surface of the outer membrane. Evidence from studies of several bacterial mutants suggests the murein lipoprotein plays an important, but not essential, structural role in stabilization of the cell envelope.

The OmpA protein of *E. coli* is a transmembrane protein that exhibits anomalous heat modifiability on SDS gels (19,26). The protein is susceptible to partial proteolytic digestion when the outer membrane is treated with trypsin. Genetic studies with mutants deficient in different outer membrane proteins suggests that OmpA protein is important in maintenance of cell morphology and outer membrane integrity. Bacterial strains with OmpA mutations have altered outer membrane transport functions including reduced amino acid uptake and rate of ferrichrome-mediated iron transport. Additionally, OmpA may have a function in F-pilus-mediated conjugation between bacterial cells.

Another major non-porin protein has been designated "protein a" by one system of nomenclature (27) and 3b by another (18). This 40K polypeptide is probably a protease which catalyzes *in vitro* conversion of the outer membrane receptor for ferric enterobactin from an apparent molecular weight of 81K to 74K. Another apparently independent function for this protein is regulation of capsular polysaccharide formation. How this protein specifically functions in this regulation is not yet clear.

Matrix porins is a descriptive name applied to a family of abundant pore-forming proteins that have similar functional and structural properties (19). As presently used, the term matrix porins refers to several constitutively expressed pore-forming proteins of *E. coli* and *S. typhimurium,* OmpC, OmpD, and OmpF, and several conditionally expressed proteins including the "new membrane proteins" NmpA-B and NmpC and Protein 2 (19,26). Additionally, LamB protein (λ-receptor) has some functional properties of a general pore, although it is a genetic and physiologic component of the specific maltose transport system.

The structure and function of matrix porins have been the subject of extensive investigations. The available evidence suggests that permeability characteristics of the outer membrane determine access of solutes to the periplasmic space and cytoplasmic membrane and that movement of hydrophilic solutes across the outer membrane is via a group of proteins which form transmembrane channels with different degrees of specificity. These proteins have been described (19) as fitting into three functional categories: (i) the family of major outer membrane proteins (matrix porins) which form general hydrophilic pores and thus serve as fixed aqueous channels allowing for passive nonspecific diffusion of solutes across the outer membrane, (ii) the pore-forming proteins with a rather specific function such as specific permeation of nucleosides (Tsx protein) or oligosaccharides of the maltose series (LamB), but they act as pores rather than carrier proteins, and (iii) outer membrane transport proteins which are responsible for uptake of specific solutes of relatively large size and present in low concentrations in the medium.

The native porin proteins have a trimer subunit structure (18) that is schematically depicted in Figure 3.

Figure 3.   Assembly model depicting trimer subunit
structure of native porin proteins.   Each matrix protein
(MP) molecule is stabilized with a triple coiled-coil
structure of lipoprotein (LP) comprised of a molecule of
the bound form (darkened) and two of the free form. The MP
is firmly bound to the peptidoglycan (PG) layer. The bound
form of LP plays an important role in the association of MP
with PG.   Three molecules of MP form a hydrophilic
diffusion pore (channel) with a diameter of 1.5-2.0 nm.

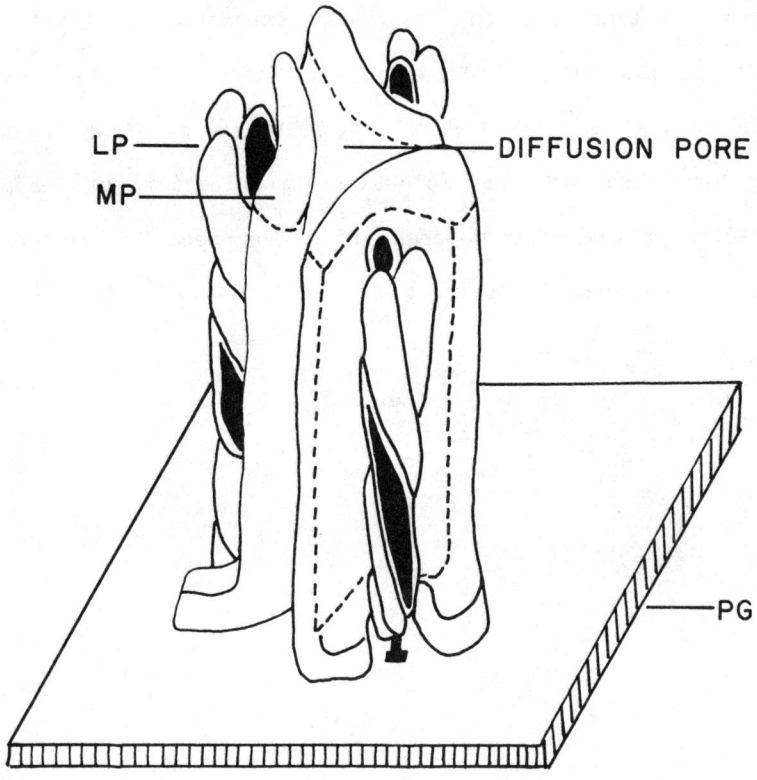

The major porins (OmpC, OmpD, OmpF, NmpA-B, NmpC, LamB and Protein 2) share a number of physical and chemical properties which include resistance to proteolysis, resistance to denaturation by SDS at temperatures below 85° C, high content of β-structure in the native state, very strong self-association, and characteristic association with peptidoglycan following extraction of the cell envelope with SDS below 85° C. A schematic cross-sectional representation of the molecular organization of major proteins in the outer membrane of a Gram-negative bacteria (19) is presented in Figure 4.

Figure 4.   Diagrammatic model of the molecular organization
of major proteins in the outer membrane of a Gram-negative
bacteria.

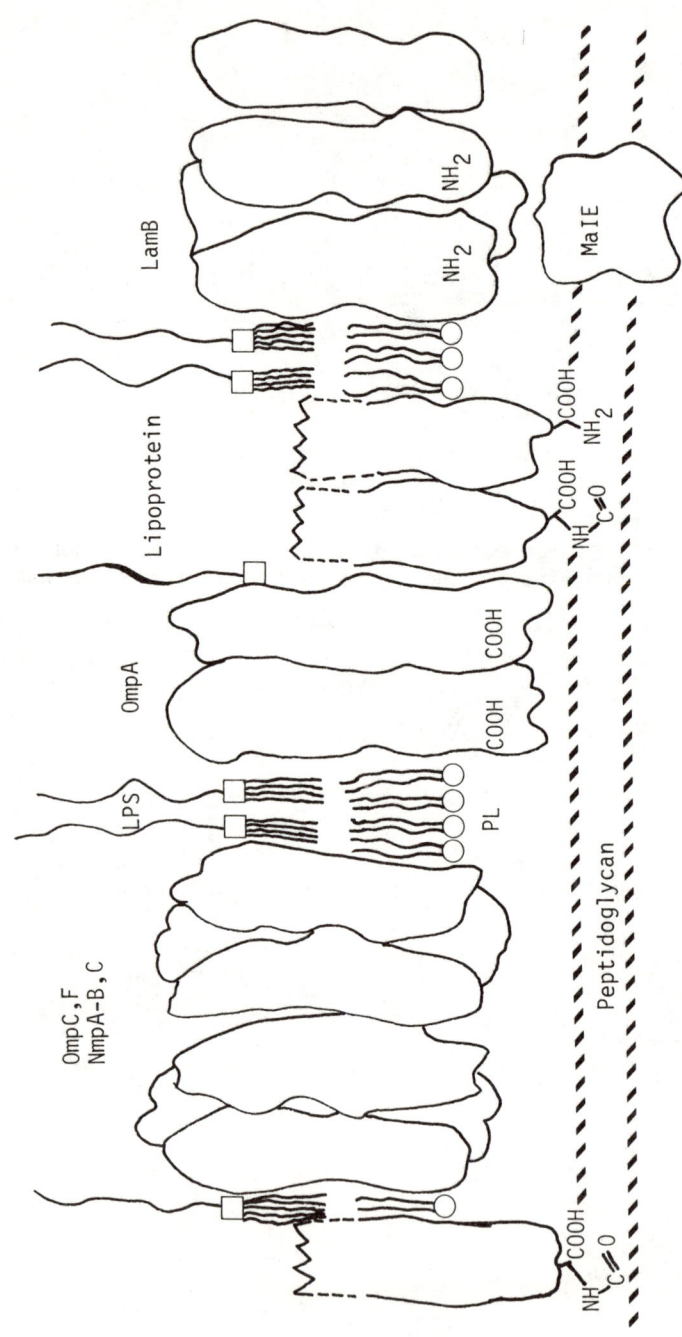

Because major outer membrane porin proteins are apparently exposed on the surface of the bacteria, it should be possible by suitable vaccination techniques to induce the production of antiporin antibody. Outer membrane protein preparations from several different genera of bacteria have been evaluated as immunogens. Porin proteins from *S. typhimurium* were effective immunogens in mice and rabbits and the active component in a passive immunization experiment was antiporin antibody (28). The O-antigenic polysaccharide chain of *S. typhimurium* covalently linked to porin protein was more effective as an immunogen than either of the subcomponents given separately (29). Immunization with more than one surface component of the organism improved vaccine efficacy. Vaccination with outer membrane proteins from *Shigella* spp. induced protection against experimental shigellosa keratoconjunctivitis (30). Studies by several investigative groups suggest that antibodies against outer membrane proteins of *H. influenzae* type b are important in providing protection against the disease (31-35). The outer membrane proteins from *Vibrio cholerae* (36,37), *Campylobacter jejuni* (38), *Pseudomonas aeruginosa* (39,40), *Actinomyces israelii* (41), *Brucella abortus* (42) and other bacteria have been the subject of recent studies.

Current Efforts and Future Directions
Related to BRDC

Many biomedical scientists are devoting increasing levels of their attention to surface-exposed bacterial antigens, in particular to lipopolysaccharides and outer membrane proteins. Serum antibodies directed against these antigens may facilitate opsonization and complement-mediated bacteriolysis and thus provide protection against natural and experimental infections. Unfortunately, in large part because of inadequate levels of research funding, but also in part because of their training and approach to the investigation of animal diseases, only feeble efforts have been made by the workers in the bovine respiratory disease area to characterize and identify the protective antigens of economically important bacteria incriminated in the etiology of the BRDC. Clearly a more molecularly-oriented approach is needed, and several very powerful tools of the modern microbiologist and immunobiologist need to be brought to bear on this disease complex. Critical to the amelioration of losses due to the BRDC is the need to define and characterize the virulence factors and protective antigens of bacterial agents causally associated with the disease. The application of the hybridoma technology for the isolation of hybrid cells secreting monoclonal antisera directed against a single antigenic site should provide opportunities to more adequately understand the relative importance of putative virulence factors and protective antigens from pathogenic bacteria (43,44). A major advantage of this technique is that it potentially allows the investigator to overcome many of the technical and scientific problems associated with the use of polyclonal antisera raised in animals with the use of complex antigens. Monoclonal antibodies have been raised against outer membrane antigens of *P. aeruginosa* and one of the monoclonal antibodies was shown to be specific for the major outer membrane lipoprotein (45). Monoclonal antibodies raised against antigens of bacteria associated with the BRDC may be helpful in identifying antigens that are important both from an immunodiagnostic and immunotherapeutic standpoint. Equipped with that information it may then be possible to use molecular cloning techniques (46) to produce the protective antigen for use in immunoprophylactic preparations.

Recent studies in several laboratories have focused attention on the possible importance of the leukotoxin of *P. haemolytica* as a virulence factor in pneumonic pasteurellosis (47-56). However, the relative roles of antitoxic and antibacterial immunity in allowing infected cattle to overcome the disease has not been determined.

The available evidence indicates *P. haemolytica* produces an exotoxin which is heat-labile, antigenic and toxic to ruminant leukocytes. Evidence from ultrafiltration and size-exclusion chromatography studies presented in one report suggests the toxin has a molecular weight of approximately 150,000 daltons (50). However, evidence presented in another report suggests the toxin has a molecular weight of 300,000 daltons or more (47). Recent studies in this laboratory indicate the leukotoxin is a glycoprotein which is unstable at high temperatures, susceptible to extremes of pH and has a molecular weight on SDS-PAGE of approximately 150,000 (57). The toxin is not hemolytic for erythrocytes from cattle, sheep, goats, swine, dogs, cats, mice, guinea pigs, rabbits, chickens, turkeys or humans (57). The toxic effects of the molecule can be neutralized with serum from cattle with a history of a shipping fever-like syndrome (57).

All serotypes of *P. haemolytica* produce the leukotoxin (57). Several studies in this laboratory have been directed at examining the relationship between extrachromosomal genetic elements and leukotoxin production by *P. haemolytica.* Bacterial strains representing each of the fifteen different serotypes and sixteen strains of biotype A, serotype 1 (the biotype and serotype most frequently isolated from clinical cases of BRDC) were examined with a plasmid screening technique and this information was correlated with the susceptibility of the strains to antibiotics and their ability to produce leukotoxin. Data from these studies suggested that *P. haemolytica* leukotoxin activity is not plasmid mediated (58). Ampicillin and penicillin resistance in the strains of biotype A, serotype 1 was apparently plasmid mediated, whereas the genetic information coding for resistance to tetracycline, streptomycin, triple sulfa and albon was chromosomal (58).

Development of an efficacious subunit bacterin for *P. haemolytica* and *P. multocida* would appear to be a worthwhile long-range goal of animal disease investigators working on the BRDC. Bacterins containing *Pasteurella* spp. alone, or in combination with other agents, are commercially available. However, many veterinarians question whether the value of these products has been adequately demonstrated. Numerous factors may impact upon the potential immunogenicity of a complex mixture of antigenic materials, not the least of which are problems related to antigenic competition between protective and nonprotective antigens, and the potential for generalized immune suppression resulting from toxic factors present in the preparation. Considerable antigenic complexity is represented by the many serotypes of *P.*

haemolytica and *P. multocida* (59–62). Although early studies suggested that immunity to *Pasteurella* infections was capsular-type specific (63,64), more recent studies indicate a somatic serotype-specific component is involved (65). The KSCN-extracted antigen of *P. multocida* type A contains some antigens common to different serotypes of *P. multocida* type A and *P. haemolytica* serotype 1 (66). The available evidence from numerous lines of investigation supports the working hypothesis that an efficacious subunit vaccine for bovine pneumonic pasteurellosis should contain, at a minimum, inactivated *P. haemolytica* leukotoxin and outer membrane antigen(s) from *P. haemolytica* and *P. multocida* or antigens common to both organisms. Which outer membrane antigens will be useful is unclear. The current status of our knowledge about outer membrane antigens of *Pasteurella* spp. is embarrassingly meager and essentially nothing is currently known about their immunogenicity.

Efforts are currently being made in this laboratory to develop methods to isolate and characterize the inner and outer membranes of *P. haemolytica* and to identify and isolate the major outer membrane proteins with a view toward subsequently testing their immunogenicity. A modification of previously described methods used to isolate inner and outer membranes from *S. typhimurium*

(67,68) was used to obtain membrane preparations from *P. haemolytica*. From three to four discrete membrane bands were obtained from each four-step sucrose gradient prepared (Figure 5). Generally, only the uppermost band had chemical and enzymatic characteristics of an inner (cytoplasmic) membrane-enriched fraction with high NADH oxidase levels and reduced 2-keto-3-deoxyoctulosonic acid levels. The two to three lower bands were identified as outer-membrane-enriched fractions based on their high 2-keto-3-deoxyoctulosonic acid levels, low or reduced NADH oxidase levels, and SDS-PAGE patterns which revealed four to six major protein bands (Figure 6), which is characteristic of outer membrane preparations from other Gram-negative bacteria (31).

Figure 5.   Outer membrane (OM)- and inner membrane (IM)-enriched fractions from *Pasteurella haemolytica* in a 30-40-50-60 percent discontinuous sucrose gradient. Fractions were analyzed for protein, pooled, centrifuged at 100,000 xg for 60 minutes and analyzed for NADH oxidase and 2-keto-3-deoxyoctulosonic acid (KDO) to arrive at tentative designations as OM- or IM-enriched fractions.   The peak designed M contained fractions composed of a mixture of OM and IM.   The peak designated IM contained predominantly IM-enriched fractions with some OM contamination.   The peak designated OM contained OM-enriched fractions.

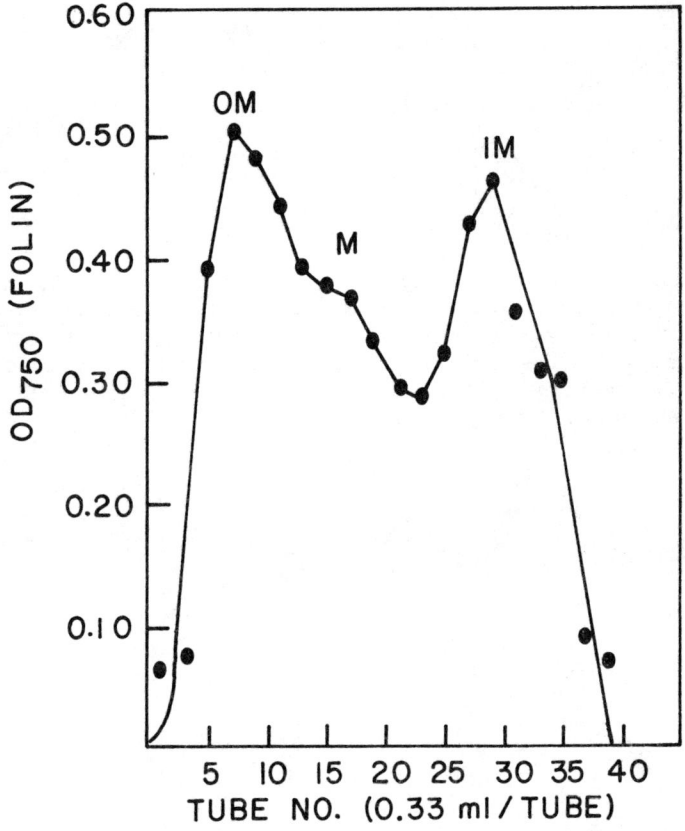

Figure 6.   Outer membrane (OM) protein profile of *P. haemolytica* on a sodium dodecyl sulfate-polyacrylamide gel. OM-enriched fractions from sucrose density gradients were pooled and subjected to treatment with detergents to enrich for OM proteins.   Lane 1 contains sarkosyl- insoluble OM proteins and Lane 2 contains Triton X-100 insoluble OM proteins.

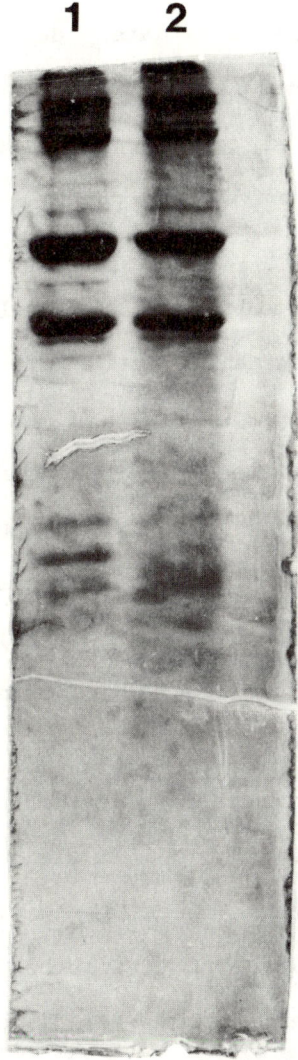

Numerous teams of investigators in different parts of the world are involved in studies of the BRDC and specifically with the "shipping fever" complex. Numerous investigators continue to isolate, identify and test the pathogenicity of novel as well as conventional agents isolated from affected cattle. Scientists working with funds from both the private and public sector continue to search for improved immunoprophylactic technologies, innovative chemotherapeutic and pharmacologic approaches, and progressive management practices to curtail losses. Notwithstanding the expenditure of considerable time, talent and capital in these studies, the economic losses associated with the condition remain at an alarming level. Alternatives to the more conventional research approaches to the BRDC have begun to provide information about mechanisms of pathogenesis and host recovery. Similarly, innovative approaches to the development of immunoprophylactic products may provide not only a useful product, but also improve our knowledge of the immune responsiveness of cattle to certain pathogenic bacteria. The use of a molecular approach to the development of a *Pasteurella* spp. bacterin would seem to be a justifiable approach in the development of methods for curtailing some losses associated with the BRDC.

Acknowledgment

The work in progress is supported in part by funds from the Texas Agricultural Experiment Station and from the Special Grants Program of the United States Department of Agriculture, Science and Education Administration, Cooperative Research (SEA-CR), Research Agreement Numbers 59-2481-0-2-070-0 and 59-2481-1-2-032-0.

The author is grateful to Drs. Yung-Fu Chang, Paul H. DeFoor and Alan B. Richards for their permission to include some of their unpublished data in this manuscript. The author acknowledges the assistance of Ms. Susan J. Renshaw in preparation of the manuscript and for the graphics work.

Published with the approval of the Texas Agricultural Experiment Station as paper Number TA 19218.

References

1. Friedman H, Voller A:Vaccines: general background and introduction, in Voller A, Friedman H (ed): New Trends and Developments in Vaccines. Baltimore, University Park Press, 1978, pp. 1-5.

2. Renshaw HW, Richards AB, Hsu T-Y:Small ruminants: immunobiologic basis for vaccination. Int Goat Sheep Res 1:132-149, 1980.

3.   Bellanti JA:Mechanisms of immunity to bacterial diseases, in Bellanti JA: Immunology II. Philadelphia, WB Saunders Co, 1978, pp. 370-384.

4.   Pasteur L:De l'atténuation du virus du cholera des poules. Compt Rend Acad Sci 91:673-680, 1880.

5.   Bellanti JA, Robbins JB:Immunoprophylaxis: the use of vaccines, in Bellanti JA: Immunology II. Philadelphia, WB Saunders Co, 1978, pp. 690-721.

6.   Jordan GW, Merigan TC:Enhancement of host defense mechanisms by pharmacological agents. Ann Rev Pharmaco 15:157-175, 1975.

7.   White RG:The adjuvant effect of microbial products on the immune response.   Ann Rev Microbiol 30:579-600, 1976.

8.   Wolstenholme GEW, Knight J:Immunopotentiation. CIBA Foundation Symposium No. 18.   New York, American Elsevier Publishing Co Inc, 1973.

9.   Beale AJ:Notes on veterinary vaccines, in Voller A, Friedman H (ed): New Trends and Developments in Vaccines. Baltimore, University Park Press, 1978, pp. 311-314.

10.   Rogers HJ:Bacterial Cell Structure.   Aspects of Microbiology 6.   Washington, American Society for Microbiology, 1983.

11.   Doetsch RN, Sjoblad RD:Flagellar structure and function in eubacteria. Ann Rev Microbiol 34:69-108, 1980.

12.   Silverman M, Simon MI:Bacterial flagella. Ann Rev Microbiol 31:397-419, 1977.

13.   Ottow JCG:Ecology, physiology and genetics of fimbrae and pili. Ann Rev Microbiol 29:79-108, 1975.

14.   Tomoeda M, Inuzuka M, Date T:Bacterial sex pili. Prog Biophy Mol Biol 30:23-56, 1975.

15.   Jawetz E, Melnick JL, Adelberg EA:Review of Medical Microbiology,   ed   14.   Los   Altos,   Lange   Medical Publications, 1980, pp. 6-31.

16.   Rogers HJ:Peptidoglycans (mucopeptides): structure function and variations. Ann NY Acad Sci 235:29-51, 1974.

17.   Wilkinson SG:Composition and structure of bacterial lipopolysaccharides,   in   Sutherland   IW   (ed):   Surface Carbohydrates of the Prokaryotic Cell.   New York, Academic Press, 1977, pp. 97-175.

18.   DiRienzo JM, Nakamura K, Inouye M:The outer membrane proteins of Gram-negative bacteria: biosynthesis, assembly, and functions. Ann Rev Biochem 47:481-532, 1978.

19.   Osborn MJ, Wu HCP:Proteins of the outer membrane of Gram-negative bacteria.   Ann Rev Microbiol 34:369-422, 1980.

20.   Inouye M (ed):Bacterial Outer Membranes: Biogenesis and Functions. New York, Wiley, 1979, p. 534.

21.   Costerton JW, Ingram JM, Cheng K-J:Structure and function of the cell envelope of Gram-negative bacteria. Bact Rev 38:87-110, 1974.

22.   Salton RJ, Owen P:Bacterial membrane structure. Ann Rev Microbiol 30:451-482, 1976.

23.   Braun V, Hancock REW, Hantke K, Hartmann A:Functional organization of the outer membrane of *Escherichia coli:* phage and colicin receptors as components of iron uptake systems. J Supramolec Struct 5:37-58, 1976.

24.   Braun V, Hantke K:Bacterial receptors for phages and colicins as constituents of specific transport systems, in Reissig JL (ed): Microbial Interactions. Receptor and Recognition, series B, volume 3. London, Chapman and Hall, 1977, pp. 100-137.

25.   Hantke K, Braun V:Covalent binding of lipid to protein. Diglyceride and amide-linked fatty acids at the N-terminal end of the murein-lipoprotein of the *Escherichia coli* outer membrane. Eur J Biochem 34:284-296, 1973.

26.   Schnaitman CA:Outer membrane proteins of *Escherichia coli.* IV. Differences in outer membrane protein due to strain and cultural differences. J Bacteriol 118:454-464, 1974.

27. Lugtenberg B, Meijers J, Peters R, Vanden Hoek P, Van Alphen L:Electrophoretic resolution of the major outer membrane proteins of *Escherichia coli* K12 into four bands. FEBS Lett 58:254-258,1975.

28. Kuusi N, Nurminen M, Saxen H, Valtonen M, Makela PH:Immunization with major outer membrane proteins in experimental salmonellosis of mice. Infect Immun 25:857-862, 1979.

29. Svenson SB, Murminen M, Lindberg AA:Artificial *Salmonella* vaccines: O-antigenic oligosaccharide-protein conjugates induce protection against infection with *Salmonella typhimurium*. Infect Immun 25:863-872, 1979.

30. Adamus G, Mulczyk M, Wikowska D, Romanowska E:Protection against keratoconjunctivitis shigellosa induced by immunization with outer membrane proteins of *Shigella* spp. Infect Immun 30, 321-324, 1980.

31. Burans JP, Lynn M, Solotorovsky M:Induction of active immunity with membrane fractions from *Haemophilus influenzae* type b. Infect Immun 41:285-293, 1983.

32. Dahlberg-Lagergard T:Bactericidal antibodies against noncapsular components of *Haemophilus influenzae*. J Clin Microbiol 17:428-431, 1983.

33. Loeb MR, Smith DH:Human antibody response to individual outer membrane proteins of *Haemophilus influenzae* type b. Infect Immun 37:1032-1036, 1982.

34. Shenep JL, Munson RS, Barenkamp SJ, Granoff DM:Further studies of the role of noncapsular antibody in protection against experimental *Haemophilus influenzae* type b bacteremia. Infect Immun 42:257-263, 1983.

35. Van Alphen L, Riemens T, Zanen HC:Antibody response against outer membrane components of *Haemophilus influenzae* type b strains in patients with meningitis. FEMS Microbiol Lett 18:189-195, 1983.

36. Kabir S:Immunochemical properties of the major outer membrane protein of *Vibrio cholerae.* Infect Immun 39, 452-455, 1983.

37. Kabir S, Skowkat A:Characterization of surface properties of *Vibrio cholerae.* Infect Immun 39:1048-1058, 1983.

38. Blaser MJ, Hopkins JA, Berka RM, Vasil ML, Wang W-LL:Identification and characterization of *Campylobacter jejuni* outer membrane proteins. Infect Immun 42:276-284, 1983.

39. Lam JS, Mutharia LM, Hancock REW, Høiby N, Lam K, Baek L, Costerton JW:Immunogenicity of *Pseudomonas aeruginosa* outer membrane antigens examined by crossed immunoelectrophoresis. Infect Immun 42:88-98, 1983.

40. Mutharia LM, Nicas TI, Hancock REW:Outer membrane proteins of *Pseudomonas aeruginosa* serotype strains. J Infect Dis 146:770-779, 1982.

41. Ayakawa GY, Williams BL, Kenny GE:Identification and preliminary characterization of a major heat-stable surface antigen of *Actinomyces israelii* by two-dimensional (crossed) immunoelectrophoresis. Infect Immun 41:11-18, 1983.

42. Verstreate DR, Creasy MT, Caveney NT, Baldwin CL, Blab MW, Winter AJ:Outer membrane proteins of *Brucella abortus:* isolation and characterization. Infect Immun 35:979-989, 1982.

43. Kennett RH, McKearn TJ, Bechtol KB (ed): Monoclonal Antibodies Hybridomas: A New Dimension in Biological Analyses. New York, Plenum Press, 1980, p. 423.

44. Tom BH, Allison JP (ed): Hybridomas and Cellular Immortality. New York, Plenum Press, 1983, p. 306.

45. Hancock REW, Wieczorek AA, Mutharia LM, Poole K:Monoclonal antibodies against *Pseudomonas aeruginosa* outer membrane antigens: isolation and characterization. Infect Immun 37:166-171, 1982.

46. Maniatis T, Fritsch EF, Sambrook J:Molecular Cloning - A Laboratory Manual. Cold Spring Harbor, Cold Spring Harbor Laboratory Publications, 1982, p. 545.

47. Baluyut CS, Simonson RR, Bemrick WJ, Maheswaran SK:Interaction of *Pasteurella haemolytica* with bovine neutrophils: identification and partial characterization of a cytotoxin. Am J Vet Res 42:1920-1926, 1981.

48.   Berggren KA, Baluyut CS, Simonson RR, Bemrick WJ, Maheswaran SK:Cytotoxic effects of *Pasteurella haemolytica* on bovine neutrophils. Am J Vet Res 42:1383-1388, 1981.

49.   Chang Y-F, Richards AB, Renshaw HW:A toxic agent derived from *Pasteurella haemolytica,* in Proceedings: Third Int Conf Goat Dis Prod 3:295, 1982.

50.   Himmel ME, Yates MD, Lauerman LH, Squire PG:Purification and partial characterization of a macrophage cytotoxin from *Pasteurella haemolytica.* Am J Vet Res 43:764-767, 1982.

51.   Kaehler KL, Markham RJF, Muscoplat CC, Johnson DW:Evidence of cytocidal effects of *Pasteurella haemolytica* on bovine peripheral blood mononuclear leukocytes. Am J Vet Res 41:1690-1693, 1980.

52.   Maheswaran SK, Berggren KA, Simonson RR, Ward GE, Muscoplat CC:Kinetics of interaction and fate of *Pasteurella haemolytica* in bovine alveolar macrophages. Infect Immun 30:254-262, 1980.

53.   Markham RJF, Wilkie BN:Interaction between *Pasteurella haemolytica* and bovine alveolar macrophages: cytotoxic effect on macrophages and impaired phagocytosis. Am J Vet Res 41:18-22, 1980.

54.   Markham RJF, Wilkie BN:Influence of bronchoalveolar washing supernatants and stimulated lymphocyte supernatants

on uptake of *Pasteurella haemolytica* by cultured bovine alveolar macrophages. Am J Vet Res 41:443-446, 1980.

55. Richards AB, Chang Y-F, Hanson TD, Renshaw HW:Interaction of goat peripheral blood leukocytes and *Pasteurella haemolytica,* in Proceedings: Third Int Conf Goat Dis Prod 3:295, 1982.

56. Shewen PE, Wilkie BN:Cytotoxin of *Pasteurella haemolytica* acting on bovine leukocytes. Infect Immun 35:91-94, 1982.

57. Chang Y-F, Renshaw HW:Unpublished data, 1983.

58. Richards AB, Renshaw HW:Unpublished data, 1983.

59. Biberstein EL, Gills MG:The relation of the antigenic types to the A and T types of *Pasteurella haemolytica.* J Comp Pathol 72:316-320, 1962.

60. Carter GR:The genus *Pasteurella,* in Merchant IA, Packer RA: Veterinary Bacteriology and Virology. Ames, Iowa State University Press, 1967, pp. 335-353.

61. Collins FM:Mechanisms of acquired resistance to *Pasteurella multocida* infection: a review. Cornell Vet 67:101-138, 1977.

62. Penn CW, Nagy LK:Capsular and somatic antigens of *Pasteurella multocida,* types B and E. Res Vet Sci 16:251-259, 1974.

63. Bains RUS:A preliminary examination of the antigens of *Pasteurella multocida* type 1. Br Vet J 111:492-498, 1955.

64. Dhanda MR:Immunization of cattle against hemorrhagic septicemia with purified antigens. Ind Vet J 36:6-8, 1958.

65. Heddleston KL, Rebers PA:Fowl cholera: cross immunity induced in turkeys with formalin-killed *in vivo*-propagated *Pasteurella multocida*. Avian Dis 16:578-586, 1972.

66. Mukkur TKS:Demonstration of cross-protection between *Pasteurella multocida* type A and *Pasteurella haemolytica*, serotype 1. Infect Immun 18:583-585, 1977.

67. Osborn MJ, Gander JE, Parisi E, Carson J:Mechanism of assembly of the outer membrane of *Salmonella typhimurium*. J Biological Chem 247:3962-3972, 1972.

68. Osborn MJ, Munson R:Separation of the inner (cytoplasmic) and outer membranes of Gram-negative bacteria. Meth Enzymol 31:642-653, 1974.

Due to illness, Dr. Renshaw was unable to present this paper at the Symposium as scheduled.

Perspectives into the Future of Bovine Respiratory Disease Research

Robert F. Kahrs, D.V.M., Ph.D.

Department of Veterinary Microbiology
College of Veterinary Medicine
University of Missouri
Columbia, Missouri 65211

Introduction

The North American Symposium on Bovine Respiratory Disease Research summarized scientific advances and practical frustrations associated with reducing pulmonic pasteurellosis. Although some dogmas of past decades have faded into oblivion and been replaced by contemporary thinking, the same questions remain and there is no assurance that today's answers will survive the test of time. Nonetheless, we are on the brink of a new era in bovine respiratory disease research. Progress will certainly be recorded in the next decade.

The presence of bovine practitioners at the Symposium provided a dimension of reality. It was reported that only 39 percent of available management knowledge is currently utilized by the beef industry and that 83 percent of cattlemen raise fewer than 100 calves a year. Thus many cattle trickle to market in small groups and are unaccessible for preconditioning. We learned from veterinarians and livestock owners that we are not doing a good job in controlling bovine respiratory disease, or in the use of available vaccines. We learned that preconditioning is a fine principle for disease control, but it has yet to be shown to be economically profitable. We were told by livestock owners that what they really need is a device for providing immediate immunity at assembly points and that rapid screening methods for the selection of therapeutic agents are required. We heard confessions that biological products need better care and handling and that there is much room for improvement in their administration. It was not mentioned that the United States is currently undergoing a crises in its biologics industry and that there are actually two industries--a regulated industry, dedicated to product quality, long-term research and product development and an unregulated industry, operating under a variety of standards. We also learned that prevention of death and disease in feeder cattle is very desirable, but in the final analysis, success of respiratory disease control programs will be measured by improved feed efficiency and demonstrable improvement in average daily weight gain.

As the papers in the North American Symposium on Bovine Respiratory Disease were presented, the old theme of multifactorial etiology of bovine respiratory disease emerged. Emphasis was placed on infective agents, host responses and the complex contributing environmental influences.

Observations

Infectious Agents of Bovine Respiratory Disease

The specific infectious agents associated with respiratory diseases are endemic and virtually ubiquitous in cattle populations. Most have mechanisms for persistence in individual animals and in populations. Most are either nonpathogenic or mildly pathogenic in simple singular infections of non-stressed, immunologically-competent, well-nourished cattle in their home environment. Most are not well-studied by contemporary standards and much could be learned by application of DNA fingerprinting, monoclonal antibodies and recombinant DNA techniques. There are still questions about the role of the major viruses in bovine respiratory disease but little disagreement remains about the etiologic importance of *Pasteurella hemolytica* in pulmonic pasteurellosis.

The Host Response

The host response to exposure and infection largely determines the outcome of infections.   In the past, this response has been described in terms of clinical signs, lesions, and detection of serum antibodies. Today the host response can be measured and understood at the cellular and sometimes molecular level and described in the language of the "new immunology," a science less than twelve years old. The immunologic response can participate in production of disease as well as in protecting the body from infection. In addition, the immunological response can be suppressed by infectious agents, drugs and chemicals, by endogenous glucocorticoids   and   by   biochemical   and   physiological responses to stress, anxiety or apprehension.   Further, the immunological response has potential of being modulated to increase   general   immunocompetence.   The   immunologic response   can   be   specifically   manipulated   to   generate resistance to specific infectious diseases and until now this vaccination approach has been the major thrust of efforts to control bovine respiratory diseases.

Environmental Influences

The emphasis on the role of environmental factors on the development and the course of bovine respiratory diseases continues.   If all cattle existed in a pastoral setting, adequately spaced and knee-deep in grass, the Symposium probably would be unnecessary.   Under these "home-on-the-range" conditions, respiratory disease would occasionally be a problem (as it sometimes is in dairy cattle) but it would not be the major concern of the beef cattle industry and the veterinary profession.   It is the marketing system and feedlot production-management system (producing 75 percent to 80 percent of slaughtered beef) that creates the environment for shipping fever and other respiratory diseases.   We have been told (and believe) that this marketing system will not change, that it is economically more acceptable to live with pulmonic pasteurellosis than to alter the deeply-entrenched tradition of multiple exchanges, frequent resale and lengthly stressful shipments prior to arrival at stocking points or at feedlots.   If this tradition ever changes, it will be for reasons other than health. Ownership from conception to consumption (totally integrated beef production) may someday occur in a few production units, but complete integration capitalizing on genetic advances

as in pork and poultry production is probably far away.
Thus the research community should not close their
laboratories in anticipation of a future lessening
importance of bovine respiratory diseases.

After this Symposium, its leaders could plan another for
1993. The stage could be the same, the actors would be the
same, and the same issues would be discussed. Hopefully,
significant advances would be reported. It is appropriate
to comment on the hopes for a future symposium from a
perspective of advising young researchers or guiding future
funding decisions.

Both basic experiments and practical field studies will
be needed to address the problem of bovine respiratory
diseases. Scientists involved will need a broad view of
the many facets of the problem. In designing experiments,
it will be necessary to narrow the focus to specific
fractions of the overall problem. Regardless of the
component selected, it will be necessary for researchers to
take a scholarly approach and keep asking *how* and *why*
things happen as they do. That means a basic-science
approach is required. Newer technology has not been widely
applied to the problem of bovine respiratory diseases.
There is a new generation of researchers on the scene, many
of them trained outside of veterinary medicine, who are

skillful in the use of this technology and the veterinary research community must welcome them. For traditionalists in the bovine respiratory research community, the biotechnology has horrendous implications. It means their research will be more complicated than ever. It means newer strains of viruses and bacteria will be identified by use of monoclonal antibodies and DNA fingerprinting. It means there will be more emphasis on understanding the complex immunologic mechanisms involved in response to respiratory infections. It means that recombinant DNA technology and molecular biology must be applied to the problem.

A new era of data-gathering is required for undertaking field approaches to bovine respiratory disease. There are field data which can provide necessary information without which basic experimentalists may be proceeding blindly. These data must be gathered in an organized, logical fashion and carefully designed surveillance programs and vaccine evaluations must be undertaken where the disease is actually occurring. The needed methodology is available in the organized discipline known as epidemiology. It has a statistical basis and a special role in situations where controlled experimentation is neither possible nor feasible.

Future Research

There are areas of study which may be profitable in the future.   Immunopathological studies on cattle are needed to determine   if   pulmonic   pasteurellosis   is   an immunologically-mediated lesion.   Studies are needed on the alleged   immunosuppression   by   BVD   virus,   on   bovine respiratory syncytial virus, *Hemophilus somnus,* and on the neglected adenoviruses,   rhinoviruses,   enteroviruses   and non-IBR herpesviruses.   The subject of immunomodulation in cattle is a fertile field for future research.   It will be necessary to study the pathophysiology of stress and detail its effects on the bovine immune system and concurrently to study and identify the action of stress-modifying drugs with the ultimate idea of a rapid-delivery system for products to reduce the contribution of stress to bovine respiratory disease.   Innovative methods must be developed to   prevent   organisms   naturally   inhabiting   the   upper respiratory tract from entering the lung. There need to be new approaches such as a biological filter, the genetic development of races of cattle with tracheas lined with supercilia or other innovations. Extensive studies are needed on anti-viral and anti-bacterial prophylactic agents and on semi-prophylactic agents to be administered after infection is established in a herd or an individual animal.

Lastly, subunit vaccines, be they chemically synthesized, genetically engineered or developed through detergent cleavage of infectious agents, must be developed to meet the burgeoning needs for safe, pure, potent and effective biologic products. A new generation of microbiologists is required to characterize known and newly-discovered infectious etiologic agents in terms of their source, their ability to colonize the upper respiratory tract and the lungs, their ability to produce toxins, the characteristics of their surface antigens and the receptor sites required by immunologic antimicrobials. Such studies should be conducted on the *Pasteurella* and hemophilus bacteria and the bovine respiratory syncytial virus, BVD, PI-3 and IBR viruses. In addition, the search for new infectious agents must continue. If we ever think we have identified the gamut of infectious agents responsible for bovine respiratory disease, we must only remember the canine parvovirus story.

Further research will unquestionably involve field studies. These are expensive and must be carefully designed and executed. But there is a potential for long-term epidemiologic studies in feedlots and for development and implementation of field techniques for unbiased evaluation of vaccines. In addition, studies will be required on the effects of various transport methods on the production of disease. Economic studies must be conducted on the financial merit of various management techniques. In addition, innovative delivery systems for administration of vaccines must be developed and immunologic and therapeutic agents must be developed so that nursing calves can be treated or vaccinated either via drinking water, by guns, or by other innovative procedures.

Certain minimal ground rules are essential for the future researcher. Research is expensive, and no project should be undertaken without careful statement of a hypothesis to be tested and statistical consultation to clarify the definitions, expedite the organization, strengthen the experimental design and obtain logical conclusions from seemingly illogical data. Future research will require a team approach, invoking knowledge, skills, experience and wisdom of people trained in a variety of disciplines.

Funding

The big question facing the future of bovine respiratory research is funding. The USDA must quadruple its budget in this area. Cattle producers must pioneer in an area they have neglected, that is, financing the research for which they clamor so loudly. They need to develop a check-off for research and need to increase their lobbying. They must understand there is no free lunch and no quick-fix. If they want quick answers for multi-complex problems, they must be prepared to support required research. The biologics industry must re-think its relationship with the research community, particularly the universities. The time is right for the development of a National Institute of Veterinary Medicine. The day when the USDA should dominate the research funding necessary to overcome a problem like respiratory disease is gone because the USDA is too plant-oriented, too heavily involved in regulatory activities and too closely controlled by agricultural politics.

Conclusion

These comments could be expanded on by a panel. Such a panel would very likely recommend nationwide studies and regional approaches to the problem of bovine respiratory disease. Future successful research will require a basic-science approach, a new reliance on quantitative epidemiology for deriving non-anecdotal conclusions from field observations and new funding structures involving livestock producers, the biologics industry and government.

Abstracts

The following abstracts of Poster Presentations were made available at the Symposium and are reprinted here.

Alternatives to Preconditioning Feeder Calves Purchased at Auctions

George T. Woods, Department of Pathobiology, College of Veterinary Medicine, University of Illinois, Urbana, Illinois 61801.

Manford E. Mansfield, Dixon Springs Agricultural Research Center, Route 1, Simpson, Illinois 62985.

Robert A. Crandell, Texas Veterinary Medical Diagnostic Laboratory, College Station, Texas 77843.

Clarence J. Kaiser, Dixon Springs Agricultural Research Center, Route 1, Simpson, Illinois 62985.

Four experiments with 293 feeder calves purchased at Illinois auctions were conducted. At the time of entrance into the feedlot, active and passive immunity with and without an antimicrobial agent in the feed were compared to controls in order to evaluate alternatives to preconditioning as recommended by the American Association of Bovine Practitioners. In Experiment 1, comparisons were made on 96 calves in four lots; Experiment 2 included 86 calves in four lots; Experiment 3 had 44 calves in three lots; and Experiment 4 consisted of 67 calves in two lots. Acute respiratory disease was treated in calves in all tests except Experiment 3. Morbidity ranged from 39 to 86 percent in experimental lots. The bovine antiserum against *P. multocida, P. hemolytica,* IBR, PI-3 and BVD viruses prevented death losses from pneumonia in Experiment 2 and reduced clinical illness in Experiment 1. In Experiment 4, intranasal IBR/PI-3 virus vaccine reduced clinical respiratory disease compared to controls. None of the preventive measures attempted significantly reduced clinical acute respiratory disease when compared to control lots.

A Profile of Lightweight Feeder Calves Vaccinated with Modified Live Pasteurella hemolytica

Charles W. Purdy, U.S. Department of Agriculture, Bushland, Texas 79012.

Charles W. Livingston, Texas A&M University Research and Extension Center, San Angelo, Texas 76901.

Glynn H. Frank, U.S. Department of Agriculture, Ames, Iowa 50011.

Joseph M. Cummins, Texas A&M University Research and Extension Center, Amarillo, Texas 79106.

N. Andy Cole, U.S. Department of Agriculture, Bushland, Texas 79012.

Raymond W. Loan, Texas Agricultural Experiment Station, College Station, Texas 77843.

Betty B. Gauer, Texas A&M University Research and Extension Center, San Angelo, Texas 76901.

David P. Hutcheson, Texas A&M University Research and Extension Center, Amarillo, Texas 79106.

A test was undertaken to determine the efficacy of a modified live *Pasteurella hemolytica* vaccine for reducing shipping fever morbidity and mortality in 100 calves purchased in Florida. Forty-one head were inoculated intradermally (ID) with 0.5 milliliters of *P. hemolytica* vaccine (A. H. Robins) in the neck region. The remaining 59 head served as controls. The following samples and observations were taken at day 0, and approximately every two weeks during the 87-day experiment: (1) nasal turbinate swabs for *Pasteurella* and *Mycoplasma* determination; (2) serum samples to determine humoral antibody against infectious bovine rhinotracheitis (IBR) virus, parainfluenza-3 (PI-3) virus, bovine viral diarrhea (BVD) virus, respiratory syncytial virus (RSV), *P. hemolytica, P. multocida,* and *Mycoplasma* sp.; (3) average daily weight gain per calf. Clinical observations (computed by a score system, including rectal temperature and feed consumed per pen) were recorded daily. The modified live *P. hemolytica* vaccine had no significant effect on average rate of gain or morbidity in the feedlot (vaccinates--83 percent versus nonvaccinates--88 percent). Two deaths due to pneumonia occurred in the vaccinates and six deaths occurred in the controls; however, the difference was not statistically significant. *Pasteurella hemolytica, P. multocida, Corynebacterium pyogenes, Mycoplasma* sp., and *Ureaplasma* sp. were isolated from both groups. Other pathogens isolated from the nonvaccinated calves which died included *Salmonella* sp., *Hemophilus somnus,* and IBR virus. Mortality was insignificant in the feedlot during the first month; however, it increased dramatically during the second month following an IBR virus outbreak. Significant serologic conversions occurred in both vaccinates and nonvaccinates to RSV, IBR virus and BVD virus. Most of the calves, both vaccinates and nonvaccinates, maintained a population of *P. multocida* throughout the experiment. *Pasteurella hemolytica,* serotype 1 was recovered from the nasal turbinates of one nonvaccinated calf during the first 58 days. Following the

IBR virus outbreak and the accompanying increased
mortality, *P. hemolytica,* serotype 1 was isolated from 15
vaccinated and 24 nonvaccinated calves.

*Airborne Particle Size and Meteorological Conditions Associated
with Respiratory Disease Incidence in Feedlot Cattle*

David K. Franzen, College of Veterinary Medicine and
Biomedical Sciences, Colorado State University, Fort
Collins, Colorado 80523.

Duncan W. MacVean, College of Veterinary Medicine and
Biomedical Sciences, Colorado State University, Fort
Collins, Colorado 80523.

Billy W. Bennett, College of Veterinary Medicine and
Biomedical Sciences, Colorado State University, Fort
Collins, Colorado 80523.

Thomas J. Keefe, College of Veterinary Medicine and
Biomedical Sciences, Colorado State University, Fort
Collins, Colorado 80523.

Dust is known to compromise the health of animals by
producing irritation and edema which may result in
pulmonary viral or bacterial infections. To elucidate the
role of air quality on the occurrence of respiratory
disease in feedlot cattle, the following parameters were
measured at a feedlot: suspended particulates in five size
fractions (>7.0μ m to <1.1μ m aerodynamic diameter) using a

467

high-volume filter apparatus, relative humidity and air temperature (hygrothermograph), and barometric pressure (microbarograph). Twenty-four-hour samples were collected four days per week from October 14 to December 18 and April 11 to May 6. Results indicate that incidence of pneumonia is directly related to the concentration of total suspended particulates and particles >7.0 μ m, when exposure to the dust occurred two weeks prior to the onset of disease (October to December only). Pneumonia was not significantly correlated to the other parameters, although temperature and pneumonia appeared to be inversely related. Upper respiratory infection was not correlated to the parameters measured. These results indicate that airborne particulates, particularly greater than 7.0μ m in diameter, can induce pneumonia after an appropriate two-week incubation period during the Fall.

The Efficacy of Liquamycin® LA-200™ in Preventing Shipping Fever

William S. Swafford, Pfizer Inc., 1107 S. Missouri 291, Lee's Summit, Missouri 64063.

Joseph M. Cummins, Texas A&M Research Center, 6500 Amarillo Boulevard West, Amarillo, Texas 79106.

David P. Hutcheson, Texas A&M Research Center, 6500 Amarillo Boulevard West, Amarillo, Texas 79106.

Eighty-eight calves (pay weight, 467 pounds) were purchased in Tennessee, grouped by weight and purchase date, and allotted to either truck or rail shipment groups. Half the calves in each shipment group were given a single IM injection of LA-200™ at 18 milligrams/pound to test its efficacy in preventing shipping fever. The transit time to Bushland, Texas, was 23 hours by truck and 122 hours by rail. The morbidity and mortality rates were high, as 63 of 88 (71.6 percent) calves became clinically ill with respiratory disease and 18 of 88 (20.5 percent) died. *Pasteurella hemolytica* serotype 1 was isolated from the lungs of every calf at necropsy. Treatment with LA-200™ reduced mortality from 12 to 44 (27.3 percent) in controls to 6 of 44 (13.6 percent) in treated animals. Treatment with LA-200™ reduced illness slightly from 77.3 percent in controls to 65.9 percent in treated calves. The reduction in morbidity and mortality attributed to LA-200™ occurred in both rail- and truck-shipped calves. The average daily gain at 28 days after arrival favored the LA-200™-treated group, 1.50 to 1.28 pounds/day. In summary, calves given

LA-200™ before shipment to an experimental feedlot had less morbidity and mortality and better average daily gains than did control calves.

The Use of a Live Pasteurella haemolytica Vaccine to Prevent Bovine Respiratory Disease

Clyde K. Smith, Ohio Agricultural Research and Development Center, Wooster, Ohio 44691.

A vaccine (PRECON-PH) has been developed using a live culture of *Pasteurella haemolytica* (PH) to prevent the development of bovine respiratory disease (BRD) in feedlot cattle and calves. The vaccine is administered intradermally in a single injection one to two weeks prior to stressing or shipping to produce a protective immune response. Safety and efficacy tests using the PH vaccine demonstrated that a single vaccination is sufficient to protect the calf against experimental stressing and challenge. Field tests of commercial cattle comparing 225 calves vaccinated with PH and 1,225 nonvaccinated calves have been conducted. The incidence of BRD among the nonvaccinated calves was 17.4 percent with 2.3 percent mortality while the incidence of co-mingled calves vaccinated with PH was 2.0 percent with no mortality. When the PH vaccine was used in field tests with a preconditioning program, the incidence of BRD was 55.2 percent among the non-preconditioned calves and 12.7 percent among the preconditioned calves. The PH vaccine has been used to vaccinate feeder calves upon arrival at the feedlot. The incidence of BRD among these co-mingled vaccinated calves was reduced 44 percent as compared to the nonvaccinated cattle and the number of treatments per case was reduced by 40 percent. The PH vaccine has been effective in prevention of BRD using both experimental and field challenges.

A Comparison of Three Therapeutic Programs for the Treatment of Shipping Fever in Weaned Calves

David Nash, Simplot Livestock Company, Nampa, Idaho 83651.

A total of 1,551 steers and 473 heifers intermittently arrived at an Idaho feedlot in October-November 1982. The transit time for the five groups of arriving cattle was less than six hours (average 3.8 hours). After processing, cattle were placed in typical feedlot facilities and observed for signs of illness. Approximately 10 percent morbidity occurred (212 calves). Sick animals were randomly assigned one of three treatments: (1) Liquamycin® LA-200™ (15-19 milligrams/pound body weight) IM + two sustained-release sulfadimethoxine (SRS) boluses; (2) 2,500 milligrams oxytetracycline IV for three days + two SRS boluses; (3) 2,000 milligrams of both oxytetracycline and tylosin IV for three days + two sulfamethazine boluses for two days + one bolus on day 3. Rectal temperatures were recorded for each animal for at least three days. Morbidity, mortality and treatment cost records were maintained. No significant differences were detected between treatment groups in regard to temperature or treatment responses. The re-treatment/death results for each group were as follows: (1) 7/1; (2) 8/2; (3) 5/2. Medication costs were higher in groups 1 and 3; however, labor expenses were not assessed during the trial and potential benefits from decreased handling in group 1 might have been realized.

The Effectiveness of Liquamycin® LA-200™ as a Therapeutic Treatment for Respiratory Disease in Feeder Cattle

A. J. Edwards, Kansas State University, Manhattan, Kansas 66505.

Respiratory diseases continue to be the number-one health problem in feedlot cattle causing about 75 percent of the sickness and 75 percent of the deaths according to an ongoing disease-incidence study. Treatments for respiratory diseases are generally aimed at using a chemotherapeutic agent that is effective against the pathogenic organisms involved and maintaining an adequate blood level in the animal over a period of time to aid in effecting a favorable response. LA-200™ has been utilized in combination with other antibacterial agents as a one-time treatment for clinically ill feedlot cattle with favorable results. The advantages to the program have been a favorable response as compared to regular three-day treatments, a reduction in amount of time spent treating animals daily and reduced medication costs in treating the sick animals.

A Comparison of Differing Levels of Liquamycin® LA-200™ with Other Therapeutic Regimens for the Treatment of Bovine Respiratory Disease

Bill W. Bennett, College of Veterinary Medicine, Colorado State University, Fort Collins, Colorado 80523.

Gary P. Rupp, College of Veterinary Medicine, Colorado State University, Fort Collins, Colorado 80523.

The efficacy of Liquamycin® LA-200™ for single-day treatment of BRD was evaluated at levels of 10, 15 and 20 milligrams/pound body weight in morbid feedlot cattle. A conventional four-day oxytetracycline regimen (5 milligrams/pound) was also tested. All treatments were administered with an initial dose of sustained-release oral sulfadimethoxine (SRS). In a second trial, 15 milligrams/pound Liquamycin® LA-200™+SRS treatment was compared to/administered with penicillin, penicillin+SRS, double-dose SRS or triple-dose tylosin. Morbidity, mortality, treatment, drug cost and labor records were maintained in both experiments. Animals that received either 10 or 15 milligrams/pound LA-200™+SRS showed consistent fever reduction. Duration of treatment favored the 15 milligrams LA-200™+SRS group as 8 percent of the animals required re-treatment (2 percent relapse rate).

Cattle administered a four-day oxytetracycline regimen had considerably higher treatment-relapse rates, and much higher labor costs. In the second trial, penicillin or penicillin+SRS groups experienced marked temperature declines. The 24-milligrams-tylosin-+-15 milligrams-LA-200™ group required a longer duration of therapy, including re-treatment, than other animals. Labor charges for the daily penicillin therapy rendered the program excessively expensive as compared to 15 milligrams LA-200™+SRS. Inclusion of 3X-tylosin or 2X-SRS also exceeded the 15 milligrams LA-200™+SRS cost. However, 2X-SRS did effect moderate efficacy improvement.

Lymphocyte Proliferative and Leukocyte Changes in Transported Feeder Calves

Frank Blecha, Kansas State University, Manhattan, Kansas 66506.

Stephen L. Boyles, Kansas State University, Manhattan, Kansas 66506.

Jack G. Riley, Kansas State University, Manhattan, Kansas 66505.

The influence of transport on lymphocyte blastogenesis and leukocyte numbers was evaluated in 40, 180 to 280 kilograms, feeder steers. Steers were allotted on the basis of weight and breed to a control or shipped group. Pre-shipment heparinized blood samples were obtained from all calves. Fourteen hours later twenty steers were transported 700 kilometers (ten hours) to a feedlot; control steers remained at the ranch-of-origin. Blood samples were obtained at unloading and seven days post-shipment. Lymphocytes were evaluated for blastogenic responses to concanavalin A (Con A), phytohemagglutinin (PHA) and pokeweed mitogen (PWM). Total and differential leukocyte numbers were determined on all blood samples. Lymphocyte blastogenic responses to Con A and PWM were lower (P<.01) in shipped steers and tended (P<.10) to be suppressed in PHA-stimulated lymphocytes at unloading. Total leukocytes, characterized by a neutrophilia, were increased (P<.01) in transported calves. These data suggest that transported calves have suppressed cellular immune functions. This immunosuppression could predispose shipped feeder calves to bovine respiratory disease.

The Use of a Live Pasteurella haemolytica Vaccine in Feedlot Calves

David P. Hutcheson, Texas A&M Research Center, 6500 Amarillo Boulevard West, Amarillo, Texas 79106.

Joseph M. Cummins, Texas A&M Research Center, 6500 Amarillo Boulevard West, Amarillo, Texas 79106.

Anthony Confer, Department of Veterinary Pathology, College of Veterinary Medicine, Oklahoma State University, Stillwater, Oklahoma 74074.

Ninety-three calves were obtained from seven different farms. Approximately half of the calves at each location were vaccinated with an experimental live *Pasteurella haemolytica* intradermal vaccine and half served as controls. Vaccine was given two weeks before shipment to an order-buyer's barn (OBB) in Tennessee where the calves were confined together for four days before shipment 1,178 miles to Bushland, Texas. Calves were bled and nasal swabs collected at the farm-of-origin (FO), arrival at OBB, arrival at experimental feedlot (FL), and at two, seven and fourteen days after arrival. Serum samples were also obtained at 28 and 56 days after arrival. Calves were weighed off truck at experimental feedlot and at all sampling periods except FO. Upon arrival and at seven and fourteen days after arrival *P. haemolytica* was isolated from nasal swabs of 22.2 percent, 34.5 percent and 14.3 percent of vaccinates and 3.2 percent, 6.5 percent and 9.7 percent of nonvaccinates respectively. No significant differences were detected for morbidity, mortality or performance for the two groups. The average *P. haemolytica* titer increased from 20.6 to 70.4 for vaccinates and 18.5 to 21.5 for nonvaccinates. The geometric mean antibody titer to *Pasteurella haemolytica* was statistically greater in vaccinates than controls fourteen days after vaccination (44 versus 4). Although a virulent *P. haemolytica* challenge was not given, the vaccine resulted in an antibody response that may have reflected improved immune status in the vaccinated group.

Chemical and Hormonal Response to Acute Physical Exertion in Beef Calves

M. R. Fedde, Kansas State University, Manhattan, Kansas 66506.

W. D. Kuhlmann, Kansas State University, Manhattan, Kansas 66506.

W. E. Moore, Kansas State University, Manhattan, Kansas 66505.

Venous blood samples were taken from indwelling jugular catheters in five Hereford steers, 150 to 230 kilograms, before, during and after a five-minute exercise bout. Animals were exercised on a large-animal treadmill ($3°$ incline) at speeds of 1.0, 1.4, 1.8 and 2.2 m· sec^{-1}. Serum was analyzed on a Technicon SMA 12/60 microanalyzer for twelve variables. Additionally, whole blood lactic acid and plasma cortisol were measured by an enzymatic assay and a radioimmunoassay, respectively. Serum $\{K^+\}$ increased by 75 percent (4 meq· ℓ^{-1} at rest to 7 meq· ℓ^{-1}) when samples were taken four minutes after the start of exercise at a medium trot (2.2 m· sec^{-1}). Significant elevations in this variable occurred even at a slow walk (1.0 m· sec^{-1}). Acute physical exertion increased serum glucose, inorganic phosphate, total calcium and sodium but caused no changes in total serum protein or chloride. Blood lactate increased at all speeds and was approximately ten times resting values at 2.2 m· sec^{-1}. Plasma cortisol did not increase during exertion; ten minutes after exertion, it was threefold higher than at rest. These chemical changes, indicative of stress, may result in a marked reduction in the electrical and contractile capability of the animal's neuromuscular system and heart and may influence a variety of regulatory or metabolic processes in other cells as well. (This study was supported in part by USDA Grant Number 59-2201-1-024-0.)

Immunity to Pasteurella haemolytica Serotype 1

Patricia E. Shewen, Department of Veterinary Microbiology and Immunology, Ontario Veterinary College, University of Guelph, Guelph, Ontario, Canada N1G 2W1.

Bruce N. Wilkie, Department of Veterinary Microbiology and Immunology, Ontario Veterinary College, University of Guelph, Guelph, Ontario, Canada N1G 2W1.

Experiments were instituted to examine stimulation of an immune response to *Pasteurella haemolytica* 1 by subcutaneous vaccination and its relationship to protection against experimental intrabronchial challenge with live organisms. Both serum and lung washings were examined for cytotoxin-neutralizing activity using bovine alveolar macrophages as the substrate; for *P. haemolytica*-agglutinating activity using an indirect (antiglobulin) microplate agglutination technique; and for opsonizing activity using ^{3}H-labeled formalinized *P.*

haemolytica and alveolar macrophages. Vaccination of calves with bacteria-free cytotoxic culture supernatant from *P. haemolytica* type 1 resulted in stimulation of cytotoxin-neutralizing activity, while vaccination with formalinized whole-cell bacterin was less effective. Both vaccines induced an immune response to bacterial surface antigens. This was detected by agglutination and opsonization. Protection against challenge was best in cytotoxin-vaccinated calves. Clinical scores in bacterin vaccinates were worse than in unvaccinated controls. In an adjunct experiment, calves vaccinated with culture supernatant from *P. haemolytica* type 11, a non-pneumonic serotype, were not protected against experimental challenge despite stimulation of a neutralizing response to cytotoxin from type 1. These calves did not develop agglutinating activity to type 1 prior to challenge. The conclusion reached is that protection against experimental challenge with *P. haemolytica* type 1 requires stimulation of an immune response to both the cytotoxin and surface antigens of the bacterium.

A Microbiologic Survey of Calf Pneumonia

William U. Knudtson, Veterinary Medical Research Institute, Iowa State University, Ames, Iowa 50011.

Mary A. Anson, Iowa Veterinary Diagnostic Laboratory, Iowa State University, Ames, Iowa 50011.

David E. Reed, Veterinary Medical Research Institute, Iowa State University, Ames, Iowa 50011.

The purpose of this study was to determine the microbial flora of lung tissue taken from 83 calves with clinical signs of pneumonia. The animals ranged from three days to one year of age and were mostly from confined dairy and small feedlot operations. Current standardized techniques were used in this study for cultivation of fastidious bacteria, mycoplasmas, ureaplasmas, viruses and chlamydiae. Single isolations were made from 18 percent of cases, multiple isolations from 71 percent and 11 percent were sterile. Major group isolations were as follows: bacteria 72 percent, mycoplasmas 59 percent, viruses 42 percent and chlamydiae 1 percent. Individual microbe percentages were as follows: *Mycoplasma dispar* 40 percent, *M. bovis* 38 percent, *Pasteurella multocida* 38 percent, *P. haemolytica* 31 percent, non-cytopathic BVD 27 percent, *Ureaplasma* spp. 24

percent, IBR 16 percent, *Haemophilus somnus* 12 percent, *M. bovirhinis* 7 percent, *E. coli* 7 percent, *Streptococcus* spp. 4 percent, *Corynebacterium pyogenese* 4 percent, cytopathic BVD 2 percent, bovine herpesvirus-3, PI-3 virus and *Chlamydia psitaci* 1 percent. There appeared to be little correlation between presence of mycoplasmas and presence of virus. The data did not support our previous contentions that viruses may predispose the lung for mycoplasma colonization.

An ELISA for Detection of Hemophilus somnus Antibodies in Bovine Sera

Randall Hubbard, Department of Veterinary Microbiology, Iowa State University, Ames, Iowa 50011.

Merlin Kaeberle, Department of Veterinary Microbiology, Iowa State University, Ames, Iowa 50011.

James Roth, Department of Veterinary Microbiology, Iowa State University, Ames, Iowa 50011.

The objective of this experimentation was the development of a specific and sensitive test for antibodies to *H. somnus* in bovine serum. An enzyme-linked immunosorbant assay was based on extracted lipopolysaccharide of *H. somnus* as the antigen and peroxidase-labeled anti-bovine Ig as the indicator to detect IgG antibodies. Use of antigen-coated polyvinyl microtiter plates allows conduct of the test in two hours with titers ranging from 0 to 1:10,240 and greater. This assay was useful in detecting specific antibodies to *H. somnus* with little or no cross-reactivity with Ag's of other bovine pathogens as well as providing insight into the humoral response to natural *H. somnus* infection and vaccination. Low to moderate titers were observed in both naturally-infected and vaccinated cattle. No correlation between antibody titer and disease resistance was observed in a herd in which *H. somnus* was contributory to clinical respiratory disease.

The Use of Human Leukocyte Interferon in Cattle During An IBR Virus Infection

Joseph M. Cummins, Texas A&M Research Center, 6500 Amarillo Boulevard West, Amarillo, Texas 79106.

David P. Hutcheson, Texas A&M Research Center, 6500 Amarillo Boulevard West, Amarillo, Texas 79106.

The objective was to determine the efficacy of human leukocyte interferon (IFN) in calves infected with infectious bovine rhinotracheitis (IBR) virus. Thirty-six feeder calves were given virulent IBR virus. Twenty-eight calves were given human leukocyte IFN on the day of and for two days after virus inoculation. Interferon was given once daily by three different routes; calves were either dosed intravenously (IV), orally or intranasally. Interferon was given at three dosage concentrations. Nasal secretions were collected daily for IFN concentrations and IBR virus excretion. Blood was collected for complete blood counts and serum was separated for interferon and IBR virus antibody determinations. Rectal temperatures, weight and individual feed consumption were recorded daily. Calves given IFN IV performed poorly; three of the nine calves died of bacterial pneumonia. All calves given IBR virus developed fever and had decreased feed intake after virus inoculation. Calves given the lowest dose of IFN tended to have less virus excretion and lower nasal secretion IFN titers than controls during IFN treatments, but more virus excretion and nasal secretion interferon after IFN treatment. Calves given IFN orally at the lowest dosage out-gained all other groups.

Antiviral Activity of Human Alpha and Bovine Nasal Secretion Interferons

Robert W. Fulton, Department of Veterinary Parasitology, Microbiology and Public Health, College of Veterinary Medicine, Oklahoma State University, Stillwater, Oklahoma 74078.

J. M. Cummins, Texas A&M Research Center, 6500 Amarillo Boulevard West, Amarillo, Texas 79106.

The antiviral activity induced by human and bovine interferon (IFN) was studied in Madin Darby bovine kidney (MDBK) monolayer cultures challenged subsequently by vesicular stomatitis virus (VSV) and infectious bovine rhinotracheitis viruses (IBRV). IFN used included nasal secretion IFN from virus-infected calves and human alpha IFN from virus-infected leukocytes. IBRV strains used as challenge virus included: (1) Cooper challenge strain; (2) an intranasal vaccinal strain; and (3) a parenteral vaccinal strain. Cultures in 24 well-tissue culture plates were treated prior to and subsequent to viral challenge with 500 IFN units. Each tissue culture well-received 10^3 PFU of each virus for one-hour adsorption. The fluids were collected 24 hours post-inoculation (PI) for VSV and 48 hours PI for IBRV. The culture fluids were frozen at $-70°$

C until assayed for plaque-forming unit activity in MDBK cells using an overlay system. Cultures treated with either bovine or human IFN had reduced viral yields for each of the IBRV strains and VSV compared to control cultures. These results indicate that these viruses are sensitive to the antiviral effects of bovine IFN and human alpha IFN *in vitro.*

Plasma Proteins and Water Balance in Bovine Lung

James F. Amend, Department of Veterinary Science, IANR, University of Nebraska-Lincoln, Lincoln, Nebraska 68583-0905.

Rebecca L. Nichelson, Department of Veterinary Science, IANR, University of Nebraska-Lincoln, Lincoln, Nebraska 68583-0905.

Vicky L. Tucker, Department of Veterinary Science, IANR, University of Nebraska-Lincoln, Lincoln, Nebraska 68583-0905.

Merwin L. Frey, Department of Veterinary Science, IANR, University of Nebraska-Lincoln, Lincoln, Nebraska 68583-0905.

Alan R. Doster, Department of Veterinary Science, IANR, University of Nebraska-Lincoln, Lincoln, Nebraska 68583-0905.

Plasma total protein concentration (TP) affects water balance in lung tissue by altering colloidal osmotic pressure (COP), a force that retains fluid in pulmonary capillary beds. We were interested in plasma protein concentration and composition (A/G ratio) as participants in regulation of interstitial water in bovine lung. We measured TP and A/G ratio, COP, lung water content, and lung tissue electrical impedance (Z) in a group of feeder-age calves. TP was determined by biuret technique, COP by a Wescor colloid osmometer, lung water by wet-dry ratio (WD), and Z by a bipolar electrode catheter and bridge circuit. TP averaged 7.4 grams/dL and COP 19.2 torr. WD had a mean of 3.8, and Z averaged 638 ohms. It was possible to define a relationship between COP, TP, A/G and plasma pH such that COP could be accurately predicted in calves from protein variables and acid-base conditions. Additional studies suggested that acidosis, elevated globulin fraction and hypoproteinemia altered COP toward increased risk of lung-water accumulation. Previous experimental infection with bovine respiratory syncytial virus, *Mycoplasma dispar,* or both agents, altered observed WD and Z. (This study was supported by USDA Grant Numbers

59-2311-0-061-0 and 901-15-179 and by the Nebraska Agricultural Experiment Station.)

Passive Immunization in Bovine Respiratory Disease

Raymond W. Loan, College of Veterinary Medicine, Texas A&M University, College Station, Texas 77843.

David P. Hutcheson, Texas A&M Research Center, 6500 Amarillo Boulevard West, Amarillo, Texas 79106.

Charles W. Purdy, U.S. Department of Agriculture, Bushland, Texas 79012.

Joseph M. Cummins, Texas A&M Research Center, 6500 Amarillo Boulevard West, Amarillo, Texas 79106.

Richard E. Mock, Texas A&M Research Center, 6500 Amarillo Boulevard West, Amarillo, Texas 79106.

Ronald D. Welsh, Texas Veterinary Medical Diagnostic Laboratory, Amarillo, Texas 79106.

Marilyn S. Rowe, College of Veterinary Medicine, Texas A&M University, College Station, Texas 77843.

The study was undertaken to correlate the antibody content of convalescent serum (collected at slaughter) and purified globulin concentrates with prophylactic effectiveness against bovine respiratory disease. Feeder calves were purchased from an order-buyer in Newport, Tennessee. Convalescent serum was collected at abattoirs in Amarillo, Texas. Hyperimmune serum was prepared by the repeated injection of adult cattle with cultures of *Pasteurella hemolytica* and vaccination, one time with IBR, PI-3, BVD, leptospiral, clostridial (seven-way) and *Hemophilus somnus* vaccines. Immunoglobulin concentrates were prepared by the polyethylene glycol or caprylic acid method. Antibody to *P. hemolytica* was measured by indirect hemagglutination, to *H. somnus* by microtiter plate agglutination and to viruses by neutralization tests. Convalescent serum administered in doses of 1500 milliliters per calf reduced respiratory disease by 60 percent, increased the average daily gain by 37 percent ($p < .05$) and resulted in a $12.36 benefit per calf. Insoluble globulin precipitates and a globulin concentrate preparation without significant antibody had no beneficial effect. A globulin concentrate with high antibody activity reduced death loss from 12.5 percent to 2.0 percent and resulted in a $28.78 advantage per calf.

Physiological Response to Acute Physical Exertion in Beef Calves

W. D. Kuhlmann, Kansas State University, Manhattan, Kansas 66506.

M. R. Fedde, Kansas State University, Manhattan, Kansas 66506.

Ventilatory and cardiovascular variables were measured in five Hereford steers before, during and after five-minute acute exercise bouts on a treadmill (3° incline) running at 1.0, 1.4, 1.8 and 2.2 m· $^{-1}$. Oxygen consumption (M_{O_2}) and CO_2 production (M_{CO_2}) were measured by collecting mixed expired gas in a balloon. Blood samples were simultaneously obtained from indwelling catheters in the aorta and pulmonary artery. Minute ventilation (V_E) increased in proportion to treadmill speed; respiratory frequency increased at the low treadmill speed (1.0 m· sec^{-1}) but did not increase further at higher speeds. The remaining increases in V_E were caused by increased tidal volume. M_{O_2} and M_{CO_2} increased ten times over resting values at a speed of 2.2 m · sec $^{-1}$. The oxygen consumption curve suggests that these animals were at or near M_{O_2} -max at this speed. The respiratory exchange ratio, R, decreased slightly at the two lowest speeds, from a resting value of 1.032, but increased at the two highest speeds. Cardiac output and heart rate increased in proportion to speed up to 1.8 m · sec $^{-1}$ but did not increase further at 2.2 m · sec $^{-1}$. Packed-cell volume increased from 26 at rest to 36 at the highest exercise level. The low level of exercise at which maximum oxygen consumption was achieved and the dramatic increase in packed-cell volume indicate that physical exercise is a significant stressor for this species. (This study was supported in part by USDA Grant Number 59-2201-1-024-0.)

Interactions of Cold Stress and Pasteurella haemolytica in the Pathogenesis of Pneumonic Pasteurellosis in Calves: I. Humoral and Cellular Changes in the Circulating Blood

N. Edward Robinson, Pulmonary Laboratory, Veterinary Clinical Center, Michigan State University, East Lansing, Michigan 48824.

Frederik J. Derksen, Pulmonary Laboratory, Veterinary Clinical Center, Michigan State University, East Lansing, Michigan 48824.

Ronald F. Slocombe, Pulmonary Laboratory, Veterinary Clinical Center, Michigan State University, East Lansing, Michigan 48824.

Six healthy neonatal calves were chilled with cold water and had a focal tracheitis induced by spraying of 5 percent acetic acid into the tracheal lumen. Leukograms, hemograms, plasma cortisol, histamine and bradykinin, and plasma solids were determined over the subsequent twelve hours. Cold stress increased plasma cortisol levels for less than one hour, but did not alter any other variable. This group of calves served as a control group for a second series of neonatal calves which received $2x10^9$ organisms of *P. haemolytica* intratracheally immediately following an identical period of chilling and acetic acid exposure. Calves receiving *P. haemolytica* became neutropenic but band neutrophils increased by twelve hours post-exposure, and plasma cortisol levels were maintained at the same or greater than cold-stress levels for all measurement periods subsequent to exposure. *Pasteurella* challenge did not influence other variables. Contrary to previous reports, these data suggest a role for the neutrophil in the initial lesions of pulmonary pasteurellosis. Corticosteroid increases occurred with cold stress and subsequent infection and may have facilitated the development of pasteurellosis. Our data provided no evidence to indicate that histamine or bradykinin is involved in the pathogenesis of pneumonic pasteurellosis. (This study was supported by USDA and Michigan Agricultural Experiment Station.)

Interaction of Cold Stress and Pasteurella haemolytica in the Pathogenesis of Pneumonic Pasteurellosis in Calves: II. Changes in Lung Function

Ronald F. Slocombe, Pulmonary Laboratory, Veterinary Clinical Center, Michigan State University, East Lansing, Michigan 48824.

Frederik J. Derksen, Pulmonary Laboratory, Veterinary Clinical Center, Michigan State University, East Lansing, Michigan 48824.

N. Edward Robinson, Pulmonary Laboratory, Veterinary Clinical Center, Michigan State University, East Lansing, Michigan 48824.

Thirteen neonatal calves were cold-stressed twice twelve hours apart with cold water hosing for twenty minutes. Ventilation, gas exchange and pulmonary mechanics were measured. Chilling increased O_2 consumption and CO_2 production necessitating increased alveolar ventilation which was achieved by increased tidal volume without increased minute ventilation. Seven calves (principals) received $2x10^9$ *P. haemolytica* intratracheally; the remaining calves (controls) received saline. Within one hour, principals were tachyneic and hypoxemic with increased minute and dead-space ventilation but no increase in alveolar ventilation. Three hours post-challenge, dynamic compliance had decreased. Twelve hours post-infection, pulmonary resistance increased and calves hypoventilated (PaCO$_2$ increased). There were no changes in lung function in the control group. Data from *Pasteurella*-exposed calves indicate that gas exchange impairment and peripheral lung injury occur very rapidly suggesting pasteurellosis is initiated in the lung parenchyma and does not extend from airway lesions. Hypoxemia and increased dead-space ventilation probably results from ventilation perfusion mismatching in injured portions of the lung. (This study was supported by USDA and Michigan Agricultural Experiment Station.)

Physiopathological Features of Acute Confinement Stress in Calves

G. L. Mason, College of Veterinary Medicine, Texas A&M University, College Station, Texas 77843.

L. G. Friedlander, College of Veterinary Medicine, Texas A&M University, College Station, Texas 77843.

A. B. Richards, College of Veterinary Medicine, Texas A&M University, College Station, Texas 77843.

J. C. Connelly, College of Veterinary Medicine, Texas A&M University, College Station, Texas 77843.

R. G. Nelson, College of Veterinary Medicine, Texas A&M University, College Station, Texas 77843.

W. L. Jenkins, College of Veterinary Medicine, Texas A&M University, College Station, Texas 77843.

The association of stress with viral and bacterial agents in the pathogensis of bovine respiratory disease is well recognized, but the mechanisms involved are poorly understood. Studies were undertaken to identify quantifiable indicators of stress in calves, and to delineate specific factors which might be involved in the development of respiratory disease secondary to the stress reaction. Calves were suddenly subjected to unfamiliar and intense confinement for 24 to 36 hours. During this time, they were denied feed and water and were forced to remain standing. Samples were collected prior to, during, immediately after and for several days following the stress period. Significant and consistent deviations of the following blood parameters were identified: hematocrit, total white cell count, differential count, urea nitrogen, creatine phosphokinase, lactic dehydrogenase, ascorbic acid, cholesterol, iron, zinc, copper, cortisol, triiodothyronine, thyroxine and fibronectin. A number of other determinations showed marginal but consistent changes. It was concluded that significant physiopathological deviations could be associated with confinement stress in cattle.

Experimental Model for Comparative Pharmacokinetic Studies in Bronchopneumonic Calves

L. G. Friedlander, College of Veterinary Medicine, Texas A&M University, College Station, Texas 77843.

G. L. Mason, College of Veterinary Medicine, Texas A&M University, College Station, Texas 77843.

J. A. Allert, College of Veterinary Medicine, Texas A&M University, College Station, Texas 77843.

R. B. Simpson, College of Veterinary Medicine, Texas A&M University, College Station, Texas 77843.

D. Nall, College of Veterinary Medicine, Texas A&M University, College Station, Texas 77843.

W. L. Jenkins, College of Veterinary Medicine, Texas A&M University, College Station, Texas 77843.

An experimental model has been developed that allows comparative pharmacokinetic studies to be conducted on antibacterial agents in normal and then bronchopneumonic calves. The system facilitates the determination of concurrent plasma and pulmonary tissue disposition kinetics. A standard procedure is followed for the evaluation of the pharmacokinetic parameters which describe the disposition of a selected antibacterial agent in calves following the intravenous injection of a single dose. The calves then have a perforated R-3603 Tygon® tubing tissue cage, a cellulose dialysis membrane sachet (volume 4 milliliters, m.w. exclusion 3,500 daltons) and a set of Spectra/Por hollow fiber bundles (i.d. 215 μ m, volume 250 μ l, m.w. exclusion, 5,000 daltons) surgically introduced into the apical lobe of the lung. Following a recovery period, the plasma kinetic study is repeated, but in this case the rate of diffusion of the agent into the fluid-filled (dextran 75 in saline) sachet or perfused fiber bundles is also measured. Finally, following the administration of betamethasone parenterally and 4 percent acetic acid directly into the tissue cage, a culture of pathogenic *Pasteurella haemolytica* (3^{-5} x 10^7 organisms/milliliter) is introduced into the tissue cage. Usually, an acute bronchopneumonia develops within 36–48 hours. The kinetic study is then repeated in the sick calves. The plasma-disposition kinetics and intrapulmonary-diffusion kinetics between normal and bronchopneumonic calves, when using a variety of antibacterial agents, can then be compared and dosage regimens adjusted accordingly.

The Experimental Production of Bovine Pneumonic Pasteurellosis:
I. Clinical Aspects

H. Alison Gibbs, University of Glasgow Veterinary School,
Bearsden Road, Glasgow, Scotland.

Edna M. Allan, University of Glasgow Veterinary School,
Bearsden Road, Glasgow, Scotland.

Alasdair Wiseman, University of Glasgow Veterinary School,
Bearsden Road, Glasgow, Scotland.

Ian E. Selman, University of Glasgow Veterinary School,
Bearsden Road, Glasgow, Scotland.

A reproducible experimental model for bovine pneumonic
pasteurellosis has been developed using conventional,
weaned, dairy-cross calves, and an infecting strain of
Pasteurella haemolytica biotype A serotype 1 *(P. haemolytica* Al)
isolated from a pathologically-confirmed incident of bovine
pneumonic pasteurellosis. Clinical findings were pyrexia,
hyperpnoea, tachypnoea, nasal discharge and reduced
appetite and were indistinguishable from those seen in
field incidents of bovine pneumonic pasteurellosis
involving recently housed, weaned, previously
single-suckled calves from September to November, a
condition usually described in Scotland as "transit fever."
In the course of the experiment, natural transmission of

the infecting strain of *P. haemolytica* A1 occurred to two control calves which developed clinical signs identical to the artificially-infected calves. All infected calves yielded large numbers of the infecting strain of *P. haemolytica* A1 in pure culture from the lower respiratory tract at postmortem, and pathological findings were typical of bovine pneumonic pasteurellosis.

The Experimental Production of Bovine Pneumonic Pasteurellosis: II. Microbiological and Pathological Aspects

Edna M. Allan, University of Glasgow Veterinary School, Bearsden Road, Glasgow, Scotland.

H. Alison Gibbs, University of Glasgow Veterinary School, Bearsden Road, Glasgow, Scotland.

Alasdair Wiseman, University of Glasgow Veterinary School, Bearsden Road, Glasgow, Scotland.

Ian E. Selman, University of Glasgow Veterinary School, Bearsden Road, Glasgow, Scotland.

Bovine pneumonic pasteurellosis has been reproduced in conventionally-reared calves using a strain of *Pasteurella haemolytica* biotype A, serotype 1 (*P. haemolytica* A1) obtained from a pathologically-confirmed outbreak of bovine pneumonic pasteurellosis. Clinical findings identical to those described in natural field cases of bovine pneumonic pasteurellosis developed in the infected calves; in addition, two control calves developed the same disease following natural infection with the experimental strain of *P. haemolytica* A1. *Pasteurella haemolytica* A1 was repeatedly recovered from the nasopharynx of infected calves and throughout the upper and lower respiratory tracts of the animals following necropsy. Seroconversion to the organism developed in all infected animals examined on days 9 and 10 post-initial infection (p.i.i.). Classical lesions of fibrinous pneumonia were found in the lungs of the animals examined on days 2 and 3 p.i.i., while by days 9 and 10 p.i.i. many areas of fibrinous pneumonia were confined by a fibrous capsule forming a well-defined nodule. These lesions were identical to those seen in field cases of bovine pneumonic pasteurellosis.

Pasteurellosis: Induction by Intrapulmonic Inoculation via a Cannula

Richard E. Corstvet, College of Veterinary Medicine, Louisiana State University, Baton Rouge, Louisiana 70803.

James R. Turk, College of Veterinary Medicine, Louisiana State University, Baton Rouge, Louisiana 70803.

Frederick M. Enright, College of Veterinary Medicine, Louisiana State University, Baton Rouge, Louisiana 70803.

Mary Lou T. Potter, College of Veterinary Medicine, Louisiana State University, Baton Rouge, Louisiana 70803.

Marian M. Downing, College of Veterinary Medicine, Louisiana State University, Baton Rouge, Louisiana 70803.

Gale W. Jeffers, College of Veterinary Medicine, Louisiana State University, Baton Rouge, Louisiana 70803.

Experiments were designed to determine whether typical pneumonic pasteurellosis could be produced in beef calves by intrapulmonic inoculation of a 20-to-22-hour culture of *Pasteurella haemolytica* type 1 (Ph1) via an indwelling cannula passed down the trachea into the lung. Animals were inoculated with either 5×10^9 Ph1 contained in 5.0 milliliters of sterile saline or 5.0 milliliters of sterile saline. At 0, 2, 4, 8, 12, 24, 48 and 72 hours post-inoculation, the lung was lavaged. Each lavage was cultured quantitatively for Ph1 and also examined for cell

502

populations. Smears of lavage sediments were stained for Phl by the fluorescent antibody technique (FAT). Animals were killed at intervals through 96 hours post-inoculation, necropsied and several sites were cultured. Lungs were examined for lesions both at the site of inoculation and elsewhere. Phl was recovered from all lavages except 0 hour in concentrations of 10^4 - 10^6 bacteria/milliliter of lavage fluid and from various sites in the infected animals. Lavage cell populations shifted from predominantly macrophages to predominantly neutrophils during the course of the experiments. FAT on lavage sediments showed many Phl with ample capsules evident, but very few organisms appeared to be cell-associated. Pneumonic pasteurellosis was produced in all of the Phl-inoculated animals. An early lesion was found at two and four hours post-inoculation, an intermediate lesion at eight and twelve hours and a late lesion at 24 through 96 hours.

Growth of Bovine Herpesvirus 1: Mouse Model

Harish C. Minocha, Kansas State University, Manhattan, Kansas 66506.

Abdeljelil Ghram, Kansas State University, Manhattan, Kansas 66506.

Boondee Atikij, Kansas State University, Manhattan, Kansas 66506.

Robyn R. Welliever, Kansas State University, Manhattan, Kansas 66506.

Infectious bovine rhinotrachetis (IBR) virus has been reported to transform mouse-embryo fibroblasts and establish a long-term persistent infection in mice (Gader, 1981). We present the first study of IBR virus propagation in mouse cell cultures. Balb C mouse lung and kidney primary cultures were inoculated with Cooper strain of IBR virus. Virion synthesis first occurred between four and eight hours after virus inoculation and maximum virus titer ($5x10^5$ PFU/milliliter) was detected in 24 hours. Cytopathic effect (CPE) in cell cultures was observed at eight hours and 90 percent of the infected monolayers showed CPE in 48-72 hours post-virus inoculation. Approximately 60-70 percent of the newly-replicated virus was cell-associated. The incorporation of radioactive precursor, ^{3}H-thymidine and ^{3}H-valine, into viral macromolecules was demonstrated into the purified virions by pulse-chase experiments. Mice inoculated with IBR virus had serum neutralization titers of 1:40 or greater and an *in vitro* cell-mediated immune (CMI) response was elicited by sensitized spleen lymphocytes. Interferon production was also observed (titer 1:30) 72 hours after *in vitro* exposure of lymphocytes to UV-irradiated IBR virus. Mouse lymphocytes required 10^{5} macrophages for maximum protein synthesis and the virus-sensitized lymphocytes demonstrated fourfold greater stimulation index as compared to nonsensitized cells. The data indicated that IBR virus may be studied in mouse cell cultures and an immune response to the virus including interferon synthesis was produced in the animal.

The Aerobiology of Calves Infected Experimentally with Bovine Herpesvirus 1 and P. haemolytica

Klaus W. Jericho, Agriculture Canada, Animal Diseases Research Institute, P.O. Box 640, Lethbridge, Alberta, Canada T1J 3Z4.

Allen R. Jejeune, Defence Research Establishment, Suffield, Alberta, Canada T0J 2N0.

The aerobiology of the tracheal and exhaled air of eight calves (four groups of two calves) was studied before, during and after exposure to aerosols of bovine herpesvirus 1 (BHV 1) and *P. haemolytica*. The purpose of this experiment was to elucidate the number of infectious agents which may reach the lung from diseased upper respiratory tract tissue (tonsil, larynx and nasal passages) and the number of infectious droplets which may be shed in exhaled air and become available for transmission to other cattle. Anderson samplers and all-glass impingers were used to sample tracheal and exhaled air. It was learned that the upper respiratory tract serves as a very efficient filter of infectious droplets in aerosol both on inhalation and on exhalation. The efficiency of this filter was significantly compromised during coughing, at which time the number of infectious droplets ($<5\mu$) were numerous in tracheal and exhaled air. The shedding of large numbers of infectious particles in exhaled air on coughing by infected cattle must therefore be regarded as an important mode of transmission of respiratory pathogens in cattle, particularly if they are reared in close proximity to each other.

Immunization Against Experimental Bovine Pneumonic Pasteurellosis

M. A. Cardella, National Veterinary Services Laboratories, Ames, Iowa 50010.

M. A. Adviento, National Veterinary Services Laboratories, Ames, Iowa 50010.

R. M. Nervig, National Veterinary Services Laboratories, Ames, Iowa 50010.

Vaccination-challenge experiments were conducted in colostrum-deprived (C-D) calves to evaluate the efficacy of *Pasteurella* bacterins and vaccines against experimental pneumonic pasteurellosis. C-D calves were vaccinated with formalin-killed *Pasteurella* bacterins and live vaccines, then challenged by intratracheal inoculation of serotype 1 *P. haemolytica* Wilkie strain A-1 and serotype A-3 *P. multocida*

507

strain 1062. Infectious bovine rhinotracheitis virus was introduced intranasally three to four days prior to the *P. haemolytica* challenge-exposure. All calves were examined for gross and histopathological lesions when necropsied at death or when sacrificed at termination of experiments, four to seven days after challenge-exposure. Clinical, hematological and pathologic responses to challenge-exposure were similar in the control and aluminum hydroxide-adsorbed *P. haemolytica* and *P. multocida* bacterin-treated calves. Pneumonic lesions were observed in the lungs of both groups of animals. In initial studies an oil-adjuvanted *P. haemolytica* bacterin effectively limited clinical and pathologic responses to challenge-exposure. Clinical responses to challenge-exposure in the calves vaccinated with live *Pasteurella* vaccines were less severe and lung lesions were generally limited to focal areas of consolidation. Vaccination of C-D calves with formalinized, aluminum hydroxide-adjuvanted *Pasteurella* bacterins has proved ineffective in reducing the clinical responses or lesions in experimentally-produced *Pasteurella* pneumonia. Clinical responses and lesions in calves vaccinated with live *Pasteurella* vaccines were less severe.

Immunological Defense Mechanisms Against Pasteurella haemolytica in the Bovine Lung

John Opuda-Asibo, Department of Veterinary Pathobiology, University of Minnesota, St. Paul, Minnesota 55108.

Evelyn L. Townsend, Department of Veterinary Pathobiology, University of Minnesota, St. Paul, Minnesota 55108.

Samuel K. Maheswaran, Department of Veterinary Pathobiology, University of Minnesota, St. Paul, Minnesota 55108.

Joel R. Leininger, Department of Veterinary Pathobiology, University of Minnesota, St. Paul, Minnesota 55108.

This research evaluated the effectiveness of three *Pasteurella haemolytica* vaccines in generating a humoral immune response in the bovine lung. The vaccines, administered parenterally to *Pasteurella*-free calves, included a live-organism preparation, a crude-cytotoxin preparation and a combined live-organism cytotoxin preparation. Pre-vaccination and serial post-vaccination lung lavages were performed using a fiberoptic bronchoscope to retrieve bronchoalveolar washings (BAWs) for several analyses. Agglutinating antibody titers in the serum and BAWs of vaccinated calves peaked at three weeks post-vaccination. Total protein, IgA and IgG1 in the BAWs of vaccinates were less than those found in the BAWs of nonvaccinates. BAWs from calves vaccinated with the cytotoxin alone neutralized *P. haemolytica* cytotoxin more efficiently than BAWs from other calves. All BAWs contained unidentified non-antibody substances that neutralized the cytotoxin. While sera from vaccinated calves were bactericidal to *P. haemolytica* in the presence of complement, no BAWs were bactericidal. ELISA is in use to determine the class of lung antibodies specific for *P. haemolytica* or cytotoxin generated by these vaccines.

Identification of Bovine Herpesvirus 1 Polypeptides Involved in Serum Neutralization

Melissa A. Lum, Veterinary Medical Research Institute, Iowa State University, Ames, Iowa 50011.

David E. Reed, Veterinary Medical Research Institute, Iowa State University, Ames, Iowa 50011.

Bovine herpesvirus 1-infected (infectious bovine rhinotracheitis virus) cell antigens were solubilized with Nonidet-P40. The crude antigen extract was separated by reaction with bovine hyperimmune serum in line immunoelectrophoresis; individual immunoprecipitates were used to immunize rabbits. Rabbit sera possessing

510

serum-neutralizing activity were analyzed by reaction with crude antigen extract in immunoprecipitation sodium dodecylsulfate polyacrylamide gel electrophoresis. An 82-92K dalton glycopeptide and a 77.5-81K glycopeptide appeared to be involved separately in inducing serum-neutralizing antibody. A non-glycosylated 108-115K dalton polypeptide and a 69-75K glycopeptide always co-precipitated and also induced serum-neutralizing antibody.

Studies on Bovine Herpesvirus 1 (BHV-1) Isolated from Trigeminal Ganglia of Clinically-Normal Cattle

Louis L. Rodriguez, Department of Veterinary Science, University of Wisconsin-Madison, Madison, Wisconsin 53706.

Jane E. Homan, Department of Veterinary Science, University of Wisconsin-Madison, Madison, Wisconsin 53706.

Bernard C. Easterday, Department of Veterinary Science, University of Wisconsin-Madison, Madison, Wisconsin 53706.

Ten isolates of BHV-1 recovered from tissue explants of trigeminal ganglia from clinically-normal cattle were studied *in vitro* and *in vivo* and their characteristics compared with those of vaccine and field strains of BHV-1.

The viruses could be distinguished by their plaque size in cell monolayers, but were not significantly different in their thermal inactivation profiles at 48° C. No temperature-sensitive mutants were found among the trigeminal ganglia isolates when they were grown at 41° C. However, differences in the virus progeny yields at 41° C were noticed between some of trigeminal ganglia isolates and the vaccine and field strains. Selected isolates had different pathogenicity when they were inoculated in young rabbits. Some of the trigeminal ganglia isolates showed different DNA pattern by restriction endonuclease analysis. The differences in the characteristics of the isolates studied is indicative of the variability among the BHV-1-producing latent infections in the cattle population. The significance of these characteristics in viral latency is discussed.

Infectious Bovine Rhinotracheitis Virus (IBRV) Infection During or at the End of a Three-Day Fast in Calves: A Difference in Virus Excretion and Interferon (IFN) Production

Jean M. d'Offay, Department of Veterinary Microbiology, College of Veterinary Medicine, University of Missouri, Columbia, Missouri 65211.

Bruce D. Rosenquist, Department of Veterinary Microbiology, College of Veterinary Medicine, University of Missouri, Columbia, Missouri 65211.

Fasting and diet changes often accompany calves during transport to and upon arrival at feedlots. The mixing and crowding of calves at this time may facilitate transmission of viruses considered to be potentiators in viral-bacterial synergism in bovine respiratory disease. In a replicate study, two groups of fasting calvs were inoculated intranasally with IBRV to determine if and how a three-day fast affected virus replication and IFN production as measured in nasal secretions. One group was inoculated 24 hours after onset of fasting and the other immediately before re-feeding. A control group was inoculated but not fasted. Overall mean IFN production was significantly higher ($P<0.01$) in calves inoculated during the fast than in either of the other groups. Highest IFN titers were recorded in the fasted calves. Mean IBRV excretion was tenfold lower on post-inoculation day (PID) 1 and significantly lower ($P<0.05$) on PID 2 in calves inoculated at the end of fasting than in the control calves. Virus excretion on PIDs 3 and 4 was highest in calves inoculated during fasting and lowest in those inoculated upon re-feeding. How fasting affects significant changes in IBRV excretion and IFN production, therefore, depends largely upon when infection occurs during fasting.

Bovine Pneumonic Pasteurellosis: Correlative Studies of Lesions and Immunity in Vaccinated Cattle

R. J. Panciera, College of Veterinary Medicine, Oklahoma State University, Stillwater, Oklahoma 74078.

A. W. Confer, College of Veterinary Medicine, Oklahoma State University, Stillwater, Oklahoma 74078.

R. E. Corstvet, College of Veterinary Medicine, Oklahoma State University, Stillwater, Oklahoma 74078.

Experimental bovine pneumonic pasteurellosis was induced in beef calves by a transthoracic challenge with *Pasteurella haemolytica* serotype 1 or *P. multocida* type 3. Challenge lesions were quantified by a lesion scoring system based on size and extension of lesions with larger scores assigned

514

to the more severe lesions. Cattle immunized with live *Pasteurella* sp. by either aerosol or parenteral routes developed high serum antibody titers to the homologous organism as determined by a quantitative fluorometric procedure (FIAX). Mean lesion scores were approximately two to twenty times higher in control than vaccinated animals. There was a significant ($p < 0.05$) correlation between high-serum antibody titers at the time of challenge and a low lesion score in four of six experiments.

Other experiments compared the immunizing effects of live *P. haemolytica* from logarithmic (six-hour) and stationary (20-to-22 hour) phase cultures. In five of six experiments, the cattle immunized with six-hour cultures had lower mean lesion scores than those immunized with 20- or 22-hour cultures. High-antibody titers as detected by the FIAX or indirect hemagglutination tests correlated ($p < 0.01$) with low lesion scores regardless of the age of the immunizing culture.

Hyoik Ryu, Department of Veterinary Microbiology, College of Veterinary Medicine, Iowa State University, Ames, Iowa 50011.

Randall Hubbard, Department of Veterinary Microbiology, College of Veterinary Medicine, Iowa State University, Ames, Iowa 50011.

Merlin Kaeberle, Department of Veterinary Microbiology, College of Veterinary Medicine, Iowa State University, Ames, Iowa 50011.

James Roth, Department of Veterinary Microbiology, College of Veterinary Medicine, Iowa State University, Ames, Iowa 50011.

The objective of this experimentation was to evaluate the ability of *Pasteurella multocida* and *Hemophilus somnus* to interfere with bovine polymorphonuclear leukocyte (PMN) function. The effect of various *P. multocida* and *H. somnus* preparations on PMN functions was examined *in vitro* by using two type A strains of *P. multocida* and one of *H. somnus* (8025). With both organisms, the ability of PMNs to ingest *Staphylococcus aureus* and iodinate protein was significantly inhibited in the presence of live cells, heat-killed whole cells or saline-extracted fractions but not in the presence of the washed, heat-killed cells. None of the preparations of the two bacteria inhibited nitroblue tetrazolium reduction by PMNs. The PMN inhibitory factors were further characterized. The *P. multocida* inhibitory factor was found to be a heat-stable capsular material of greater than 300,000 molecular weight. The *H. somnus* heat-stable saline supernatant extract contained two materials with differing effects. The material that inhibited iodination of protein was found to be less than 10,000 molecular weight while the material that inhibited *Staphylococcus aureus* ingestion was greater than 300,000 molecular weight.

Plasmid Patterns of Pasteurella haemolytica Isolated from Cattle

Robert E. Briggs, College of Veterinary Medicine, Iowa State University, Ames, Iowa 50010.

Glynn H. Frank, National Animal Disease Center, Agricultural Research Service, U.S. Department of Agriculture, Ames, Iowa 50010.

Epidemiological studies of *Pasteurella haemolytica* in bovine respiratory disease have revealed that serotype 1 is the predominant serotype recovered from pneumonic lung. Plasmid patterns may offer a means to further subdivide *P. haemolytica* serotypes. Plasmids of *P. haemolytica* were isolated from 90 pneumonic bovine lung isolates and 400

517

field nasal isolates by methods described by Kado and Liu (1981). They were separated by agarose gel electrophoresis, stained with ethidium bromide and observed under UV illumination. The lung isolates included serotypes 1 (81), 2 (2), 6 (3) and 11 (2). The nasal isolates included serotypes 1 (325) and 2 (75). Serotype 1 isolates included at least four plasmid patterns with three predominating. No plasmid patterns were found exclusively in nasal or lung isolates. Serotype two isolates included at least three plasmid patterns. Serotype 6 isolates did not contain plasmids (although an ovine isolate did). Both serotype 11 plasmid patterns were different. No identical plasmid patterns were found among different serotypes. Within serotypes 1 and 2, identical patterns were found from isolates obtained from cattle in different areas of the U.S. Plasmid patterns can be used to subdivide serotypes 1 and 2. There is evidence that these plasmids are relatively stable and widely distributed in the U.S. Many isolates of *P. haemolytica* carry no plasmids.

Isolation and Partial Characterization of Plasmids and Bacteriophages from Isolates of Pasteurella haemolytica

Alan B. Richards, Texas Agricultural Experiment Station and Department of Veterinary Microbiology and Parasitology, College of Veterinary Medicine, Texas A&M University, College Station, Texas 77843.

Loyd W. Sneed, Texas Veterinary Medical Diagnostic Laboratory, College Station, Texas 77843.

Harland W. Renshaw, Texas Agricultural Experiment Station and Department of Veterinary Microbiology and Parasitology, College of Veterinary Medicine, Texas A&M University, College Station, Texas 77843.

Extrachromosomal genetic elements have been shown to code for factors associated with bacterial pathogenicity in many species and could possibly play a role in the pathogenicity of *P. haemolytica*. The presence of inducible bacteriophages and plasmids was therefore studied using the methods of Lwoff (1953) and Portnoy, Moseley and Falkow (1981), respectively. The bacterial isolates were also tested for drug resistance and the ability to cause bovine leukocyte cytotoxicity. A bacteriophage common to all isolates was observed in UV-induced bacterial cultures and the bacteriophage was classified as a group 5 phage (Tikhonenko, 1970). Bacteriophages isolated from a particular bacteria appeared incapable of undergoing an infectious lytic cycle in any of the other bacterial isolates. Eight bacterial isolates contained three distinct plasmids with the molecular weights of 2.7, 3.2 and 3.4×10^6 daltons. Two isolates had two plasmids correlating to the smallest and largest of the other three plasmids, while five isolates had no detectable plasmids. Plasmid and drug-resistance patterns suggest a causal relationship between the smallest and/or largest of the three plasmids and bacterial resistance to ampicillin and penicillin. All bacterial isolates caused a leukocyte cytotoxic effect on bovine leukocytes.